The Twilight of Cutting

The publisher gratefully acknowleges the generous support of the Hull Memorial Publication Fund of Cornell University.

The Twilight of Cutting

AFRICAN ACTIVISM AND
LIFE AFTER NGOs

Saida Hodžić

UNIVERSITY OF CALIFORNIA PRESS

University of California Press, one of the most distinguished university presses in the United States, enriches lives around the world by advancing scholarship in the humanities, social sciences, and natural sciences. Its activities are supported by the UC Press Foundation and by philanthropic contributions from individuals and institutions. For more information, visit www.ucpress.edu.

University of California Press
Oakland, California

Library of Congress Cataloging-in-Publication Data

Names: Hodžić, Saida, 1977– author.
Title: The twilight of cutting : African activism and life after NGOs / Saida Hodžić.
Description: Oakland, California : University of California Press, [2017] | Includes bibliographical references and index.
Identifiers: LCCN 2016036910 (print) | LCCN 2016038727 (ebook) | ISBN 9780520291980 (cloth : alk. paper) | ISBN 9780520291997 (pbk. : alk. paper) | ISBN 9780520965577 (ebook)
Subjects: LCSH: Female circumcision—Political aspects—Ghana. | Female circumcision—Ghana—Prevention. | Non-governmental organizations—Social aspects—Ghana. | Feminism—Ghana.
Classification: LCC GN484 .H64 2017 (print) | LCC GN484 (ebook) | DDC 392/.109667—dc23
LC record available at http://lccn.loc.gov/2016036910

25 24 23 22 21 20 19 18 17
10 9 8 7 6 5 4 3 2 1

For Nadia

CONTENTS

Anthropologists Say

Why do you want to study *female genital cutting*?

Why do *you* want to study female genital cutting?

Are there NGOs in Africa?

You can study NGOs or you can study female genital cutting, but you can't do both.

You don't need to do this. You can always change your project, you know.

What will you do if they invite you to watch?

Why don't you do research in Bosnia instead?

You know, I started doing research on FGM as well. There is nothing new you can say about it.

I hate your topic! I actually wanted to study it too, but [a senior feminist anthropologist] told me not to. Nobody will take you seriously.

PREFACE

COMING TO QUESTIONS

I came to this project not because of an affective response to cutting but because of an affective response to anthropology. When in 1999 a campaign against female genital mutilation (FGM) made headlines in Germany, where I then lived, I was disappointed that I first heard about cutting from the newspapers rather than in my anthropology classes. I witnessed the moral panic that cutting provoked without being able to name or understand either cutting or the confluence of racism, liberal concern, and humanitarian care that it animated. So without the tools that my anthropology education should have given me, I went about developing them elsewhere.

My youthful disappointment in anthropology stemmed from a deep faith in its objectives, many of which I hold on to despite the discipline's sanctioned omissions, as well as regulatory norms and structures of feeling that foreclose as much as they enable, all of which too often presuppose that ethnographic authors' backgrounds are more similar to the readers' than to the ethnographic subjects'. As I recall, it also puzzled me how a practice said to be so central to the societies that performed it was not considered central to the discipline predicated upon the study of these societies.[1] It bothered me that anthropologists were not more visible in public debates and, when they were, that responses to dominant discourses were largely informed by ethnographies of circumcision, not by ethnographies of contemporary activism against FGM.[2] If anthropology failed at this, I thought, it was failing itself. I learned over time that certain anthropologists were researching contemporary anticutting campaigns but largely without the imprimatur of the discipline.[3]

Feminism, in the form of women's rights activism, was newly compelling and provided avenues for questions but not answers. At a conference on FGM and asylum I met German activists who spoke of transnational activism and their dynamic collaborations with nongovernmental organizations (NGOs) founded by African women. I was intrigued. But these activists talked about their work as that of enlightenment (*Aufklärung*), and the African organizations with which they collaborated were not offered a seat at the table.[4] I wanted to know what they were doing and what they had to say.

I had never imagined myself an Africanist anthropologist. My Africanist classmates in Germany had bad hair, wore hemp clothes, and were comfortably at home in the anthropology club. They traveled to Africa and were interested in sustainable development projects that empowered local communities. I am more like them now, but my global mobility was born out of duress. I was a refugee from Bosnia with a bad passport whose presence in Germany was, according to the state, merely tolerated or suffered (*geduldet*).[5] At the time I was writing my master's thesis on changing citizenship laws, was interested in political activism, and was close to other immigrants whose research revolved around issues closer to home or, rather, to the awareness of the fracture and the impossibility of home.

The German anti-FGM campaign brought cutting close to the worlds I inhabited: anthropology, women's rights activism, displacement, and feminist advocacy to expand, in reference to FGM, the laws that governed which asylum seekers would be allowed to stay in Europe. Cutting really was close to home, but saying something worthwhile about it required leaving. To provincialize the idea that FGM is an African problem that demanded Western enlightenment in its various guises, whether activist or critical, I wanted a shift in perspective. I sought an analytical detour in a doctoral program where another kind of anthropology and transnational African studies was possible and where gender studies had an institutional home.

To challenge Western reason, it does not suffice to analyze cutting as a culturally specific phenomenon or to criticize anti-FGM campaigns from the vantage point of the West. The latter involves "left-allied critical assessments of any putatively progressive project," as Wendy Brown and Janet Halley put it (2002a: 2), be it humanitarian or feminist. Even this kind of critique is often unwelcome in public culture and is met with such responses as "How can doing good be wrong?" "They are at least doing something," and "They have good intentions." But while it is true that the current political environment in the United States does not welcome this kind of critique, the analytical left that provides it does not readily embrace a questioning of its own suppositions, methodologies, and sensibilities. The central question I raise is why, after three decades of African anticutting campaigns, is there a critical vocabulary that can shred the neocolonial, racist gaze inherent in Western anti-FGM discourses but not one that can account for the subtle imperial formations that structure the lived experiences of Africans, on and off the continent, who are involved in efforts to end cutting or are subjected to those efforts?

That this question is salient was made clear when Wanjiru Kamau-Rutenberg, a political scientist at the University of San Francisco, campaigned against the racist humanitarianism of Raëlians (cultists who believe humans are descended from aliens) and their Clitoraid campaign, which was ostensibly aiming to save cut women's pleasure. Kamau-Rutenberg wrote that feminists should instead support African women "engaged in domestic campaigns to end the practice of female circumcision within our communities," but locating African campaigners proved difficult.[6] Because she wanted to offer African women's initiatives "public recognition for their diligent and good work that too frequently goes unrecognized," she sought suggestions from her blog readers, many of whom are feminist academics. The readers mentioned the Waris Dirie Foundation; Tostan; Foundation for Women's Health, Research and Development (widely known by its acronym, FORWARD), and Global Women Intact, organizations that had several things in common: they were heavily publicized and operated in the global North or, in the case of Tostan, were run by an American woman living in Senegal. Herein lay the difficulty: how to generate "public recognition" for domestic initiatives in Africa that received so little attention that they were virtually unknown to critical scholars?

This ethnography begins where that conversation ended but follows a different path, taking Ghanaian efforts to end cutting as a point of departure and focusing on NGOs that have organized campaigns against cutting since the 1980s. Although cutting *is* waning in Ghana, albeit unevenly, I turn to these NGOs not as solutions, which is how they are interpellated by their Western supporters, but as sites of "problematization" (Foucault and Rabinow 1997). My purpose in exploring Ghanaian campaigns, their regional and transnational encounters, and the forms of governmentality they produce is not to charge them with answering "How do we end cutting?" but to account for their work, their historicity, the life worlds and subjectivities they engender, and the modes of reflection, immanent critique, and disidentification they set in motion.

Since the mid-1980s African NGOs have been engaging in new forms of enterprise and activity regarding female genital cutting. African concerns about cutting have spurred new institutions, discourses, and scientific and political projects, bringing about unexpected social transformations both intended and unintended. Cutting is waning not only in Ghana—support for the practice is ending across the continent (UNICEF 2013). Yet this waning is disavowed by discourses that portray cutting as intractable. What does it mean that while cutting is ending, the discourse of "intractable FGM" is on the rise? And what kind of a feminist anthropology is needed in such a moment?

Ghanaian NGOs engaged in ending cutting have traversed regional boundaries, as the imperative to end cutting has been constitutive of Africa's relationship to the global North for nearly a century. African women, and at times men, have been brought into the fold of Western debates about cutting as the authorizing voices that Gayatri Spivak calls the "native informants" (1999: 6)—subjects who are denied normativity and autobiography—but they have also, within and to the side of these interpellations, pursued their agendas and organized initiatives to end cutting.[7] They have not done so entirely on their own terms—advocacy against cutting has been from the outset a collaboration of Africa and Europe, and later the global North. These collaborators are particular kinds of friends, as Tsing points out: those "who work with the enemy in wartime" and "who are not positioned in equality or sameness" (2005: 246).

Recent African histories of ending cutting are important and need to be reckoned with. I do so to shed light on the dynamics of objects and people in motion and challenge the "as-if" character of constructions of cutting as immutable, the public celebrations and co-optations of African "grassroots" activism, and the critiques of neocolonialism that fail to account for its contemporary vectors, material underpinnings, and governmental forms, all of which, I will argue, entangle Africa and the global North. Rather than treating cutting as an African problem to be debated within the perimeters of Western moral and critical publics, this book examines how cutting becomes materialized as an African problem in which the West has long been implicated. I want to explore how the question of cutting mediates Africa's relationship to the global North as well as Ghana's relationship to its citizens. My approach to challenging conceptions of cutting as an object of Euro-American moral self-fashioning and a property of Africa, Islam, and lack of enlightenment is to attend to the intersections of "here" and "there" while taking the multiplicity of African perspectives on cutting as an object of concern.

What Is Your Name?

That's a Muslim name.

Yes, it is.

But you are Christian.

Of course she is a Christian. How can she be a Muslim?

I am not a Christian.

Then what are you?

Welcome! I am happy to meet a white Muslim! I have never met a white Muslim before. I am very happy.

Ask her! Ask her! You want to know, so ask her.

Did you see how he said your name? Saida? Ha, ha, ha. He does not dare ask you if you are a Muslim. Ha, ha, ha. A foolish man.

I will call you Sadia. That's our Ghanaian name.

Introduction

GOVERNMENTALITY AGAINST ITSELF

"She should have been given a death sentence!" Hope exclaimed, referring to the arrested circumciser.[1] We were sitting on the stairs outside the Ghana Association for Women's Welfare (GAWW) building, craving a reprieve from the dampness and lethargy of office life. This was January 2004, and Accra was enveloped in sandy, hazy dust from the Sahara that the harmattan dashed upon the city. Workdays were slow; Mrs. Mahama, the director, was out of town on business, and Hope and Musa, the NGO's two steady employees, had little to do. Hampered by a slow Internet connection and separated from the bustle of central Accra by a few miles, they were waiting out the hours and days until Mrs. Mahama returned. I often sat outside with them, taking a break from reconstructing GAWW history in the NGO's archives. Together we waited for Samira, the fruit seller, to come by and chat about this and that.

On this day the quiet was punctured by a radio announcement that the Bawku Circuit Court had sentenced a seventy-year-old woman to five years in prison. For GAWW, which was dedicated to anticutting campaigns, the widely publicized sentence was welcome news. GAWW was instrumental in Ghana's criminalization of cutting in 1994, as well as in the proposed stricter measure that Parliament would soon debate. Hope's insistence that "they should have given her more"—if not a death sentence, then "at least thirty years in prison"—testified to intensified public desires for the greater punishment of all those involved in cutting. Yet, while Hope felt vindicated and outraged, Musa was troubled. He disagreed with the sentence and shook his head vehemently. "Five years are too much, especially considering that she is an old woman," he said and asked Hope: "Could you send your mother to prison like that?"

I found myself puzzled: Why did Musa, who had helped advance the criminalization of cutting, contest and oppose the sentence of a circumciser? That was not an exception but the rule among those who exercised governmental power in an effort to alter the conduct of Ghanaians, but the majority, as I learned over time, lent greater weight to this question.[2] Musa is one of many who fetishized law but not punitive rationality, that is, governmental power that relies on practices of imprisonment (Foucault 1984: 337). Other NGO and government workers were also initially enthusiastic about law enforcement but later changed their minds. Although situated early in my fieldwork, and early in the nascent African and global embrace of the "Zero Tolerance against FGM" paradigm, this moment is one I returned to time and again, as Musa and Hope's conversation exemplified how Ghanaians handled the desires to end cutting. While Hope's desire for the circumciser to receive a death sentence embodies the strident public discourses against FGM, Musa's contestation of punitive rationality is at the crux of less visible but widespread perspectives and is central to the ethnographic puzzles and analytical questions this book explores.

In recent decades, much ink has been spilled in debating how "we" should think about cutting and position ourselves toward the desires to end it. However, the political concerns and ethical dilemmas that need serious attention are not those of Western subjects but of African women and men, on and off the continent, who are most engaged in and affected by the efforts to end and regulate cutting.[3] Are efforts to end female genital cutting a problem, and, if so, what kind of a problem are they and for whom? For whom is the *ending* of cutting a problem and why? In this book I seek to redefine answers to these two questions from the perspectives of Ghanaian lifeworlds. At times a third question surfaces: "Is cutting itself a problem and, if so, what kind of a problem?" In Ghana governmental campaigns have mobilized and transformed rural women who have been cut; NGO workers who have traversed the villages and towns in their quest to end cutting; nurses, health volunteers, and civil servants who have formed watchdog committees to prevent cutting and punish perpetrators; researchers who produce so-called facts about cutting; circumcisers, some of whom have stopped cutting and some of whom have been imprisoned; as well as educators, priests, imams, doctors, lawyers, journalists, politicians, big women and small girls, chiefs, and soothsayers.

The critical responses of these actors to anticutting campaigns did not take shape in direct opposition or resistance to them. There are no "backlashes" that anthropologists and historians have widely discussed and come to anticipate (Shell-Duncan and Hernlund 2000b: 33). Cutting has been ending in many districts, dramatically so in areas where sustained, decades-long campaigns have taken place. Although official discourses stress the underground resistance to NGOs, both the general public and the subjects of NGO interventions embraced the cultural reforms, public health campaigns, and legislative changes. Behind this embrace is not resistance to NGO advocacy but critiques of what it leaves unaddressed and refusals to institutionalize governmental meanings. While power, as Achille Mbembe writes, "attempts to institutionalize its world of meanings as a socio-historical world and to make that world fully real, turning it into a part of people's common sense" (1992: 3), social worlds structured by governmental rationalities think, feel, speak, and act in reference to them without being overdetermined thereby. Neither the agents nor subjects of NGO interventions are fully enveloped in the governmental logic entailed in anticutting campaigns, but they are always in conversation with it.

In Ghana the waning of cutting has been accompanied by critical responses to the colonial order of things and its afterlives in the liberal governance of everyday life.[4] Anticutting campaigns entail and reinforce what Elizabeth Povinelli calls "the late liberal distributions of life and death, of hope and harm, and of endurance and exhaustion across social difference" (2011a: 5). The campaigns reflect which lives are valued and cared for and which are considered such a threat to the body politic that they deserve only surveillance, "sensitization" (educating those considered ignorant), and harsh punishment. Of concern in the governance of groups that practiced cutting in northern Ghana and among migrants in the South are not just the laws and policies that institute punitive rationality and give birth to desires for capital punishment such as Hope's but more subtle and insidious forms of governing—those that distribute limited lifesaving measures but not wealth or resources and that substitute concern for care. This governance is minimalist in that its exercise of democracy is reduced to voting (see Comaroff and Comaroff 2012) and its exercise of biopolitical public health measures is reduced to lifesaving (see Redfield 2013). In addition, the state also rests on performances of such minimality, such as when it claims not to have money to supply gas for police vehicles, as I will show in chapter 7.

The subjects of NGO campaigns—cut women and circumcisers—accommodate NGO platforms but critically and creatively question this form of governance, which takes without giving and punishes without caring. But

NGO workers and civil servants charged with implementing the resulting laws, policies, and sensitization projects also find themselves in a double bind. They are impelled to align themselves with problematizations of northern Ghana that posit cultural pathology and patriarchy as the main sources of the region's impoverishment and suffering. Their very authority is predicated upon "knowing villagers without aligning themselves closely with them" (Pigg 1997: 276). Indeed, subject positions offered to governmental workers hinge on repudiating villagers and their ostensibly abject traditions. The governmental workers are asked to surveil and sensitize the villagers to the undesirability of cutting and to turn themselves into citizen-enforcers of law and order. And they do. But the governmental workers then find themselves deeply torn. The governance they are asked to embody offers them a seductive place in modern Ghana but does not feel right for very long.

This is not a dilemma they discuss publicly. Whereas in the global North discussions of cutting require a public performance of cultural sensitivity, even when private feelings are less nuanced, in Ghana public discourses require taking a tough stance and an unabashed embrace of statist moderni-zation theories. GAWW and its umbrella organization, the Inter-African Committee on Harmful Traditional Practices Affecting the Health of Women and Children (IAC), are not only particularly irreverent about the value of tolerance but turn their refusals of tolerance into a mark of distinc-tion. Campaigners have little space for *publicly* articulating complex feelings, critical thoughts, or ambivalent perspectives. When in 2009, I pushed, prod-ded, and cajoled Martin Abilba, the Bolganaba (Gurene for chief of Bolgatanga), the capital of the Upper East Region, to comment on the critical perspectives on anticutting campaigns, perspectives that I knew by then were oblique, he said that none existed. "People actually bought the idea" that cutting needed to end because it "was obsolete," he said, equating the aboli-tion of cutting with its framing as an anachronism and critiques of cam-paigns with wholesale resistance. The notion of cutting as obsolete renders in a popular idiom what is otherwise officially known as a discourse about "harmful traditional practices." This codification of harm has become an unquestioned consensus in Ghanaian public culture. For those who govern northern Ghana, cutting and other "harmful traditional practices" said to subjugate women and children and destroy rural livelihoods are the primary frame of reference for development blueprints. The Bolganaba was amused by my questions and added: "The dissidents you are looking for, they are in your country," by which he meant the United States. "What I saw in New

York!" he laughed and shook his head. "Your freedom or your democracy is democrazy, no more democracy. It's democrazy." The chief shared the reformist spirit of NGOs and had traveled to New York with Dr. Adjei, the director of Rural Help Integrated (RHI), a Bolgatanga-based anticutting NGO that was one of my main research sites and vantage points. The chief saw my questions as radical and dissident, suggesting that those who governed Ghana, and northern Ghana in particular, could not afford to have qualms about the ending of cutting.

But for NGO workers and civil servants at the frontiers of governance, those tasked with the everyday practices of rule, living with such misgivings is part of the job and integral to their subjectivity. Governmental workers are impelled to reposition themselves against cutting, everything that it stands for, as well as the people associated with it. And they do so. But they also have critical responses that are voiced not in public protests or debates but in a different key: in indirect speech and in practices of living. They gather their force from sensibilities, that is, entanglements of thought, affect, and habitus, which are not easily located in stable ideologies or discrete cultural formations. These sensibilities are at the interstices of social and governmental logics and in consonance with tacit principles on which society is built, such as the ethics of relationality and mutual responsibility.

To understand the governmental workers' critical responses and sensibilities, my analysis reorients anthropological discussions about social control of the political away from a model that posits an originary separation of "society against the state" (Clastres 1989; see also J. Scott 2012, 2014) and toward an understanding of the social as already entangled with the governmental. In Ghana a variety of people are compelled to participate in the governance of self and others. Social theorists would understand these entanglements of the social and governmental as an outcome of the specifically neoliberal bureaucratization of everyday life (see Hibou 2015). The critical impetus of such work notwithstanding, it wrongly conceives everyday life before neoliberalism as somehow free from bureaucracy. An understanding of power that follows from considerations of the social as outside and preceding governance posits an external structure that is *imposed* upon people and communities whose options are then limited to acquiescence or resistance (see Sharma 2008: 97). Anthropologists studying development and governmentality have offered a way out of this binary framework. Aradhana Sharma thus writes that "communities are neither given nor cohesive, but are constantly remade through modern governmental practices, such as development, census, and voting, which provoke multiple, shifting, and antagonistic identifications" (154). And they have been remade for a long time—the "prior" time is itself a governmental artifact (see Povinelli 2011b).

I might add that governmental worlds are also profoundly social and that the subjectivities, affiliations, and positionings of NGO workers and civil servants are also remade through the interventions they stage. As Ilana Feldman writes, "Bureaucratic life is everyday life" (2008: 233), and governmental worlds are profoundly social and encultured. Rather than understanding governmental workers as fundamentally different from their rural and urban constituents, I emphasize that they share both social and material worlds (see Sharma 2008: 113).[5] At the same time I show that modernizing processes demand that NGO workers and civil servants disidentify from these shared worlds and instead construct themselves as temporally, morally, and civilizationally *ahead* of them.

We should think of the forms of contestation that emerge in this context as "governmentality against itself." Governmental workers and subjects of interventions are not engulfed by governmental power, as theorists of bureaucracy would suggest, claiming that "nothing escapes or can escape organization" (Lefebvre 2010: 159); as João Biehl writes, "Rationalities play a part in the reality of which they speak, and this dramaturgy of the real becomes integral to how people value life and relationships and enact the possibilities they envision for themselves and others" (2013: 580). But while governmental reason shapes lifeworlds, lifeworlds are not fully defined by governmentality. All the ethnographic chapters that follow highlight their interdependence and interplay. Rather than seeing NGO workers and civil servants as unidirectionally imposing governmental norms onto their rural subjects, I show that they equally subject themselves to them. All those involved in and affected by anti-cutting campaigns are in dialogue with prescribed forms of meaning and subjectivity but have critical perspectives on the power that regulates life and invites participation while offering little nurture or care.

This analysis also leads me to advocate learning about the social by examining social engineering and governmental practice. It is often posited that "we must first understand" something cultural before trying to change it. As I will show, this dictum serves as the basis for both governmental practice and opposition to the zeal of reformers. In anthropology it has served as a pillar of analytics and politics alike; hence, the ethnography of the cultural meanings of cutting is put into the service of political opposition to repugnant discourses. The operating assumption here is that anthropology holds the key to the workings of culture and society. It is thought that social engineers—development experts, humanitarians, state bureaucrats, and others—do not have anthropologists' intimate knowledge of historical contexts and cultural and political formations, and as a result the interventions of social engineers fail and/or do harm. As Gosselin writes, those "working to end excision often do not have the benefit of this knowledge," referring to cultural meanings and social dynamics (2000: 193). I suggest that we must interpret otherwise and analyze social dynamics as already imbued with governmental knowledge and practice. Politically speaking, the argument that "we must first understand" can neither put interventions on hold nor prevent other forms of damage and violence. Rather than halting anticutting campaigns, anthropology has become *further* entwined with them. Those in charge of Ghanaian NGO and international UN campaigns have been attracted to anthropology and have brought it deeper into the fold of governance. Dr. Adjei, the RHI director, trained himself in ethnographic fieldwork methods; GAWW sponsored survey research in Ghana's North and among migrants in Accra; the World Health Organization hired Bettina Shell-Duncan to carry out anthropological research; while the UN Population Fund and UNICEF contracted Ellen Gruenbaum to evaluate their campaigns and assist in their design. Anthropological taxonomies and sensibilities thus continue to be entangled with governmental practice.

I will show that NGO governmentality is awkward, frictional, and ruptured: it does not operate as a programmed, rationalized, or lubricated machine but is haphazard, contingent, and performative. This is another governing dynamic that is both "tenuous and effective" (Feldman 2008: 13), for it has substantial effects and produces new formations of subjectivity, rule, and dissent. NGO interventions have breathed life into the state and entrenched existing social divisions but have also set in motion popular critiques of scarcity, vulnerability, and sovereign violence, that is, violence implicated in the character of law itself (Agamben 1998; Benjamin 1986). Challenging the fallback position that ties failure to harm, I propose that it was precisely NGOs' *mis*readings of rural frameworks that produced these unintended consequences (see chapter 4). The encounters between NGO and popular understandings of cutting, bodies, and a host of related notions—from blood, health, poverty, discipline, and imprisonment to gender, sexuality, ethics, and the state—allowed rural Ghanaians to accommodate NGO platforms as well as to critique what they leave unaddressed. Finally, the very success of NGOs' attempts to turn civil servants into particular kinds of "native informants"—citizen–law enforcers—instigated a confrontation with hegemonic discourses and challenged governmental rationality from within.

These are the ethnographic endpoints, and my analysis traces the conditions of their emergence in social and governmental lifeworlds. Exploring the "less dramatic durabilities of duress that imperial formations produce as ongoing, persistent features" of postcolonial life (Stoler 2008: 192), this book examines the genealogies of anticutting campaigns and the forms of rule, subjectivity, and positioning they instantiate. I focus on historically situated practices and taxonomies that problematize cutting as a harmful tradition and the surprising results of intimate encounters between NGO workers and villagers.

ETHNOGRAPHY OF PROBLEMATIZATION: REASON, AFFECT, PRACTICE

My analytical object is problematization, defined as an inquiry into "how and why certain things (behavior, phenomena, processes) become a problem," as Foucault wrote (Bacchi 2012: 1), and become objects for thought and regulation (Foucault and Rabinow 1997: 117). I examine how cutting becomes an object of intervention, that is, how Ghanaian NGOs and those who enter into their orbits problematize cutting by constructing it as a particular kind of problem—a "harmful tradition," ignorance, and "persistent resistance" to interventions and to law—and trace the genealogies, permutations, and effects of this problem making. An analysis of problematization is not deconstruction but a somewhat more programmatic approach to examining social and governmental objects. If deconstruction questions categories and concepts, problematization analyzes their historical contexts of production and traces their contextual operations. I examine the conditions of possibility and historical processes by which Ghanaian NGOs produce FGM as a problem in order to eliminate it, exploring their discursive processes and practices.

Departing from conceptions of problematization as an activity of those who govern, I consider it also an activity of the governed. While both Rose and Rabinow ascribe "the elements of thought, intention and calculation" (Rose 1999: 4) and "thinking as an activity" (Rabinow and Rose 2003: 12) only to the West and the institutions of "modern government" that emanate from it, I contend that thinking as an *activity* is not limited to agents of governmentality. Subjects of NGO projects have critical perspectives of their own about the causes of their problems and the adequacy of available governmental solutions. These knowledges and perspectives are in turn thoroughly informed by sedimented and emerging governmental discourses and practices.

Problematization is bundled with the distribution of capital and with larger geopolitical forces that underwrite how cutting is understood and regulated. The production of knowledge about cutting, strategies for intervention, and their evaluation are co-constitutive with the socioeconomic and political orders at global and national scales. This point is underexplored by anthropologists who denounce the study of ethnos, culture, place, or people and focus instead on the anthropos (Rabinow 2005) or "how practices of government put the social and biological life of the human in question" (Inda 2005a: 11). In efforts to end cutting, culture, ethnos, place, and people are central to governmental problematizations, and therefore I treat them not as analytical categories but as ethnographic objects. I show how and why coding harmful traditions hinges on problematization of culture as a site of regulation and reform. Similarly, the cultural reasons and meanings of cutting are also the subject of intense debate among those who want to end it, both in Ghana and internationally. I examine how the colonial and modernist reason positing the study of meaning as necessary for interventions has become a governmental dogma, and show how it has been inflected by anthropology. Anthropological reason, the ethnographic style, and feminist politics have been entangled with governmental efforts to end cutting from colonialism onward. Hence, my analysis of problematization turns our gaze back at ourselves and examines how anthropology and feminism have informed and been informed by both imperialism and anti-imperialism alike.

There are additional theoretical consequences to understanding how constructions of "a place and its people" are central to the very operations of government. The targets of governmental intervention are not simply humans whose life is in question. When people are defined as problem populations in need of management or reform, they are always already marked by categories of social differentiation—be they race, class, gender, citizenship, ethnicity, or place—and their humanity is often put in question. In Ghana, as I will explain shortly, efforts to end cutting hinge on constructing northern and poor migrant neighborhoods (called *zongos*) as sites of noncitizenship and disorder. In international governmental discourses the place of interventions is either "Africa"—a racialized signifier of violence, liminal humanity, and lack—or African and Muslim migrants, who are figured as suspicious and threatening quasi-citizens. These understandings have social and material consequences for those who govern as well as for those who must inhabit these categories.

The governmental recognition of northern Ghana as extremely poor has been central to the intensifying of NGO operations in the region. Funded by a host of donor agencies, NGOs were able to seamlessly insert themselves into the regional body politic, producing new economies, social relations, and fields and forms of governmental activity. Their effects are palpable in new regional economies (where hotels, catering agencies, volunteer work, workshop venues and conference centers, research and monitoring infrastructures, etc., spring up to serve the NGOs) and in the conceptual sedimentation of discourses about cultural pathology and patriarchy as the sources of the region's problems. The latter shape the character of interventions as well as the subjectivities of NGO and government workers, who must align themselves with such discourses.

One purpose of studying problematization, as Carol Bacchi puts it, is to "make politics, understood as the complex strategic relations that shape lives, visible" (2012: 1). The stakes of problematization are high—the way that the causes of poor health, lack of law enforcement, or the disavowed ending of cutting are defined shapes the design of subsequent policies and projects. By understanding cutting as a "harmful traditional" practice "resistant" to interventions, NGOs mobilize "sensitization" and criminalization as remedies. To sensitize, in the language of NGOs and the government, means to educate those considered ignorant; sensitization is seen as a necessary first step toward development. In practice, this means apprising people of how their own behaviors and practices are harming them. Those subjected to sensitization are ambivalent about it; they do not reject such projects but see them as irrelevant to their real problems.

Problematization works upon the senses rather than disembodied reason and thought. Affect, sensations, and performativity are central to the problematizations of cutting and efforts to regulate it. I therefore understand governmental problematizations as terrains not simply for the will to know but also for the will to feel and incite those feelings in others. I will show that governmental affects come in myriad forms. Those produced at sensitization workshops take on such hegemonic forms as repugnance, shame, and alarm. But "sensibilities" are also invoked by those who critically contest and oppose dominant governmental practices; they include a medley of historical characters, from regional colonial administrators to anthropologists, Ghanaian civil servants, and cut women and circumcisers.

My main contribution to theorizations of problematization is to detach it from reason, the West, and the focus on agents of governmentality. Attending to the affective, performative, unfinished, haphazard, and excessive dimensions of problematization, this book challenges theorists who take governmental rationality at face value and further rationalize it by declaring it a property of scientific, Western modernity (Inda 2005b; Rabinow 2005; Rose 1999). NGOs and their collaborators construct themselves as rational by way of performative acts that oscillate between projecting irrationality onto others and authorizing their interventions by reference to science. I want to show that rather than *being* rational, governmentality performs and *distributes* rationality, with important political consequences for all involved.

So Did Cutting End? The Politics of Knowledge and Performance of Rationality

Studying problematization means departing from second-order questions and categories. Discussions of cutting often begin with seemingly definitive facts: a map, a census, a demographic or epidemiological factoid, a statistical account, a generalized anthropological statement about meaning and values. In addition, those who plan and fund anticutting campaigns demand answers to predetermined questions: Has cutting ceased or is it still happening? Are NGOs failing or successful? What does cutting mean? The acts of asking and answering these questions have entangled knowledge and politics since colonial rule (see chapter 1), intensely so in recent decades. When ethnographic questions so closely resemble those posed by donors and governmental agents, anthropologists need to ask why and take a detour. This book addresses different questions, because not only is cutting plural and contested, so are its endings, and so is the knowledge about them. My analytical goal is to inquire into the practices and effects of raising some questions about cutting but not others. I ask how the facticity of cutting and its endings is constructed and how, why, and to whom it comes to matter. What are the stakes of claiming that cutting has or has not stopped? Who measures this and to what ends? Why do NGOs discuss the meanings of cutting? What are the institutions that produce and deploy knowledge about cutting? What regimes of rule, technologies, politics, and economies does the construction of knowledge about cutting articulate?

As I will show, cutting is waning in Ghana, however unevenly and incompletely, but its endings are in question and intensely contested. Epidemiology is used to bolster public discourses that insist that rural communities continue to practice cutting *underground* and that they *resist* anticutting campaigns. I shall suggest that notions of *underground resistance* and *failure* are bolstered by a performance of scientific rationality. In addition to responding meta-analytically to this performance, I also construct some provisional facts of my own in chapter 2. I do so because the argument that the endings of cutting are contested has also been appropriated and now serves to mark northern Ghanaians as unruly and untrustworthy. If a critical analysis does not make its own assertions, it may inadvertently reproduce and reaffirm this discourse.

My goal is to illuminate from Ghanaian vantage points the relationship between the performance of scientific rationality and the desire for punitive rationality and "zero tolerance." Two questions have been central in the recent history of governmental will to truth, in Ghana and globally: How many people practice cutting and who are they? Is cutting harmful and what makes it harmful? The search for answers to these questions redistributes rationality and care along existing geopolitical divides. Cutting, it is said, persists because Africans, on and off the continent, stubbornly hold on to it. Population statistics about the rates of cutting are constructed in ways that maximize the numbers of "at-risk" girls, and epidemiological evaluations of the harms of cutting combine governance by evidence and governance by alarm to cast cutting as a "killer of women and children" (Hodžić 2013: 86).

At stake here are rearrangements of care. Campaigns against cutting, as well as their constitutive techniques—legislation, search for evidence (of rates, of harms), public health education—legitimize themselves in the name of care for cut women and concern for and protection of their daughters. But from the vantage point of Ghana we see the tensions produced by the injunction to extend care to those who are simultaneously constructed as irrational, noncitizens, and less than human. The Ghanaian mobilizations and contestations of liberalism starkly reveal liberalism's latent violence, its ongoing collusion with Malthusian ideologies of modernization, and the readiness to sacrifice the few for the larger public good.

Problematizing Place and People

Organized efforts to end cutting in Ghana began with the founding of GAWW in 1984, but the project of ending cutting has everything to do with the nation-state's pride in its modernity and its construction as a beacon of postcolonial Africa. Since cutting was not practiced by the country's majority groups but only by those at the socioeconomic and political margins—cutting is largely northern and rural and is *thought of* as foreign and Muslim—the state welcomed NGO advocacy and charged the chiefs with "modernizing the custom" (see chapter 2). Ghana was the first sub-Saharan African country to win independence from Britain, and its president, Kwame Nkrumah, was the leader of the pan-Africanist and nonaligned movements. Nkrumah invited black revolutionary leaders to the country and welcomed the diaspora, extending to African Americans the right of residence and turning Ghana into "the vision of black modernity" that symbolized "the prominence of Africa in global affairs" (Gaines 2006: 23). After Nkrumah's fall and decades of economic and political struggle capped off by austerity measures, Ghana again became a global beacon at the turn of the millennium, now as a neoliberal donor darling (Chalfin 2010; Piot 2010) that welcomed foreign investment, "projected a commitment to gender issues and gender equity" (Manuh 2007: 130), and promoted global visions of women's rights (Hodžić 2011). In 2009 Ghana was the first African country Barack Obama visited as president and was touted as "one of America's best friends in sub-Saharan Africa and a small outpost of stability, democracy and civil society in an often-volatile part of the world."[6]

This picture fractures upon closer investigation. Ghana no longer makes claims about being a beacon of critical black consciousness (Hartman 2007; Pierre 2013; Holsey 2008), and the residues of nonaligned politics are barely visible on streets that bear the names of Nehru, Nasser, and Tito. Since 2011 Ghana's status as a donor darling has been in jeopardy, and in 2014 Ghana accepted a bailout from the International Monetary Fund, which required further austerity measures. Many NGOs have lost funding, as have many state agencies. The discrepancy between the country's self-image and its impoverishment is routinely satirized in everyday life: urban Ghanaians refer with rueful irony and clicks of the tongue to "this, our country" and jokingly revise the slogan that Ghana is a gateway to Africa to "get away from Africa" (see also Droney 2013).

Some things remain consistent: the nation-state maintains that it cannot accommodate female genital cutting and must repudiate it. Ghana readily passed laws against cutting; in this, too, it took the lead among independent African nations. Despite these efforts, the country was embarrassed in 2000 when a Ghanaian woman, Adelaide Abankwah (real name: Regina Danson) was exposed as having made fraudulent claims about her fear of cutting (she portrayed cutting as brutal punishment for premarital sex) in her application for asylum in the United States. Ghanaians are uneasy about the charges of backwardness that perpetually afflict their country, and the Abankwah case was seen as a testament to how readily Americans believed tales of extraordinary African violence (Kratz 2007). When a chief from Danson's hometown of Biriwa testified in New York City, he felt the need to defend Ghana's honor against such discourses by stating that "Ghanaians are civilized people who do not practice human sacrifices."[7] Ghanaian responses to the Abankwah case highlight the double cost of constituting Ghana and Africa by reference to "FGM": while Ghana struggles to maintain its global self-image, internally it displaces the "savage," as the Biriwa chief put it, onto the North of the country.[8]

In Ghana's political culture public discourses superimpose notions of harmful and stubborn tradition onto northerners, who are imagined to practice cutting, whether they have done so or not. Ghana's North and South have been entangled through centuries of migration and incorporation, but one would not get that impression from popular and governmental discourses. As Bayo Holsey found when studying the aftermath of slavery in the coastal cities of Elmina and Cape Coast, the image of the North is mediated in reference to cutting and savagery. "Following the European discourses . . . coastal residents attribute the North's impenetrability to an imagined hostility of its inhabitants toward civilization" (Holsey 2008: 94), a hostility that is seen as embodied in female genital cutting and the northern rejection of Christianity. The Upper East Region has the highest rates of what the census refers to as "traditional religion," and all of northern Ghana is now subject to intense evangelical crusades (Goldstone 2012). After watching a popular TV show on the subject of cutting with her hosts, Holsey noticed that it was used to "erect a moral cordon": "The next day, many people continued to discuss the program and similarly commented on the 'barbarism' of the practice and at the same time were quick to say that only people in the North do such things; they do not" (2008: 94). Holsey and I are not alone in this analysis; much recent anthropological work addresses stigmatized representations of northern Ghana, such as those regarding infanticide (Awedoba and Denham 2014) and witchcraft (Crampton 2013). In popular and political cultures the North is the country's Other: it is seen as hot, violent, unruly, and either animist or Muslim. In fact, I was regularly congratulated for getting by in the North, which is seen as inhospitable to the comfortable life a white person is presumed to desire.

This rhetoric sometimes acquires a violent nationalist bent, as media and other public discourses figure northern Ghanaians as criminal. Northern Ghanaians have long been marked by other terms of nonbelonging: Muslim, immigrant, and slave. Indeed, when the first northern Ghanaian, Hilla Limann, won Ghana's presidency (under extenuating circumstances), a popular song accused former president Jerry Rawlings of "kill[ing] the royal persons and ma[king] a slave heir" (Obeng 2002: 95). Today northern Ghanaians often serve as scapegoats for the increasing number of roadside robberies and car hijackings, which are then discursively established as reasons for retribution, violence, expulsion from the state, and formal exclusion from Ghanaian citizenship.

The notion of constitutive and relational marginality (Tsing 1993) helps illuminate this ethnographic context. As the nation's Others, ethnic groups that have practiced cutting are figured not as outside the polity altogether, since they are made hypervisible by governmental knowledge production and subjected to state and NGO rule, but as outside citizenship and the polity proper. Hence, the groups at the margins of the state serve a constitutive function for Ghana's conception of itself as progressive by embodying what Tsing calls "a *displacement* within powerful discourses on civilization and progress" (Tsing 1993: 7–8)—they are the ones the Ghanaian state labels unruly and against whom it defines itself as modern and governable. It has long been argued that imperial and colonial powers produced the idea of traditional Africa in order to define themselves as modern. Yet colonialism also partitioned the spaces within its colonies, doubling this effect (Mamdani 1996). As a result southern and urban Ghanaians as well as the Ghanaian state look to northern Ghana as its long-standing Other, figuring it as a site of "disorder" (Comaroff and Comaroff 2006a) within aspirations for the rule of law, stability, and order. To be clear, northern Ghana is not abandoned in the sense of being left alone—women and men targeted by NGOs are subjected to intensified governmental attention born out of liberal and modernist concern. NGOs and the state incorporate the region into the body politic under neoliberal management (Brown et al. 2006: 35) that combines the region's visibility and recognition with the simultaneous exclusion of its peoples from economic benefits, as well as from normative notions of citizenship and modernity.

Ghanaian anticutting campaigns actively reinforce this imaginary of northern Ghana. GAWW, RHI, and others also reinforce statist definitions of development as teleological progress and organize their campaigns accordingly.

NGO leaders and workers always differ from their subjects in class and sometimes in ethnic affiliation and religion. Both GAWW and RHI were founded by southern Ghanaians who came from groups that did not practice cutting historically and to whom cutting was thus foreign. Moreover, the point of campaigns is to emphasize the differences between NGO workers and their subjects, not to bridge them. NGOs rule over rather than mobilize rural subjects or, more specifically, the NGOs mobilize civil servants, chiefs, and educated volunteers to rule over other peasants and migrants.

GAWW's early leaders, Gloria Aryee, Marjorie Bulley, and Emma Banga, were members of Ghana's cultural and political elite: they had privileged access to higher and international education, Accra's high society, and state power structures. Yet I find it difficult to refer to them as elites without questioning this very term and its anthropological deployments; many of us are no less elite than the people we characterize as such. GAWW leaders were not wealthy and they shared the destiny of the country. The NGO had started at the tail end of the "Rawlings chain" years, named for the collarbones made visible by starvation resulting from the country's economic collapse. In 1984, when GAWW was founded, Ghana had just accepted structural adjustment policies, currency devaluation, and inflation. Aryee, a high school principal, and Bulley, a university librarian, subsisted on allowances from the IAC of up to US$150 a month, supplementing their civil servant salaries when these were insufficient for sustenance.

In later years IAC funding dried up, Aryee and Bulley retired from their jobs and GAWW activities, and a new crop of people began running the organization. They are northern women and men from more humble backgrounds who are now living in Accra. Their work with GAWW coincided with Ghana's neoliberal boom; after the 2000 election that set the country on a neoliberal course, funding flowed in for both the government and NGOs. Nonetheless, NGO money was rarely earmarked for staff salaries, so allowances were squeezed out of project funds and per diems; it is only NGO directors and employees of donor-NGOs who at times find ways to appropriate funds for substantial personal benefit. GAWW's sole employees were Musa, the accountant and youth project manager, and Hope, the secretary. For Edna, a part-time GAWW worker, NGO work was a second, after-hours job without a formal salary, and Mrs. Mahama had been seconded to the NGO by the government from her former job as a public health nurse. RHI workers' steady salaries were unique among the NGOs in Bolgatanga, because of the unusually adequate long-term funding Dr. Adjei had secured from the UN Population Fund. Martin, Olivia, Gina, and other RHI workers lived on salaries of US$50 to US$150 a month, depending on their rank, thus earning as little as laborers and as much as public school teachers.

While people like Musa and Hope understand themselves as workers, NGO leaders are more likely to understand themselves as activists. But they do not imbue activism with the aura of an idealistic, political calling devoid of pragmatic pursuits, nor do they deny that their activism is entwined with what has been called "governance feminism" (Halley et al. 2006). Members of the Ghanaian women's movement, for the most part, do not label themselves in any way, but the Ghanaian feminist anthropologist Takyiwah Manuh calls them gender workers (2007), and I have heard them occasionally refer to each other as gender activists, gender advocates, feminists, and gender persons.[9] While GAWW started as an association to which its members volunteered their work, RHI began with Dr. Adjei's informal lectures about reproductive health; over time both grew into professional NGOs, contemporaneous with the NGO boom in Ghana at large.

Regional, ethnic, and class divides structure the work of these NGOs, and some people are more attuned to them than others. Dr. Adjei, an Akan man who lived and worked in Bolga for thirty years as a medical doctor, researcher, and NGO director, was particularly adept at bridging differences. Due to the undesirability of the remote Upper East Region, few doctors posted to Bolga ever arrived, and even fewer stayed very long, but Adjei settled down and founded a clinic and an NGO. He is an "articulated" subject (Choy 2005; Langwick 2008) who knew just how to deploy his national and international stature and regional knowledge. He had studied and taught around the world and displayed his many diplomas on his office walls. But he also knew how to mobilize the signifiers of local appropriateness—he took the Bolganaba with him to New York and was admired for it. "You know, Dr. Adjei has just returned from New York where he received an award," I was told time and again when I first arrived.

Some Things Must Be Said: Positionings

Although cutting usually maps onto the coordinates of class, ethnicity, and the rural-urban divide, it also spills outside them. A scholar from the Upper East Region who works at the University of Ghana pulled me aside at the end of our conversation in his office and told me that one of his sisters was cut against their middle-class family's will:

We were all opposed to it. We asked why. But she couldn't say why. I still don't understand why she did it. She certainly wasn't forced to it. She isn't weak willed either. She did this against the family's wishes, and she married a man the family didn't want her to marry. But here is somebody with secondary education who decides to do it.

A middle-class woman who is cut is an aberration. I was never able to ask NGO workers and civil servants whether they were cut because they volunteered that they were not early in our conversations. Any urban woman from Wa, Bolgatanga, Bawku, or Navrongo must preemptively declare that she is not cut and that she knows nothing of it, lest she be associated with cutting and its shame. *Some things must be said,* because the FGM discourse interpellates subjects, who must position themselves in reference to it. Ghanaian women feel the imperative to disavow cutting as a prerequisite to situating themselves within modern Ghana. By contrast, in the global North, feminist critics of the FGM discourse must denounce the practice in order for their critique to be heard, especially if they were born in Africa (see Nnaemeka 2005a). Consider Scheper-Hughes's words: "I don't 'like' the idea of clitoridectomy any better than any other woman I know. But I like even less the Western 'voices of reason' . . . on this topic" (1991: 27).[10] Or Gruenbaum, who states what is objectionable about cutting so that her subsequent analysis can be heard: "Clearly, the health of women and girls is seriously harmed" (1996: 462). Such rhetorical moves have unintended consequences: by denouncing the medical harms of cutting, scholars also reify them. But my main point is that while Western feminists must distance themselves from supporting cutting in order to legitimize their criticisms and situate themselves within the realm of acceptable moral debate, Ghanaian women must distance themselves from intimate experiences with cutting. For urban women this means saying that they are uncut. For rural women in Bongo it means saying that their daughters are not cut or that they will not allow their daughters to get cut. For the last generation of cut women it means facing shame that cannot be deferred or projected onto others. However, they can, and sometimes do, remain silent about their experiences and claim that they were not cut.

Cultures of governance also require specific statements about cutting. While UN agencies and Western NGOs must prove that their care is genuine and distanced from imperialism, Ghanaians must continually reconstruct their own modernity and distance from a practice that marks them as backward. This, too, is an effect of positioning.

Thus far I have portrayed efforts to end cutting as an ethnographic object that is separate from anthropological and feminist analysis. In the following section I want to highlight that efforts to end cutting have both constituted and been constituted by anthropology and feminism alike. Examining African concerns about cutting over the last century leads to the presence of Europeans and the inflection of debates about cutting by feminist political zeal, anthropological reason, and ethnographic sensibility.

In 1984 Marjorie Bulley, Gloria Aryee, and Bertha Antsui traveled from Accra to Dakar, Senegal, where, together with activists from other parts of Africa, they founded the Inter-African Committee for Traditional Practices Affecting the Health of Women and Children, widely known as the IAC. The IAC was envisioned as an umbrella organization with national chapters or affiliates, which were eventually established in twenty-eight African countries. In Dakar, when the question was posed, Aryee declared herself president of the new IAC chapter in Ghana, and Bulley became secretary. They named the organization the Ghana Association for Women's Welfare, or GAWW, and immediately threw themselves into the work of advocacy, quickly turning GAWW into one of the IAC's favorite chapters.

This would be one way to tell the story, and it is how the IAC and its supporters like to tell it—a story of African grassroots organizations striving to eliminate cutting in Africa. But scratch the surface and other histories come into view, complicating the imaginary of purely local African initiatives. In 1977 diplomats and activists living in Geneva had founded the NGO Working Group on Traditional Practices Affecting the Health of Women and Children. The group was the precursor to the IAC and was a joint African-European construct that involved the participation of people from around the world. Rather than drawing public attention to the potentially contentious question of cutting, the IAC used the notion of "traditional practices" and sought to placate African governments by framing cutting as an obstacle to health and development, which became a mainstay of arguments by the IACs and GAWW.

Managing IAC's public reception meant paying attention not only to terminology but also to the people who were the public embodiment of the organization. From its inception the working group had two coordinators, one African, the other European. The first coordinators were Isabelle

Tévoedjrè, a professor of literature who lived in Geneva as the wife of a Beninese representative to the UN, and Margareta Linnander, a Swedish woman employed by Save the Children International. Together they traveled throughout Africa, mobilizing support for advocacy against cutting and setting the stage for the 1984 Dakar meeting. When Tévoedjrè returned to Benin, where she founded the IAC national chapter, Berhane Ras-Work, the wife of an Ethiopian diplomat, replaced her. Ras-Work was elected the first president of the IAC in Dakar, and she has continued to be the face of the organization, as well as its president.

As I sifted through GAWW archives in Accra, initially maintained by Marjorie Bulley but no longer under her meticulous librarian's care, I found faxed correspondence, reports, plans, schedules, notes, and letters exchanged by GAWW and the IAC head office. In the early years the majority of GAWW funding came from the IAC; both Ras-Work and Linnander lived in Geneva, where they lobbied for money that was then distributed on the continent. Save the Children, and in particular the Swedish chapter, Rädda Barnen, was a frequent donor for many years; GAWW archives are replete with documents and reports written for them. Linnander, the link between Save the Children and the IAC, has been praised for diplomacy and sensitivity, as well as her "continual avoidance of publicity" (Sanderson 1995: 26). Her position within the IAC was understated but authoritative; the correspondence in the GAWW archives shows Linnander clearly in charge of much of the decision making about the kind and amount of funding GAWW would receive. Over time Ras-Work turned her position as a "native informant" into an asset and took control of the IAC.

If we follow Jomo Kenyatta, the Kenyan political leader who would later become an anthropologist and then the first president of independent Kenya, on his journey to imperial England in the 1930s, another history comes into view. After a colonial crisis about female circumcision in Kenya Kenyatta was invited to testify in London before Parliament's Committee for the Protection of Coloured Women in the Crown Colonies, which was focused on how to end circumcision.[11] As he later writes in his book, Kenyatta gave "the Gikuyu's point of view" and believed that his contribution put the brakes on the movement to criminalize circumcision ([1938] 1965: 126). Kenyatta also attended a 1931 conference on African children held in Geneva under the auspices of the Save the Children Fund; during that conference several European delegates called for laws criminalizing circumcision. Kenyatta was content that they did not prevail: "General opinion was for education which would enable the people to choose what customs to keep and which ones they would like to get rid off" (127).

This story has two important features. One is that the Save the Children Fund is the same organization whose members later cofounded the NGO Working Group and then funded IAC campaigns, serving as one of the network's main donors. The history of Western entanglements with efforts to end cutting is not always so linear and is certainly not continuous, but the past and the present are held together by durable connective tissue. The second is that Kenyatta's opposition to colonial violence and dispossession was entangled with his political testimonies about circumcision and his subsequent anthropological analysis. He stressed that many educated Gikuyu defended circumcision but that his point was not to defend it but to spread an understanding of its character as "the very essence of an institution [initiation] which has enormous educational, social, moral, and religious implications" (128). Like regional colonial officials themselves, Kenyatta described initiation as a "condition sine qua non of the whole teaching of tribal law, religion, and morality" (128). Thus the first professional ethnography of cutting was born from a transcontinental political encounter and deployed anthropology to reshape the function of knowledge in governmental politics. In turn, African and Western debates against cutting were inflected by anthropology from their inception.

This point was missed by feminist anthropologists in the 1990s when they established the basis for the discipline's reluctance to seriously contend with contemporary efforts to end cutting. As Scheper-Hughes wrote, Egyptian and Sudanese women ought to "argue this one out for themselves" (1991: 26; see also Gruenbaum 1996). The problem is, the Sudanese have not been arguing this one out solely by themselves for more than a century (Abusharaf 2006b; Boddy 2007), nor have other Africans. At a time when Western publics became repulsed by the specter of FGM, anthropologists were repulsed by FGM discourse itself, with its neocolonial racism and injunction to "draw the line" between cultural and ethical relativism. The solution? For some, a self-imposed silence of thirty years (Hale 1994). For others, the injunction that *everyone* stop writing about cutting. Scheper-Hughes urged: "Hands off! Enough is enough! ... We have to ask ourselves (again and again, it seems) why we choose (and why we choose to award) the topics that we do in light of who we are and how we are positioned (individually, culturally, and politically) vis-à-vis those we turn into the objects of our study" (1991: 26).

Its progressive impulse notwithstanding, the command "hands off" too easily let anthropology off the hook. The construction of cutting as a problem has been a joint, transcontinental enterprise that has implicated both anthropology and feminism for nearly a century. For if, as Saba Mahmood suggests, the question of how to practically transform the lives of Muslim (and African and other postcolonial) women "is not ours to ask" (2005: 36), neither is it a question we can write ourselves out of. My analysis does not aim to answer the liberal dilemma ("Do we have the right to intervene?") but to put ethnography to use to transform what can be said about cutting and liberal governance alike, if we do not write ourselves out of power-knowledge formations.

Mahmood writes:

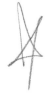

> If there is one lesson we have learned from the machinations of colonial feminism and the politics of "global sisterhood," it is that any social and political transformation is always a function of local, contingent, and emplaced struggles whose blueprint cannot be worked out or predicted in advance.... And when such an agenda of reform is imposed from above or outside, it is typically a violent imposition whose results are likely to be far worse than anything it seeks to displace. (2005: 36)

Local, above, outside, imposition—these terms assume stable cartographies of peoples and places that are fundamentally separated, as well as power structures that work by way of "vertical encompassment" (Ferguson and Gupta 2002: 982). Absent from this imaginary are the co-constituted character of much of the world, the character of governmental power that does not act upon stable subjects but produces them (Butler 1993), as well as the complex agency of transnational collaborators, understood, again, in Tsing's terms as operating across difference (2005). I suspect that Mahmood would agree with these points, which is precisely why I draw attention to her. I do not take these formulations as representative of her larger theoretical understandings of place, power, and agency but as representative of a much larger anthropological discourse that postulates a fallback position for opposing not only FGM discourses but neocolonial feminism at large. This position recognizes neocolonial elements in contemporary campaigns by their characteristics as imposed from above, bound to fail, and producing greater violence and harm. In contrast it sees meaningful and successful social transformation as local, emplaced, and self-motivated. Or, as Scheper-Hughes puts it, citing Kenyatta as a native informant, "the attention given to the subject by outsiders (even the most balanced and well-intentioned ones) may do more harm than good" (1991: 27).

In more general terms, what I call the *fallback position* states that the local and the social are sites and sources of meaningful social change and that governmental, statist, development, and, especially, outside interventions are prone to failure and to doing more harm than good. We should think of this fallback position as an anthropological and feminist safe place that readily generates consensus against the zeal to reform the global South: no one will be offended by an argument made from this position, and everyone will recognize anthropology within it. To express a variant of the fallback position is to express anthropological sensibility. And not only anthropological—feminist theory also pays its respects to this position's distance from the intersections of liberalism and feminist neocolonialism (captured by the shorthand terms *global sisterhood* and *global feminism*) by critiquing efforts of white men trying to save brown women.

The problem is that the fallback position has both political and analytical limitations. Politically it misses its target: not only have campaigns against cutting been thoroughly collaborative but global feminists have absorbed the anthropological objection exemplified in arguments such as Mahmood's. They agree with every word and utter such statements themselves; after all, they would say, they support African grassroots initiatives.[12] At the conference I mentioned earlier, German activists (some of whom are anthropologists by training) discussed the necessity of culturally sensitive campaigns proceeding from within Africa. And if there was one thing they all agreed on, it was their opposition to the racist sensationalism and neocolonialism of the earlier generation of Western feminists; the main theme of backstage conversations was the participants' objections to Fran Hosken's activism and Hanny Lightfoot-Klein's book *Prisoners of Ritual* (1989). Hence, not only would Western activists not recognize themselves as the targets of anthropological and feminist critique, they actively subscribe to it, perform it, and, at times, co-opt it. As do Western governments, a point to which I return later.

The analytical limitations of the fallback position emerge from the same problem. Critical feminist anthropology has not been able to explain how cutting could end, and few have written about contemporary developments in anticutting efforts and their consequences (Shell-Duncan and Hernlund 2007; Shell-Duncan et al. 2011, 2013; Abusharaf 2006a; Gruenbaum 2009). Anthropologists have had much to say about "the facts attached to this widespread custom in order to have some idea why the African peoples cling to this custom," as Kenyatta put it long ago ([1938] 1965: 128–29), but much less to say about how and why they *do not*. Many anthropologists anticipate that cut women will "resist" campaigns, and understand the unintended consequences of NGO interventions primarily through the idiom of failure.

Scholars also believe that Western women and men are the primary agents of campaigns and that Western discourses and affects therefore need to be the primary target of analysis and critique. This leaves the actual efforts to end cutting on the continent unexplored, including the attendant politics of governmental knowledge—despite titles promising such analysis (Nnaemeka 2005b). I attend to the multiplicity of African positions on cutting, their instrumentality in global governance, their myriad effects on social life, as well as the relationship of punitive rationality, social science, and epidemiological knowledge.

What is more, other scholars who rely on the fallback position and the postcolonial feminist analytics of white women's burden of formulating arguments against globalist feminism—whether these are about cutting, veiling, violence against women or others—cannot account for the compound imperial formations that exist either in the contemporary moment or (as I will venture later) in the past. And they know this: many who retreat to the fallback position would, in a different, theoretical conversation, agree about the limitations of conceptions of an unmediated locality and the model of power the position entails. The central difficulty, as I see it, is this: anthropological sensibilities and abilities to address topics such as anti-FGM campaigns have not kept pace with the theoretical developments in the discipline. My goal is to bring these closer together. This cannot be done from a hands-off position, with its correlative injunction that freezes critical feminist anthropology while the rest of the world is on the move, as are deployments of anthropological knowledge for anticutting campaigns.

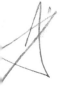

Writing otherwise about cutting and interventions against it means confronting contemporary vectors of power, inequality, violence, and imperial formations *head on,* examining them as ethnographic objects. In doing so, I attempt to redraw the cartographies of existing debates by allowing analytical questions to emerge from the social and governmental lifeworlds of the subjects of anticutting campaigns. Rather than simply contributing to existing debates about cutting, these questions lead us in unexpected directions. The chapters that follow stage an encounter between lived social and governmental worlds and anthropological and feminist theory about the interstices of social and governmental worlds, intersections of activism and governance feminism, and the importance of decoupling the analysis of unintended consequences of NGO interventions from the analysis of failure. My goal is to expand the tools for studying (post)colonial formations and developing decolonial analysis by foregrounding a critical appreciation of *sensibility*.[13]

To that end, I lay out my analytics, or conceptual "tracks" (Pigg 2005: 45). Pigg writes:

> I noticed that AIDS workers were not simply engaging in this "frank and open" discussion but actually were doing a great deal of work to create the very discursive ground that would make this possible. It was as though they had been funded to run a railway, and to do so by planners who somehow believed that the job merely involved managing arrivals and departures when, in fact, it first involved the laying of the tracks. (2005: 45)

In what follows, I delineate the premises of my approach. Here I have sketched out the specific ways in which *African* does not mean separate from the West but signifies their intertwining. Thus abstracted, this is not a new argument, and indeed many an element of my approach is already a stone set by others. I am simply rearranging them in a new route. Mine is an analysis "from the South" (Comaroff and Comaroff 2012) that foregrounds ethnography's unfinished character (Biehl 2013) and interruption of theoretical certainties. But first I emphasize my alternative analytics and clarify how my work departs from the common approaches and overdetermined debates about cutting that may appear to resemble my own.

After Relativism

This book is haunted by relativism, since female genital cutting has served as one of the primary objects for public and interdisciplinary debates about this anthropological principle. Whereas for anthropologists, relativism aims to unsettle, dissipate, and transform, its public and cross-disciplinary uptake is often reduced to comparison and adjudication. Across the disciplines cutting has been the privileged object of public and classroom debates regarding the limits of liberalism, multiculturalism, and tolerance and the inherent dilemmas of human rights. "Scholarly debate," Audrey Macklin observes, "has been preoccupied with the question of whether FGM should be tolerated" (2006: 217). Relativism becomes a performance of multicultural liberalism. Thus asking whether we should tolerate purports to settle and consolidate objects, political principles, and ethical values, while the very performance of debate produces thinking and feeling liberal publics and subjects who question. The framing of relativism as adjudication ("Rites vs. rights," "Is FGM a human rights violation?" "Where do we draw the line?" and even "Do we have the right to intervene") thus goes hand in hand with the production of those who adjudicate as questioning subjects, and whose democratic education, citizenship, rationality, thoughtfulness, and care are shored up in the process.

Relativism also operates by direct comparison and evaluation; cutting is set against the designer vaginas and male circumcision of today and against clitoridectomy-as-cure of yore. Comparison is meant to place African and Western practices on a level playing field but ultimately separates them by juxtaposing "their" cutting against "our" cosmetic surgeries. This kind of relativism also reduces commensurability to physically similar acts, thereby failing to imagine forms of commensuration that may be more relevant, such as the cultivation of subjectivity and sociality through discipline and pain. Consider the insights gained by Saba Mahmood's correlation of Egyptian Muslim women's piety not with Christian prayers but with the self-discipline of a "virtuoso pianist who submits herself to the often painful regime of disciplinary practice as well as to the hierarchical structures of apprenticeship" (2005: 29).

The modality of my analysis should not be misunderstood for either adjudicative or comparative relativism or for anthropological relativism. In Africanist anthropology relativism is an honored tradition of questioning Western reason, though it stops short of the task it sets itself. This relativism accepts what Latour calls the authority of Western "tribunals of reason" that render judgments about the irrationality of Others from a position of self-ascribed rationality. Relativism not only grants the West the authority to set the normative scaffolding upon which to evaluate African practices but also endorses the epistemic structure of accusation that positions anthropology on the defensive, rather than questioning the authority of the court. The conclusion is that Africans "are not so much illogical as simply *distant* from us" (Latour 1987: 190). Latour's ultimate point is that social scientists should question how science constructs itself as rational, rather than accept the fallout of its self-ascribed authority to adjudicate rationality. For me, the question is also how the distribution of rationality functions as a tool of governance.

Anthropological relativism tries to show that Africans are smart, creative, reasonable, agential, and yes, human. That they are people with history, not, pace Hegel (as Africanists often point out), outside it. That they are not simple, close to nature, unchanging, isolated. That they have magic does not mean that they lack science or rationality. That African women are not victims of patriarchy. But who needs that proof? Listen to the words of Ama Ata Aidoo's characters in her prose poem *Our Sister Killjoy*:

> '. . . You know how here in the western hemisphere, they still want to believe that the only thing Black people can do is to entertain them? Run, jump, and sing? Of course, we Africans have never really succumbed to their image of the Nigger . . .'
>
> '. . . But you can see how by remaining here someone like me serves a very useful purpose in educating them to recognise our worth . . . ?'
>
> 'Educating whom to recognise our worth, My Brother?' I asked.
>
> 'The people here,' he said.
>
> 'Where?'
>
> 'Here, in the West.'
>
> 'You mean white people?'
>
> 'Well . . . yes . . .'
>
> 'But they have always known how much we are worth. They have always known that, My Brother, and a whole lot more. They may not consider it necessary to openly admit it . . . that's another matter. They probably know it strategically unwise to. My Brother, if we are not careful, we would burn out our brawn and brains trying to prove what you describe as "our worth" and we won't get a flicker of recognition from those cold blue eyes. And anyway, who are they?' (Aidoo 1977: 129–30)

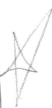

Aidoo's character Sissy objects to providing proof of African worth and reminds the expatriate "famous doctor" that history provides proof enough: the West is well aware of what it gained from exploiting Africa. Yet the burden of proof remains and is acutely felt by migrants in the West and by northern Ghanaians in the south of the country. Public discourses about FGM exacerbate it, and this is one of the reasons why scholars of Africa participate in tribunals of reason—*somebody* has to challenge the accusations of irrationality and lesser worth. But this is a self-appointed position, and it risks reinscribing the self-ascribed rational position of the West. Meanwhile, writing about Africa without offering a defense of the value, worth, and humanity of Africans is misread as complicity with the opposite view, the view of the continent in a perpetual state of lack (Mbembe 2001: 8). A continent minus. A continent that needs to catch up (Comaroff and Comaroff 2012: 12). This danger of misreading notwithstanding, I want to disengage from such proofs, so as not to affirm the entitlement of an audience that demands them. It is one thing to write for an audience that cares much but knows little—we all have more to learn. Something different and more sinister is at stake here:

accepting the demand for the proof of humanity, I suggest, negates this humanity in its very performance.[14] If scholars have to work so hard to preempt notions that Africans are lacking, lagging behind, or less worthy, it means that at some level they disbelieve African coevalness or are allowing Western publics an entitlement to this disbelief.

There is more to this problem, as even critics of liberalism are not free from its associated anxieties. Liberal democracies, writes Povinelli, are "haunted by the specter of mistaken intolerance" because they "know that in time their deepest moral impulses may be exposed to be historically contingent, mere prejudices masquerading as universal principles" (Povinelli 1998: 578). Anthropologists and feminist theorists of liberalism alike are hyperaware of this anxiety, whether they feel it as their own or anticipate it in the larger public, and expend much effort on its negotiation. The anxiety-prevention model demands that we perform a critical distance from any suggestion of intolerance; it is as if trigger warnings were insufficient and the triggers had to be anticipated far in advance, as well as cushioned and ameliorated.

I do not deny that what the West thinks about Africa matters, but I want to raise the question of what we do when we make it matter and suggest that we need not make it matter more than it already does. Rather than ascribing to the West an external authority and an epistemic and moral position that sets itself apart from the object it is concerned about, I insist that such a position is untenable. The point is not to argue that, with respect to the complex problems that are said to trouble Africa, the West is, as relativists claim, the same but that it is implicated. The West is always already entangled in the governance of Africa and is implicated in very specific ways in the governance of cutting, including its endings and nonendings alike. This book traces these implications.

To be clear, my attempts to refuse performative proofs of African rationality are not acts of tacit complicity with (neo)colonial discourse; rather, they constitute a critical take on the dominant modes of refuting this discourse. What happens when we proceed from the vantage point that takes African rationality as a basic supposition that needs no proof? How might this alter our practices of reading, learning, and writing? I see it as opening up space for analyzing how and why the constructions of rationality and irrationality, humanity and abjection, operate in the contemporary governance of cutting. So questions of rationality are not off the table but are themselves ethnographic objects that are constitutive of Ghanaian NGO governance as well as of the global forces that produce Africa and Africans as objects of intervention.

Rather than relativizing the harms of cutting, I show how ideas about these harms are constructed, understood, and acted upon and how they mobilize and redistribute care, violence, and rationality. I proceed from Ghanaian vantage points to reveal how multiple perspectives on what is harmful about cutting emanate from embodied lifeworlds. Subjects of NGO interventions do not relativize the harms of cutting but resituate the historical emergence of harm. These perspectives matter in everyday life and are part and parcel of reflections that hold local value and materialize action. I strive to think alongside them, or write "nearby," as Trinh puts it (Chen 1992: 87; Trinh 1989), to illuminate how Ghanaians mark the violence of history and sovereign violence, as well as to examine their erasure in liberal constructions of governmental power.

FROM THE SOUTH

This book puts into action what Jean Comaroff and John Comaroff refer to as "theory from the South" (2012), which for me is a type of analysis, rather than theory, a point to which I return shortly. Rather than seeing the postcolonial South as a passive terrain merely impacted by forces that originate in the West, or global North, or as sites for extracting raw data that can feed theories produced elsewhere, the Comaroffs suggest that "it is the global south that affords privileged insight into the workings of the world at large" (2012: 1). Bringing into the present the established argument that colonies were laboratories for "untried practices of governance and extraction, bureaucracy and warfare, property and pedagogy" (2012: 5), the Comaroffs understand the postcolonies as also "harbingers of history-in-the-making" (2012: 13). For me, this wording formalizes and invigorates the existing anthropological impetus to consider the ethnographic lifeworlds we study not as sources of information for preexisting questions and debates but as sites where both our questions and insights are transformed and reconfigured. Insights gained from Ghana shed light on wider African and Euro-American processes of governance and reorient theoretical debates about them.

For me, "from the South" is not a theory in the sense of an explanatory framework that orders the world, provides interpretive lenses, or shapes answers to my questions but an analytics that accounts for my points of departure, modes of inquiry, and scales of analysis. As a methodological principle, this means that my analysis proceeds from Ghanaian social and governmental worlds and follows concrete encounters across different sites. Ghanaian campaigns against cutting are important to understand in their own right, as they reveal not only the contours of governmental practices but also the surfaces they rub up against and the textures of subjectivity and experience that are reshaped in encounters that span regions and continents. But the campaigns also offer privileged insight into the constitution of contemporary global governance and its articulations with (neo)liberalism, feminism, and anthropology alike. Governmentality, too, is a South-North collaboration that is multidirectional and at times surprising. I read Achille Mbembe's argument that "the peculiar 'historicity' of African societies, their own *raisons d'etre* and their relation to solely themselves, are rooted in multiplicity of times, trajectories, and rationalities that, although particular and sometimes local, cannot be conceptualized outside a world that is, so to speak, globalized" (2001: 9) to include the practices of governance.

That the global South is a site of theoretical insights and an anchor of critical thought is particularly consequential for my engagement with feminist theory. Feminist diagnoses of the present often proceed from the vantage point of the global North and cannot account for the multiple guises and plural histories of the present. Analyzing *from* the South leads me to reexamine the epistemological certainties of feminist critique and reconceptualize its consequences. As governmental practices do not travel unimpeded (Tsing 2005), neither should the theories that account for them. I will suggest that histories of the (neo)liberal present, including such phenomena as governance feminism and its intersections with NGOs and activism, appear in a different light when analyzed from the South. They are less overdetermined than critics contend, leaving space for understanding how governmental power works through subjects and is reconfigured in that process.

Analyzing from the South is another way of saying that contexts and subjects matter and not just as background. Critical theory "is immanent in life itself" (Comaroff and Comaroff 2012: 48), as is problematization. Rural and urban Ghanaians alike, the subjects and agents of NGO projects, have critical perspectives on the present that are not only locally consequential but can transform the registers of scholarly critique, its foci, and its affects.

In the Way of Theory: Ethnography's Unfinished Business

By saying that "from the South" is an analytics, I also want to draw attention to some of the inherent tensions between ethnography and theory. In recent years anthropologists such as João Biehl (2013) and Janelle Taylor (2005) have provoked the discipline to rethink the form and value of ethnography, urging us to recognize that ethnography's force takes shape not as a contribution to theory but as being "in the way of theory." What is ethnography in the way of theory? True to form, Biehl begins his explanation by way of an ethnographic vignette. When Biehl told Geertz that he was tired of the question "What is your contribution to theory?" and asked Geertz how he would respond, "Geertz replied without missing a beat: 'Subtraction'" (Biehl 2013: 573). This statement is more than a provocation. To say that ethnography subtracts from theory can mean that it chisels something off theory, such as certainty or encompassment. As Biehl puts it, "Anthropologists are always fighting reductionist and hegemonic analytical frames even as we struggle to articulate and theorize the conditions of our subjects' becomings" (586).

Positioning ethnography in the way of, and against, theory does not situate it outside theory but in a particular relationship to it—not one of subordination, equivalence, or complementarity but one based on ongoing skepticism of master narratives and refusals to neatly order the world and issue final judgments. Ethnography compels us to question the epistemological certainties of theory work. Rather than foreclosing questions, positing schemas, or claiming that all is said and done, ethnography is a confrontation with surprise, uncertainty, and the messiness of everyday life. Ethnographic encounters are subjective and intersubjective, they are attuned "to the relations and improvised landscapes through which lives unfold" (Biehl 2013: 583).

Affirming ethnography's quality as being in the way of theory is Biehl's self-professed political move. Theory orders the world, Gregory Bateson, Pierre Clastres, and Gilles Deleuze and Félix Guattari have long argued, while ethnography is committed to instability. This, of course, is a performative statement, a call for an ethnography of instability. We need to acknowledge that anthropologists have long ordered the world, especially that of former colonies, and that we continue to do so in writing and by naming—Biehl, too, names ethnographic subjects *ours*. Disciplinary norms demand that we impose order precisely on those intersubjective encounters and "open-ended, even mysterious, social processes and uncertainties" (2013: 590) that are the lifeblood of ethnography. This is particularly the case with subject matter that is for many profoundly unsettling, such as female genital cutting. In this book I steer between the imperative to impose order and the ethnographic desire to attend to the world in flux, the world that moves on. As a result the sensory pull of my ethnographic memory and the materiality of fieldwork are often in tension with analytical scaffolding; at times I leave things unfinished so I can return, revisit, and encounter them anew.

Mine is an excessive ethnography that is marked by an aesthetics of formal surplus and close-up depictions of governmental encounters and reflections upon them. I strive to attend to the complexity, surprise, and excessive quality of social worlds that overflow analytical frames. This type of ethnography lingers on the haphazard, the contingent, the unpredictable. It follows fragments and splinters, conceived not as cultural particulars but as shreds of partial connections of a world linked through friction (Tsing 2005). It does not strive to moderate, restrain, contain, purify, or comfort. It leaves some things open, others closed, some unsettled, and others provisionally adjudicated.

Excessive ethnography is not a celebration or a political coup. I refuse to impose final order on situations of flux and uncertainty because it seems to me the right thing to do, but I neither forget the conditions of possibility in this approach nor take them for granted. Declaring the virtue of the unruly and the uncontained is itself a form of privilege that is not afforded to all. For those who have to obey, pass, and assimilate, overt unruliness is not an option. Unruliness, as I show in chapters 1 and 2, is an accusation leveled at northern Ghanaians by the governing apparatus that tries to manage and contain them, not something they can proudly declare. Feminist ethnographers also know this firsthand; for more than a century they have written dozens of unruly ethnographies that were dismissed and disparaged by the discipline (Visweswaran 1994).

Against Certainty: Feminist Theory and Desire for Law

Given that anticutting campaigns are characterized by NGO-ization and single-issue politics, feminist critical theory would see them as constituting bad feminist attachments and forms; campaigners would be seen not as feminists proper but as "feminist bastards" (Hodžić 2014). In particular campaigners would be castigated because they partake of governance feminism (Halley et al. 2006), which not only depends on state-centered and donor-funded forms of power but also has "an overwhelming investment in the power of the criminal law."[15] For leading feminist theorists the desire for law is both misguided and dangerous, and "left legalism" (Brown and Halley 2002b) has become a subject of scrutiny and critique. These theorists emphasize that the recognition and protection offered by law come at the cost of regulation, exclusion, and punishment. Rather than leading to social transformation, liberation, or more power for women, legal advocacy results in what has been called "carceral feminism" (Bernstein 2014).

Proceeding ethnographically and from the South, this book tells a different story about the feminist desire for law and its effects. My goal is not to vindicate the feminist fetishization of law, much less to celebrate it, but to show how Ghanaians wrestle with it and curb its excesses. I focus on how people—NGO workers, police officers, nurses, chiefs, rural men and women, circumcisers, cut girls—live with the law, and I demonstrate that they are never fully enveloped by it and that they work on the law as much as the law works on them. Ghana has been at the forefront of two global waves of criminalizing cutting, outlawing it in 1994 and expanding the scope of liability and punishment in 2007. GAWW wrote both pieces of legislation in collaboration with feminist lawyers, nudged them through passage, and then worked on their enforcement, mobilizing passions for law and order as well as sowing distrust and fear. The people subjected to these laws did not want them, but governmental workers enthusiastically embraced the law and the opportunities to serve as citizen-enforcers. However, after participating in arrests, they changed their minds; the last time the law was formally enforced was in 2004. By digging beneath the desire for law, the power ascribed to it, the technologies and haphazard circumstances of its enforcement, and the eventual turn against punishment and sovereign violence, I want to excavate the lived effects of governance feminism that critique alone cannot account for. There is more to the law than the maintenance of imperial order and collusion with repressive forces. This book is an invitation to consider governance feminism and NGO-driven campaigns against cutting not as bad objects but as ambivalent and complex ones.

My theoretical aim is to expand the analytico-affective grounds of feminist analysis of governance feminism and legal advocacy. I agree that Ghanaian campaigns have instituted a punitive rationality that converges with the regulatory forces of the state, as well as with neoliberalism and imperialism, but my approach differs in tone and affect. While critique situates itself outside its objects, I do not inscribe a fundamental difference between scholars and activists, critics and workers, those who are entitled to a secure position on the left and those whose politics are lived and ambivalent. I here take a cue from Wendy Brown's question "And how did we become cops anyway?"—a question she posed not in reference to governance feminism but to building curricula for women's studies and gender studies and our own regulatory and policing power as professors (Brown 1997: 85).

My departure from feminist critique does not represent radical disagreement but a difference in vantage points, the affective tenor and scope of our conclusions, and the terrain upon which they are crafted. I do not aim to refute arguments about punitive rationality or to assuage fears about the repercussions of carceral feminism but to cast them in a different light. Or rather, to bring them closer. To breathe the same air.

Feminist legal scholars studying governance feminism have taken up ethnography as a method but not crucial aspects of ethnographic sensibility, such as the commitment to proximity and thinking *with,* or the postcolonial feminist commitment to writing nearby. As Trinh puts it, this is a form of speech "that does not objectify, does not point to an object as if it is distant from the speaking subject . . . that reflects on itself and can come very close to a subject without, however, seizing or claiming it" (Chen 1992: 87). These are more than positions—they are affective dispositions and they matter. Rather than writing critique from a distance—moral, affective, epistemological, political, and geopolitical—I explore what emerges in close-up encounters, those of NGO workers and their subjects, as well as my own. What emerges is disidentification—"a strategy that works on and against dominant ideology," trying to transform its logic *from within* (Muñoz 1999: 11)—and immanent critique, produced by both agents and subjects of governmentality and put into action by them.[16] Urban Ghanaians and international scholars alike criticize NGO corruption, nepotism, and state indifference, but those whose lives are ruled by NGOs in one way or another articulate *lived* critiques of NGO governmentality. These critiques are trenchant but often quiet and barely perceptible; they resonate locally because they are words to live by—in tune with politics and the poetics of living. They respond to and refute some of the fundamental premises of NGO governance of northern Ghana, namely, that tradition is what hurts and that violence is justified when committed in the name of modernity and empowerment.

Writing nearby does not mean collapsing analysis and politics (see Mahmood 2005) or performing affective neutrality. I was neither politically neutral nor unaffected by the NGOs' projects. I was disheartened by the extent to which NGO-state governance not only entails blaming and shaming rural populations but is structured by this principle; meetings and workshops dominated by discussions of "harmful traditional practices" are the mainstay of development projects in the Upper East Region. As I will show, there is nothing pretty in this mode of governance (although the encounters generated by it are intensely social, amiable, and at times comic and lighthearted). Nor was I in favor of the criminalization of a practice that I learned was desired, in however complex ways, by those subject to it, and I was even less in favor of a revised law that would imprison cut girls and women themselves. But while I do not disavow my feelings, they are not the endpoint of my analysis. I am not a spectator waiting for a show to please me, who then writes a critical evaluation when it does not. The NGOs I write about have higher stakes in their projects and their social worlds than I do; I am connected to their world but not determined by it—they stay and I am a visitor. But I am also a visitor who takes the perspectives and complaints of NGO subjects seriously, and this multitude of perspectives is precisely the challenge that feminist ethnography brings to single stories and too-certain theories.

Some anthropologists work their way of out of this conundrum by writing sympathetically about NGO workers. Thomas Yarrow, for instance, turns to NGO workers' life histories and testimonies to argue against the understanding of NGOs as "resources that elites exploit to their own advantage ... whereby educated Africans exploit their positions of social privilege for personal gain." By doing so he wants "to counter the widespread assumption that for African NGOs moral discourses are nothing more than a charade behind which selfish acts of accumulation and aggrandizement are concealed" (2008a: 335). I fully agree with this view but find that it does not sufficiently challenge populist criticisms of NGOs. Pointing to the complexity of NGO workers is a widespread strategy that constitutes ethnographic sensibility but inadvertently misplaces the locus of critique on individuals. The point is not that NGO workers and civil servants are good people with good intentions just doing their jobs, and struggling to survive, though all this is true. Nothing in this book suggests otherwise; of course they are complex people with good intentions. But the limitations of this type of individualizing gesture are evident if we take seriously the anthropology of humanitarianism, which begins by situating good intentions and good people as constitutive of the problem to be addressed (and the common liberal solution to it), rather than figuring them as the solution or the locus of alternative hermeneutics.

I do not relativize or ameliorate what is potentially offensive and unsympathetic about NGOs and their workers but emphasize their *positioning*. I situate them in historical and global contexts of governance, showing that NGOs reauthorize colonial discourses that are not theirs to begin with. People are not fully enveloped by governmental forces and discourses, and can disrupt the modalities of governance that subjectify them, but opening up space for seeing just how they do so requires us to refrain from patching

while they may reproduce these discourses, it was not theirs or similar the ruptures revealed by close-up ethnographic description. Rather than suturing through relativizing and writing sympathetic accounts of individual lives and commitments, I want to reveal the governmental workers' positioning and the intensity of forces that pressure them. NGO workers and subjects alike are compelled to identify with ideologies of modernization, law, and order by devaluing and disidentifying with tradition—which is primarily projected onto rural subjects and is something the governmental workers have to disown. In doing so, they also have to distance themselves from kin and, ultimately, from themselves. And this leads me to the ultimate point of my analysis, which is to determine just how people in the Upper East Region exist in the face of interpellations that work not just upon them but through them. This is where complexity lies. That NGO workers and civil servants turn away from the exercise of power and from the subject position of citizen–law enforcers, as I show in the final chapter, means *much more* because being on the side of the law is one of the few viable subject positions accorded them within the nation-state and the global order alike.

From the South as a Scale

An ethnographic analysis from the South necessarily rethinks the normative ethnographic scope and scale of Africanist anthropology. It takes a cue from the classical conviction that the locus of anthropological study is not its object, that "anthropologists don't study villages (tribes, towns, neighborhoods . . .); they study in villages" (Geertz 1973: 22), and that consequently "where an interpretation comes from does not determine where it can be impelled to go" (23). But while this classical model distributes semiotics cross-culturally, it places theorizing in the North. When the interpretation is impelled to move, it moves to the world of ideas, whether to support or challenge them (in Geertz's example, sheep raiding tells us something about revolution). Taking "*from* the South" seriously unsettles the distribution of interpretative force. Accordingly, "the South" is a vantage point, not a locus of study; an analysis from the South is not confined to it but *is* grounded in it, including its world of ideas and reflection. From the South does not mean connecting a non-Western place and people to Western ideas but connecting place to place and ideas to ideas or, rather, tracing connections between places that are already mediated by ideas and governmental knowledges.

Specific sites and loci are my points of departure for an analysis of encounters, relationships, connections, and frictions of governance that span regions

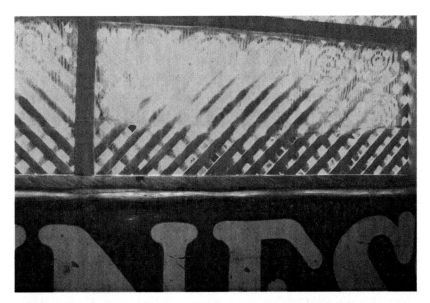

FIGURE 1. Observer observed: children peek in for a glance from outside the village bar.

and continents. Villages and NGOs are not what I study, but they are vantage points for tracing vectors that span regions and continents, past and present. Analysis "from the South" moves the anthropologist along with the objects. I explore and mediate encounters between people and places, encounters that make people, places, and the knowledge about them.

Anthropologists might object to the resulting categories of my analysis— at times I write about Africa (not just Ghana) and Ghana's North (not the Frafra ethnic group). I here take a cue from James Ferguson, who highlights the problems with an anthropology that shies away from writing about "Africa" in favor of more specific categories (2006). I do so because there is no Ghana that is not already a part of Africa and the postcolonial present. What is more, public and governmental cultures themselves operate across scale. As Ferguson writes, "The world is (perhaps now more than ever) full of talk, not of specific African nations, societies, or localities, but of 'Africa' itself" (2006: 1). Committed to the primacy of specificity, Africanist anthropology understands such discourses as sweeping and misguided generalizations, and contests them by appealing to cultural and contextual particularity. One upshot is that, as Ferguson puts it, "the discipline that contributed more than any other to what V. Y. Mudimbe . . . has termed 'the invention of Africa' has had almost nothing to say about 'Africa'" (2006: 1). Another consequence I want to stress is that the commitment to particularity inadvertently reifies the colonial mapping of ethnic groups and statist constructions of locality, thus naturalizing them as primary sites of identification and analysis. We cannot understand the intensity of moral concerns about and within Africa without attending to phenomena that cross regional and national borders. As I will show, Ghanaian and regional public cultures diagnose the present as a moment of a moral crisis, and the resulting moral panics, as well as the critical responses to them, are informed by translocal phenomena.

Within Ghana governmental problematizations of both cutting and "lack of development" hinge on certain understandings of the country's North. This is another category of governance that anthropological analyses see as illegitimate. Most studies conducted in the region use the ethnic group as a primary referent, even though the ethnic group is not a primary node of subjectivity or affiliation.[17] However naturalized the ethnic group may be, there is nothing self-evident about it; its salience is a product of colonial governance and has been both reinforced and contested by anthropologists (see chapter 1). For example, there are no Frafras unadulterated by the colonial taxonomies bolstered by anthropological reason. Ghana's North is also a product of colonial governance that endures in the contemporary political imagination. We have much to gain from addressing it head on and not merely as a construct but as a product of sedimented histories that structures the lifeworlds of people in the region. The imaginary of Africa and Ghana's North in the worlds of development agencies and NGOs has concrete effects on how people are governed, on forms of rule, subjectivity, and meaning. As Ferguson writes, Africa is real, it has "a mandatory quality" and it is "a category within which, and according to which, people must live" (2006: 6). Expanding the scale of analysis does not mean forgoing but reframing what a contextualized analysis and privileging of the specific look like when we trace the vectors that constitute place and people.

My goal is not to represent anyone, much less to claim representativeness: Africa does not stand for the world, Ghana does not stand for Africa, the Upper East Region does not stand for northern Ghana, one village in the Bongo District does not stand for the entire district, and the women and men I got to know and with whom I conducted research do not stand for all of Bongo and Bolgatanga, or for Frafra or for northern, Ghanaian, or African women and men. Rather than considering them as microcosmic instantiations of something larger, I trace how they are *incorporated* into social and governmental worlds. The NGOs I analyze received funding not because there was something particularly Ghanaian about their work but because they belonged to a cluster of African NGOs trying to end FGM. To locate their work within the structures of governance and their entanglements with lifeworlds, I explore how they construct and materialize people as being of a place, as belonging or not belonging, as being proximate or distant—or, as is often the case, as physically and ethnically proximate but affectively and morally distant.[18]

Transnational Vectors: Is the Global North Evolving toward Africa?

It is often presumed that anticutting discourses and campaigns are Western and imposed on Africa, but in actuality the European Union and the United States are in many ways "evolving toward Africa" (Comaroff and Comaroff 2012) or at least trying to do so. Activists and governments alike are looking to Africa for solutions and want to emulate African strategies. When in early 2013 the U.K. Department for International Development announced that it was dedicating thirty-five million pounds to the cause, Efua Dorkenoo, then of Equality Now, suggested that "to eliminate FGM," the U.K. needed to "follow Africa's lead," pointing to success stories of decreased rates of cutting on the continent.[19] A few years earlier the Dutch government had also announced a plan "to visit African countries in 2010 in order to learn from successful campaigns to combat female circumcisions," referring to this process as "reverse development cooperation."[20] African countries were also said to possess superior statistical knowledge: at the launch of a new national campaign, "Say No to FGM," which targeted African immigrants to the Netherlands, the Dutch deputy health minister said that her government did not know how many Somali and other migrant women were mutilated, whereas the national statistics from African countries were "more reliable" and provided a "clearer picture of the situation." These constructions of the discovery of African strategies disavow longstanding entanglements of the West in anticutting campaigns, as well as the violence inherent therein.

To some the discovery of Africa meant a newfound source of culturally sensitive and culturally appropriate campaigns. As the Dutch minister of development cooperation put it:

I am looking for non-repressive means of securing opportunities for girls and women and ensuring their safety. What I mean is an approach like the one adopted in Senegal. A respectful approach that enables people to draw their own conclusions about female circumcision, and lead their own opposition to it.[21]

The professed desire for anticutting campaigns to be nonrepressive and empowering flies in the face of overt exercises of power in anticutting campaigns, both in Africa and in the global North. As I will show, Ghanaian and other IAC campaigners insist that Westerners are too soft, that cutting is mutilation and should therefore be dubbed "FGM" not "FGM/C," that it is not culture but violence, that its subjects need to be surveilled rather than cared for and sensitized rather than empowered, and that those who refuse sensitization should be incarcerated. RHI's more culturally sensitive and liberal-sounding campaigns are also deeply hierarchical, but the implications of these power relations are not in the least straightforward (chapter 4). Although an ethnography of deliberate intolerance cannot but provoke a sense of liberal panic, my goal is not to assuage it. Rather, I contextualize it and, instead of smoothing it over, leave it unsettled and delineate its fissures in order to reveal its surprising effects. In contrast to Ghanaian campaigns that are overtly hierarchical and often repressive, governments in the global North couch their anti-cutting policies as empowering, nonrepressive, and African-sourced , but these policies are in practice far more violent.

While the Dutch hoped to learn from Africa, the United States wants to learn from the United Kingdom and from the Inter-African Committee's "Zero Tolerance" policies. Two Democratic members of Congress, Joe Crowley of New York and Sheila Jackson Lee of Texas, proposed additional legislation against cutting (which is already a crime under federal law), titled the Zero Tolerance for FGM Act of 2015 (in a congressional subcommittee since February 2015). The IAC's concept of "zero tolerance" is a multilayered global product that also defies the discovery of pure African solutions. The concept was imported to Africa from the United States, where it serves as a penal ideology and practice that calls for prosecuting crimes without consideration of mitigating circumstances and for automatic and severe punishment. In 2003 the IAC repurposed this concept, and Zero Tolerance to Female Genital Mutilation Day has since become the network's most resonant global export. It has been adopted by the United Nations, and international NGOs and governments have seized on it for staging events that demonstrate their tough stance and punitive power. One upshot has been a concentrated focus on calls for greater surveillance and criminalization of African migrants living in the global North. In February 2015, for instance, British police and the U.K. Border Agency carried out an operation at Heathrow airport, arresting and then immediately releasing a Zimbabwean woman on her way to Ghana, with the stated intention "to raise awareness ... to coincide with the International Day of Zero Tolerance of FGM."[22] Regardless of the outcome, the spectacular arrest made FGM a tangible threat, not only to immigrant girls seen as at risk but also to the self-definition of the United Kingdom and Europe.

The proposed Zero Tolerance for FGM Act is a response to the Western iteration of the "underground resistance" discourse and addresses the perception that immigrant African and Middle Eastern parents are intent on circumventing U.S. law and taking their daughters to their home countries to be cut. Similar laws prohibiting international travel for purposes of cutting are already in place in western Europe, where they have been put in the service of surveillance, punitive rationality, and a demonstration of Fortress Europe–style state sovereignty by way of border control. Crowley wants the United States to follow the lead of the United Kingdom, where, he says, "the government, in collaboration with FGM survivors, is taking strong action." The United Kingdom is indeed among the world leaders in a particular style of intervention: those that construe African and Muslim immigrants as a threat to their children and the national body politic and that subject them to surveillance. Immigrants are scrutinized by social services, teachers, medical authorities, and legal institutions, while their daughters are urged to disidentify with their parents. Similar processes are underway in the European Union, Canada, and Australia.

In the United States passionate anti-FGM politics are now supplanted by the desire for facts: the amendment proposes a study of the domestic prevalence of cutting. And given multicultural democracy's recognition of its "specter of mistaken intolerance" (Povinelli 1998: 578), the image of the anti-FGM activist is no longer a white feminist from the West but an African woman—ideally, a survivor of the practice. Thus the voice of Jaha Dukureh, a Guinean-born immigrant who runs an NGO in Atlanta aimed at drawing attention to the dangers of cutting, has been the most prominent in raising awareness of the ostensibly rampant *underground* performance of cutting on U.S. soil. Existing (and important) feminist theorizations of African women as agents, not victims, do little to illuminate the construction of an African activist who serves as a privileged "native informant" and legitimizes proposed legislation. Dukureh was identified as the potential face of legal advocacy by the *Guardian*'s campaign to end FGM, which was begun in 2014. Soon after being trained in London and promoted by the *Guardian*, Dukureh joined hands with the American NGO Equality Now and Representative Crowley to petition for the study on prevalence. Analyzing the search for facts "from the South" reveals, as we shall see in chapter 3, that this search leads not to evidence-based governance but to increased surveillance and criminalization.

That the global North looks to Africa is not something to be celebrated. By importing zero tolerance to FGM, the global North adopts the IAC's motto but fails to import the checks on the excesses of liberal violence that are immanent in Ghanaian and African governmental lifeworlds. While Ghanaians at first glance embrace zero tolerance policies and laws, in practice they also put constraints on them (see chapters 6 and 7). Meanwhile the global North's self-congratulatory tone of "following Africa's lead" is particularly jarring, insofar as it treats Africa as an inspiration for ruling African migrants through oppressive logics that figure them as suspicious, untrustworthy quasi-citizens and unwanted members of the polis.

Fieldwork in Governmental Worlds

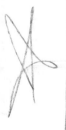

My main fieldwork sites and vantage points for my analysis of translocal encounters were two NGOs, GAWW and RHI. While this gave my research a more formal and programmatic structure, Ghanaian NGO worlds traverse public and private, formal and informal, social and governmental forms. NGO workers socialized during the day, not after hours. So I joined them in banter, intrigue, and serious conversations, shared snacks of bananas and groundnuts in Accra and *toubani* in Bolga, and watched lives unfold over time. I immersed myself in the daily rhythms of these workers and joined them at meetings, workshops, and public health outreach campaigns in urban and rural areas. We traversed various corners of the Upper East Region, and I followed them to the Northern and Upper West regions and Accra, as well as to Geneva and Washington, D.C. Between 2002 and 2009 I spent one year in the Upper East Region, primarily in the Bolgatanga and Bongo districts, and half a year in Accra, with the bulk of fieldwork taking place between October 2003 and October 2004.

GAWW put female genital cutting on Ghana's governmental agenda: the NGO had educated and "sensitized" nurses, teachers, police, Parliament members, other civil servants, and some groups that practiced cutting; GAWW was also the main force behind the criminalization of cutting in 1994 and in 2007, and in some cases it was behind enforcement of the law. They were also responsible for incorporating education about cutting in Ghana's reproductive health policy and medical training curricula for nurses. RHI described its approach as community based and designed projects that addressed rural women and men by way of public health outreach programs. GAWW is still operational, having survived a change of leadership at the turn of the millennium, but RHI closed its doors in 2007 when Dr. Adjei retired.

I observed how both organizations engaged in the making of regulatory mechanisms: emergent legislation, the production and mobilization of medical knowledge, and the codification of cultural meanings of cutting. I sought out and examined legal memoranda, prison registers, and court transcripts. I visited government offices and studied their registers of NGOs, policies, and reports. To understand the aftermath of NGO interventions, I reversed my ethnographic positioning for a part of my fieldwork—I relocated to a village in the Bongo District, where, rather than taking the NGOs as points of departure, I investigated how NGO projects land and reverberate in social and political life. This shift in ethnographic vantage point enabled me to reframe my analysis from within the larger predicaments and experiences of the subjects of NGO interventions. Although I am conversant in Frafra-Gurene, I relied on help from two research assistants for all interviews that were not conducted in English. My analysis also draws heavily on more than one hundred in-depth interviews and life histories I conducted with NGO workers and volunteers, civil servants, government and donor officials, chiefs, politicians, "ordinary" men and women (cut and uncut), and former circumcisers.

Since anticutting interventions are translocal, an ethnography of their problematization has definite beginnings but an uncontained form. This project began as my own encounter with the limits of anthropology and feminism, and although Ghana was my main point of departure for a transnational and historical analysis of encounters, my ethnographic terrain was not restricted to *the* field (in the singular, with a definite article) that constitutes an elsewhere—a confined space-time marked by deliberate, professional, and secure passages across social and geographical distance. Both questions and objects followed me wherever I went, to the here and now of life, writing, and teaching. My research was on an "awkward" scale (Comaroff and Comaroff 2003), tracing the rhizomes in which Ghanaian efforts to end cutting are nodes of a larger global phenomenon. Because of the analytical frame I imposed on it, this book is more focused on Ghana than the field-work itself would have demanded.

Tracing the genealogies of current campaigns meant going to Ghana's National Archives in Accra, as well as the British Colonial Archives in London. Understanding Ghanaian public and governmental cultures meant reading and analyzing news media and popular culture, as well as government documents. I also followed debates about government regulations of cutting in other African news media, both by using databases such as AllAfrica and by keeping tabs on IAC meetings, reports, and documents. Throughout the years I kept abreast of UN and Western feminist interventions against cutting by means of their media presence, as well as by reading their documents and observing their public events—all the while keeping an eye on how these projects reposition African efforts to end cutting and how they draw on anthropological knowledge and feminist discourses.

I did not arrive in Ghana with intimate knowledge of the country, so I was learning not only about my specific research questions but also about social rules, norms, tastes, cadences, silences, moods, and rhythms. At the same time I was also unforgetting forms of sociality and being that I had grown up with but had since cast aside. As this was the fourth country in which I was making a home, I was learning by osmosis and absorption. A migrant learns not by asking questions or having the freedom to make mistakes but by being alert to the social cues and open to the world around her—whether on *tro-tros* (vans that are the main means of public transportation), in markets, Accra's highlife bars, or at home. I lived with Ghanaians from all walks of life (university professors, NGO workers, villagers) and different ethnic groups. Many were transnational subjects: some had studied abroad and some had worked in Nigeria before being expelled during the bilateral crisis in the 1980s; my Accra hosts were a German Ghanaian couple, and in Bolga I lived with an Indian Canadian NGO worker. This book is not about any of these people, but they inhabit many of its pages.

CHAPTER SKETCHES

This book's narrative progresses from the historical appearance of cutting as an object of governance to the exploration of the logics and techniques of contemporary NGO interventions and their surprising effects on formations of subjectivity and disidentification with the political order and sovereign violence.

Chapter 1 (Colonial Reason, Sensibility, and the Ethnographic Style) analyzes the history of efforts to regulate and criminalize cutting in northern Ghana in order to examine the durable traces those efforts left on the present and to expand and retool postcolonial feminist analysis. I want to account for the forms of knowledge, affect, and ordering of the world and desires to change it that stretch from colonialism to the present. I show that imperial interventions entailed opposition from within by regional officers posted to what is today northern Ghana and whose politics were shaped by a white man's burden to protect the natives from other white men and women. By looking back at the larger British governance of northern Ghana, I show how violence and dispossession were enmeshed with the feminist will to knowledge, anthropological taxonomies, and benevolent appreciation of cultural difference and its codification for purposes of securing colonial rule. This entanglement gave rise to a conflict among colonial officials whose form and logic evince enduring forms of power-knowledge and sensibility that live on in present governmental campaigns and scholarly analytics.

Chapter 2 (Making Harmful Traditional Practices) examines the Ghanaian problematization of cutting as a "harmful traditional practice" and contextualizes it within governance discourses and policies that conceptualize poverty in northern Ghana as an effect of harmful traditions. Here I show that the codification of harmful traditions is embedded in the larger frameworks of modernization and development that have shifted over time. The national discourse of harmful traditions is the primary mode of problematizing northern poverty; this discourse draws on neoliberal technologies of recognizing scarcity while shifting the responsibility for it to northern Ghanaians and their traditions. I suggest that anticutting campaigns use this notion to mediate the fraught relationship between Ghana's North and South and the place of the North in the Ghanaian polity. I argue that the public embrace of this problematization results from the construction of northern Ghana as a counterpoint to southern civilization and modernity and as a site for displacing postcolonial lack, shame, and disorder.

Chapter 3 (When Cutting Did and Did Not End) examines how it is that the discourse of FGM lives on, despite the demise of cutting. Although cutting is on the wane in Ghana, the discourse of its "intractability" is used to produce suspect citizens and to legitimate punitive rationality. In this chapter I show how social science is mobilized to support claims that rural communities resist anticutting campaigns and continue to practice cutting underground. This chapter also refracts the endings of cutting through the lens of nostalgia: former circumcisers long for the ancestral benevolence that cutting secured for them, and uncut Ghanaians bemoan the disappearance of the traditional patriarchal values they believe cutting upheld.

In chapter 4 (Mistaken by Design: Biopolitics in Practice) I turn to practices of persuasion as techniques of governance and examine how RHI addresses rural publics in the Upper East Region. Through an ethnography of public health educational film screenings, I try to understand how RHI's work is persuasive, even though it eschews translation and mobilizes misrepresentations. Rather than interpreting these as indicators of a lack of knowledge or tying them to failure, I suggest that they constitute deliberate, tactical refusals of translation. Medical anthropologists tend to emphasize and critique what is *said* in public health and development interventions and how it is said, but I want suggest that what is *done* and how power is *materialized* matters much more. My analysis of the place of knowledge in NGO interventions shows that NGOs like RHI know how to make knowledge matter, and NGOs also recognize that more than knowledge is needed for the production of authority. Claims about the harms of cutting become "true" when presented in visual spectacles that materialize governmental power and set the conditions and constraints on which knowledge about reproduction, health, and society is socially productive.

For women who have stopped cutting, the success of interventions against cutting in northern Ghana is also an index of a troubled economy and consequent bodily vulnerability. In chapter 5 (Blood Loss and Slow Harm in Times of Scarcity) I recast the aftermath of governmental achievements in light of the perspectives of rural women in the Bongo District who were targeted by NGO and state interventions. Taking their concerns about lack of blood as a starting point, I explore how they problematize harm and make sense of the end of cutting. Cutting is now seen as unworthy of blood loss and as a critical event that generates a lifelong susceptibility to illness. Cutting had to stop, they say, given how the struggles of the contemporary moment have meant that women can no longer afford to lose blood. Furthermore, while NGOs and the state seek to isolate cutting in a hermetically sealed world of rural northern Ghanaians who resist change, these women link the end of cutting to national and pan-African concerns and idioms, joining a chorus of voices that criticize national blood shortages and emphasize the associated failures of biopolitical care.

After adopting its Constitution of 1992, Ghana criminalized cutting not once but twice. In chapters 6 and 7, which should be read together, I investigate the intimate relationship of violence and law by analyzing, respectively, the associated efforts to reform and enforce the law against cutting. Chapter 6 (The Feminist Fetish: Legal Advocacy) illuminates how GAWW's advocacy for more severe legislation functions as an early instantiation of the logic of zero tolerance to FGM. I attend to Ghanaian advocates' reckoning with both the power of law and the tensions within feminist liberalism, namely, those between protection and punishment, and freedom and violence. In chapter 7 (Against Sovereign Violence) I reveal that the collusion between feminism and sovereign violence is contested, even when it seemingly wins the day, and that NGO workers and civil servants themselves turn "against the state" (Clastres 1989) in the form of what I refer to as "governmentality against itself." By way of an ethnography of the arrest, trial, imprisonment, and pardon of two circumcisers I show that civil servants and NGO workers' participation in law enforcement eventually brings the fetishization of law into crisis and leads to a disidentification, not only from sovereign violence but also from the imperial order of things.

You will get this question, my Gurene-language teacher tells me. *Zaam zaam fu yese la tinkana?* (Please, which place do you come from?)

First you answer: I come from abroad. *Mam yese la solemitiŋa.*

They will then ask: Which part of abroad? *Fu yese la solemitinkana?*

I say, Bosnia.

He disagrees: Don't tell them you are from Bosnia. They will not know about Bosnia. Say Germany. Or America.

He was right about most of the villagers. But in Accra, Bolgatanga, and Bawku I met more people who spoke my mother tongue than I had ever met in the United States. They told me:

I studied in Yugoslavia. That was a long time ago, when things were good.

I studied in Belgrade.

I studied in Zagreb.

I was in Srebrenica, with the UN Peacekeeping forces.

At a workshop at the University of Ghana, a professor sitting next to me handed me a note, asking:

Da li si iz:

a) Hrvatske?

b) Srbije?

c) Slovenije?

A Bosnian in Ghana is less thinkable than a Croat, Serb, or Slovene.

Others said: *Zdravstvuj! Kak pozivajes?*

Harasho, spasiba. But I don't actually speak Russian.

You don't speak Russian?

No, my parents' generation learned Russian in school. I learned English.

I see. I studied in Russia.

Oh, you are from Bosnia! I want to go to Kosovo. There are such opportunities there for preaching. I want to go on a mission there. The entire region is very interesting to me.

Young men rattled off the names of soccer players.

Ah! Bosnia-H-e-r-z-e-g-o-v-i-n-a! Salihamidžić! Ibrahimović! Džeko!

The Black Stars coach is from Serbia. Do you know him? Plavi?

Halihodžić is the coach for Ivory Coast.

1

Colonial Reason, Sensibility, and the Ethnographic Style

Colonialism is not a history that arrives on a ship, as Ortner puts it (1984), determining historical agency sui generis. Nor is cutting an initially immutable or stable practice that colonialism suddenly transformed. The history of practices of cutting is plural, discontinuous, and fragmented; it is a history of ongoing regulation, change, and intervention. Significant transformations have been documented by scholars analyzing the twentieth century. Migrant groups, such as the West African Zabarma, who migrated to the Sudan more than a century ago, have had to contend with social pressures to alter the kind of cutting they practice (Gruenbaum 2001); meanwhile some Sudanese adopted the British-propagated "intermediate operation," which the Sudanese now refer to as "government circumcision" (Boddy 2007: 196); and in the Chad, girls from nonpracticing groups adopted cutting on their own, acting on desires to "experiment with modernity" (Leonard 2009: 93). However, practices of cutting, interventions aimed at eliminating them, and larger historical forces have been intertwined for much longer.

Take the passages from the hadith (the sayings of the prophet Muhammad) that are much talked about in scholarly and political debates: "Um Atiyyat al-Ansariyyah said: A woman used to perform circumcision in Medina. The Prophet (*pbuh*) said to her: Do not cut too severely as that is better for a woman and more desirable for a husband."[1] This saying is frequently cited in debates about whether Islam requires cutting (Fluehr-Lobban 2013: 97; Gruenbaum 1996) and in efforts to understand when and where cutting began; the passage is taken as evidence that Muslims practiced cutting in the seventh century and that it arrived in Africa from Saudi Arabia (see Gruenbaum 2001: 45).[2] I turn to this saying to highlight something of an entirely different order, which is that as early as the seventh century, cutting existed simultaneously with attempts to regulate it. In this case a religious authority was trying to modify and reduce the extent of the cut. We should assume that this was neither the first nor the last time before colonialism that authoritative historical figures weighed in on whether or how cutting should be practiced. That little is known about how cutting was lived and regulated between the seventh and late nineteenth centuries is a reflection of disciplinary formations and omissions rather than the stability of an unregulated set of practices.

My turn to *colonial* history as the precursor of contemporary interventions is motivated by their intertwined logics and the durable traces colonialism left on the present.[3] My aim is to analyze and expand existing understandings of what exactly these traces are. I will suggest that they are surprising and not at all as obvious as existing feminist and postcolonial scholarship suggests they are. My goal is to point to the limits of what has become a taken-for-granted analytics in prevalent critiques of neocolonialism and to suggest that they unwittingly extend colonial reason and sensibility into the present.

"Imperialism is a will to dominate that haunts us even today," writes Nnaemeka (2005b: 7). That is true, but this definition sheds light on only the more obvious forms of imperialism in Western anticutting discourses and campaigns such as the Clitoraid campaign titled "Adopt a Clitoris" sponsored by the Raëlian Church. Clitoraid was raising funds for clitoris reconstruction surgeries at a "pleasure hospital" the Raëlians wanted to build in Burkina Faso by offering African women's clitorises for metaphorical adoption (see preface).[4] To critics of efforts to save Africa, be they scholars, activists, and/or subjects of feminist and humanitarian interventions, the campaign mobilized in the name of saving African women was obviously neocolonial. Critics started a countercampaign and questioned the exploitative and racist sensationalism that objectified and commodified African women's genitals and offered them for figurative ownership. Kamau-Rutenberg's emerged as one of the critical scholarly voices in the African and diasporic blogosphere and public culture that question the premises of humanitarian interventions and the terms under which Africa becomes an object of Western attention (Wainaina 2005; George 2013).[5] The Raëlians' adoption strategy was particularly jarring; although common in humanitarian organizations (Bornstein 2001), it crossed the threshold of acceptability when it was applied to the genitals of African women. Kamau-Rutenberg writes:

> Nobody's genitalia should be talked about in the way that Clitoraid is talking about African women's genitalia. In fact, no part of anyone's body should be up

for adoption in this way that reminds us too much of the slave trade (Oh no, I went there!). Seriously, what does it mean to "adopt a clitoris"? Does that mean you own said clitoris or are you just fostering it for a little bit? Do you get to name it? What are the implications for the person whose clitoris is being adopted?[6]

Both ownership and objectification of women's (and men's) genitals were precursors of colonialism in the era of scientific racism and constitutive of it. Colonial officials and ethnographers stationed in what is today northern Ghana did not write much about genitals, given their commonly expressed disdain for nudity, but the pictures they took and bodily drawings they made reveal their fascination with and objectification of local subjects. The governmental ethnographer Captain R. S. Rattray took pictures "showing the method of tying the penis" and a nude reclining woman (Hawkins 2002: 77, 247), while the National Archives in Accra are replete with drawings of bodily and facial scarification. And if we accept that colonial rule has itself been predicated on blackness as genitality, the colonial conquest had both land and genitals as its targets (Fanon 1967).[7] There is much to be said for a symbolic analysis of the colonial order and its conceptualization of Africa as a virgin territory. Anne McClintock (1995) has shown that female genitals make their appearance in colonial maps. The same symbolism is mobilized in anticolonial movements, such as in Ngũgĩ wa Thiong'o's *The River Between* (1965), which depicts the struggle over female circumcision between the Gikuyu and Scottish missionaries; on the book's cover the shape of the ridge divided by the struggle is also vaginal.[8]

Ghanaian campaigns against cutting evince less obvious forms of imperial debris, and my intention is to examine their surfacing in governmental practices (see Taylor 2005). To do so I need to retool postcolonial feminist analysis and question the stability of the alliance of theory and a form of critique we might call critique from a distance. Anticutting campaigns are often understood through the critical lens of Gayatri Spivak's famous indictment of the colonial paradigm of white men saving brown women from brown men. It is well known that in India and elsewhere, the British turned women's liberation from tradition into an excuse for colonial rule (Mani 1998: 2), thus turning the "woman question" into a justification for their colonial civilizing mission (Chatterjee 1989). Scholars apply this critical lens to contemporary anticutting campaigns and understand them as neocolonial instantiations of the "white man's burden medicalized" (Morsy 1991), as well as, in broader terms, the saving of African women from African men by Westerners— including by white and African American women (Nnaemeka 2005c). This scholarship rightly points to the racialized neocolonialism inherent in Western feminist preoccupations with saving African women's genitals; campaigns are replete with patronizing, narrow concerns void of larger analyses of African gender relations and subjectivities, geopolitical inequalities, imperial formations, and feminism's own imbrications in them. As Nnaemeka writes, "The problem with this circumcision business is that many Westerners who plunge into it do so thoughtlessly" (2005a: 37). However, an unintended effect of this theorizing and its focus on Western discourses is that entire areas of critical inquiry have been cordoned off, leading to misconceptions of power relations that have structured both colonial and contemporary anticutting campaigns. Among other things, it prevents us from understanding that imperialism entailed opposition *from within,* such as the anti-interventionist logic of regional officers stationed in what is today northern Ghana, a logic that was shaped by a white man's burden to protect the natives from *other* white men and women.

The widespread reception of Spivak's critical phrase as a platform for feminist analysis gives an illusion of completeness of inquiry into histories of the postcolonial present. Certainly, white men and women were central to anticutting debates and interventions during colonialism: missionaries posted to Kenya tried to ban it (L. Thomas 2003; Kanogo 2005), British parliamentarians debated criminalization across the empire, and two British nurses trained Sudanese midwives in alternative forms of the operation (Boddy 2007). But the postcolonial present is more complicated, and the cast of characters has multiplied many times. In addition to imperial feminists, colonial officials and missionaries, and anthropologists, anticutting campaigns now include African feminists, both diasporic and continental; other activists who are women of color; and regional governmental reformers. As I stressed earlier, recent advocacy against cutting is also an African-European-American collaboration; the Swedish NGO worker Margareta Linnander cofounded the Inter-African Committee on Harmful Traditional Practices Affecting the Health of Women and Children (IAC), and in Ghana, IAC members such as the wife of the Dutch ambassador lobbied for the Ghana Association for Women's Welfare (GAWW) to receive funding from the Dutch Embassy. The Ghanaian advocacy is also internally fractured, as middle- and upper-class Ghanaian women and men, often from the South, as well as northerners who have migrated south, have been the main advocates against cutting. Similarly, urban NGO workers are trying to save rural northern women from cutting, which also means from themselves.

In this chapter I want to show that the presence of white people is an insufficient basis for analyzing imperial formations, and I will highlight instead the continuing reverberations of a colonial *logic*—in both interventions and critical opposition to them. I agree with Ann Stoler's assessment that the field of contemporary postcolonial studies is "overconfident in its analytics and its conceptual vocabulary, too assured of what we presume to know about the principles and practices of empire that remain in the active register" (2008: 192). I strongly suspect that Spivak would agree that what she originally wrote about colonial rule in 1820s India cannot be uniformly applied to the 1930s Gold Coast or to postcolonial Ghana. I will provide some specific examples of continuities, building on Lata Mani's work (1998), but my purpose is to question what we really know about colonial campaigns against cutting and their contemporary afterlives. Feminist criticism has rarely availed itself of existing historical analyses (L. Thomas 2003; Kanogo 2005; Boddy 2007), and this situation is compounded by the limits of analytical imagination. Too often scholars fail to differentiate between debates and practices, whether colonial or postcolonial. As Stoler writes,

> Academic debates about the lessons of empire . . . have been contained and constrained by the framing of issues and arguments against which critique has been posed. In the rush to account for the nature of imperial practices today and their similarities or differences from earlier European and U.S. imperial interventions, a very particular vocabulary has seized hold of our intellectual and political space. (2008: 192)

How do we make space for new arrangements of anthropological and historical study and critical analysis? The charge is to revisit the question of how colonialism informs contemporary governance and political and analytical sensibilities. By portraying complexities of colonial rule, my purpose is to set the stage for analyzing enduring forms of power-knowledge and sensibility that live on in present governmental campaigns and scholarly analytics. This requires questioning the assumption that colonial political debates seamlessly led to or accurately reflected policies and practices of rule, as well as paying attention to the less perceptible residues of imperial formations that structure both anticutting interventions and the work of their opponents. I want to account for the forms of knowledge, affect, ordering of the world, and desires to change it that stretch from colonialism to the present. This chapter will first shed light on specific logics of colonial power in anticutting campaigns of the Gold Coast, as Ghana was then called, and point to their complex afterlives.

At the heart of British colonial debates about cutting was a tension between two opposing camps: the humanitarian-feminist camp, which wanted to criminalize cutting and thereby liberate African women from the custom perceived as detrimental to Africans' reproduction and population growth, and the administrative-ethnographic camp, which opposed imperial reformist zeal and argued that African women did not need that form of liberation. These camps were gendered, classed, and ordered by the hierarchies of imperial rule. The first included British parliamentarians, among them aristocratic and middle-class women and men based in London (Pedersen 1991), and the second included British male administrators posted to Africa such as those governing the Northern Territories of the Gold Coast; these men often had military backgrounds. They positioned themselves differently with respect to cutting, the woman question, and the very purpose of colonial governance.

The critical paradigm of white men saving brown women from brown men cannot explain why British women at the center of the empire wanted to save African women from African men and from themselves, whereas British men posted to the Gold Coast were trying to save local societies from the British women and men at the imperial center. The imperial will to dominate was opposed from within, using a specific logic. By labeling the first position feminist and the second ethnographic, I want to draw attention to the afterlives of this colonial situation in contemporary campaigns and scholarly analyses, both anthropological and feminist.

COLONIAL INQUIRIES: THE DESIRE FOR FACTS

The first colonial interventions to end cutting in what is today northern Ghana were not couched in such terms. In concert with the minimal, rather than the biopolitical or welfare, logics of colonial rule of this region, the British did not sponsor widespread campaigns against cutting. They, did, however, inquire into Ghanaian practices. The terrain of the colonial debate was knowledge about cutting and arguments about the feasibility of legislative and other efforts. The imperial quest for knowledge was thought of as a precursor of potential campaigns but ultimately constituted the extent of the campaign itself.

In the spring of 1930 British concern about what they termed "circumcision," reached the Gold Coast by way of a circular letter titled "Native Customs Calculated to Impair the Health and Progress of the less Civilised Population in Certain parts of the Empire." Preceded by missionary and governmental experiments with regulating circumcision in Kenya, these concerns had traveled to London before landing on the shores of the Gold Coast.[9] In late 1929 London-based members of Parliament, including the "nation's most strenuous defender of women's rights," Eleanor Rathbone, who was "determined to improve the status of women in the empire" (Pedersen 1991: 657), and a newly minted humanitarian, the Duchess of Atholl, formed the Committee for the Protection of Coloured Women in the Crown Colonies. At the time the governing Labour Party embraced the pursuit of native rights and racial equality, and these women demanded that the British government "be held responsible not merely for equal rights between races but also for guaranteeing equal rights between Black women and Black men and for 'protecting' women from 'barbaric' practices" (656). I must note how this endeavor was circumscribed, given that the campaigns for British and colonized women did not proceed along the same tracks: Rathbone and other members of Parliament advocated for social welfare such as family allowances in Britain but not for women in the colonies. Rather, Rathbone and her colleagues made African female circumcision a political priority and campaigned for its prohibition.

One essential point in understanding the colonial history of cutting is that the British government's zeal to end it has been overestimated. Atholl and Rathbone's campaign was not met with widespread enthusiasm by the political establishment, and their committee work and parliamentary speeches never turned into policies. Despite prolonged and passionate debates in Parliament and in the press about the harms of cutting, the colonial government took no concrete steps toward ending the practice. In Kenya, a settler colony that was one of the epicenters of anticutting interventions, the primary agitators for ending the practice were missionaries, not the colonial administration (Kanogo 2005; Pedersen 1991). And as Janice Boddy's sole historical ethnography of colonial efforts to end and regulate cutting shows, the regional British administrators were ambivalent about intervention (2007). When two Scottish nurses in the Sudan, the sisters Wolff, started reformist campaigns at their midwifery school and tried to transform infibulation into clitoridectomy performed under hygienic conditions, they received little funding from colonial administrators (Boddy 2007: 186). The nurses were stigmatized for their lower-class origins and occupation and faced "bureaucratic indifference" as well as contempt from the male administrators (258). They were seen as at once performing the empire's civilizing function and as being too close to everything that was impure and abject, given that midwifery touched upon the bodily and gendered aspects of health, being, and morality that post-Victorians considered abhorrent and vile. Meanwhile the Sudanese midwives they trained received only modest stipends after "years of wearisome struggle" (225). Despite the professed interest of the British in coupling the civilizing mission with securing the reproduction of Sudan's laboring classes, which the British believed was threatened by infibulation, the fundamental character of their rule did not change. They ruled "in the name of humanity, eugenics, and of the increase of the population," but these were more subjects of ideological debate than governing practice.[10] The woman question here was women's and men's talk, primarily among the colonizers. This discrepancy between colonial obsessions with cutting as an object of debate and concrete campaigns to end it is mimicked today by the contrast between the plethora of contemporary Western anti-FGM discourses and the far lesser investment of resources and money in anticutting campaigns, in particular those in Africa.

Nonetheless, in the 1930s Atholl persisted in making circumcision, which she came to label mutilation, an issue that the colonial administration could not ignore. The committee's work instigated investigations into the extent of circumcision across the empire. In a letter to colonial officers the secretary of state denounced the ceremonies that "amount practically to mutilation and are in any case the cause of intense physical suffering, increased difficulty and danger in motherhood, and an appallingly high rate of infant mortality" and asked for information about the extent of the practice.[11] After receiving this inquiry, the director of medical and sanitary services and the acting colonial secretary, both stationed in Accra, demanded reports from officials in Tamale, the colonial capital of what the British termed the Northern Territories, which today comprise the three regions of northern Ghana. The Tamale-based administrator in turn requested information from the district chief executives and the few medical officers stationed across the region. In a flurry of exchanges during the next three years, these British men wrote reports about circumcision, debated whether to try to end it, and primarily argued against interventions by highlighting how *not* to go about them. As they exchanged letters from 1930 until 1933, their debate became more polarized. While the London-based administrators advocated for campaigns against cutting, regional officers took a relativistic position.

Their reports are instructive not only for what they say but also for their underlying taxonomies of governance and sensibility—the intersections of affect and politics that informed what kind of knowledge they deemed necessary. The colonial officers were given a few prompts for what they were to address: "I am to ask you to submit a report on the *prevalence* of the practice of the circumcision of females on attaining the age of puberty in the Northern Territories, *its effect on the birth rate* and whether it involves *any cruelty and hardship* to the girls," read a letter sent from Accra to Tamale.[12] While questions about prevalence and effect on the birthrate constitute a desire for medical and epidemiological facts related to reproductive governance of the population, the question of cruelty and hardship to the girls signals the humanitarian interest in the woman question. In their reports colonial officers went beyond these specific demands for knowledge and provided more detailed ethnographic descriptions.

Saying More Than Required: Letters from the Northern Territories

A penchant for ethnography was inscribed in the very character of colonial rule and was given administrative credence with the formalization of indirect rule as a principle of governance. The 1930s saw the publication of an ethnographic account of the Northern Territories by the first professionally trained anthropologist, Captain R. S. Rattray, author of *The Tribes of the Ashanti Hinterland* (1932). He was based primarily in Tumu in what is today the Upper West Region, and his work was soon followed by Meyer Fortes's 1937 fieldwork in Tongo in the Upper East. But British officials and army officers stationed in the Northern Territories had been writing ethnographies since their arrival in the region at the turn of the century (Cardinall [1920] 2012; Northcott [1899] 2011). Colonial officers charged with answering questions about cutting tried to follow suit and provided more ethnographic detail than was deemed necessary or useful.

The acting commissioner of the Northern Province, stationed in Navrongo, wrote in a neutral, dispassionate, and levelheaded tone that performed objectivity and facticity. Rather than reporting about a specific act of cutting, he generalized about how the cutting is usually done, stating the following to the chief commissioner of the Northern Territories in Tamale on September 1, 1930:

Excision of Girls

With reference to your telephone message I have the honour to report as follows:

1. The excision is done publicly—the girls usually being about 14 years of age—sometimes up to 18 years of age.

2. It is done after the harvesting of the early millet—about July or August or about November when the main crop has been gathered.

3. Many girls like to be excised and go of their accord to the native Doctor—others are taken by their mothers. Mothers are jeered at if they have daughters who are not excised and girls who are not excised are said to be treated as males.

4. No reason for the operation other than that it is customary. It is said to have no effect on child birth, pregnancy or infant-mortality and does not affect desire for sexual intercourse.

   If not excised girls are sometimes called "Dirty".

5. In the operation 1–2 Fluid ounce of blood are lost.

6. Deaths from the operation reported are rare.

7. A large crowd attend the operation. Sometimes girls are excised in batches—sometimes singly.

8. It is a disgrace to scream from pain when or after being operated on. The old women present yell and shout in order to drown the cries of the girl.

9. Girls sometimes dance after the operation to show "sang froid". Girls are quite naked when operated on. All beads and clothing being removed.

10. The operation appears to be practically universal among the bush people of the Northern Province. The exception being the TALANSIS who do not practice it.

11. Christians are not excised.

12. In the Wa District the age for excision said to be seven or eight years but statement lacks confirmation.

13. Doctor REID of Zuarungu is conducting an enquiry to ascertain certain fact in regard to child birth and infant-mortality. According to him a fair proportion of the women of these tribes are not excised.[13]

In this letter the acting commissioner offers a generalized, quasi-scientific, and objectivist account of cutting as a uniform operation. He deduced the rules of the practice about which he had read only a couple of reports, extrapolating general principles governing when, how, on whom, and why cutting was practiced. In contrast Dr. Reid, the medical officer stationed in Zuarungu, the colonial capital of what is today the Bolgatanga District, highlighted the ritualized qualities of the act of cutting.

Dr. Reid wrote the most detailed reports of all. One was an ethnographic description of two sets of publicly performed "operations," as he called them, accompanied by photographs of one procedure taken by the agricultural officer. The second was an epidemiological report based on his investigation of "100 consecutive women who attended the Zuarungu Hospital during the month of August and September, 1930." Like other medical doctors posted to the Gold Coast who "dabbled in amateur anthropology," as Akyeampong, Hill, and Kleinman put it somewhat derisively (2015: 4), Reid was drawn to ethnographic description and was particularly taken by the first, more ritualized, and skillful operation he witnessed, providing a three-page description. He began:

> I had the opportunity on the 24th July, 1930, of witnessing the operation performed on three girls, ageing apparently 13 to 16 years, the eldest one being already married.
> The operation took place at midday outside the wall of a compound, about 100 yards away from the main road passing through Zuarungu. There were present about 50 native onlookers of both sexes and of all ages, besides the operator and his half-dozen assistants.
> The girls had not been prepared surgically in any way except that all clothing, rings, armlets, anklets, beads and other adornments were removed; they thus quite naked.
> The operator (PAKUGUGA) was a man of about 30 years of age.[14] He had learned the technique of the operation from his father and grandfather; thus the practise is familiar. His fees were 6d for single girls and 1/- for married women.

On the pages that follow, Reid describes with great precision the position of the men and women who held the girls, the circumciser's moves, the treatment of the wound, the subsequent washing and dressing of the girls, the water and flour water given to them, as well as the bestowing of canes, which "the girl must carry . . . whenever she leaves the compound so that all people may know that she has just had the operation performed on her." Given the level of detail with which Reid describes these actions, it appears that he was standing nearby, perhaps only a few feet from the circumciser and the cut girls. Like the medical officer at the African Hospital in Tamale, Reid had much to say about the procedure. Both expressed concerns about the nudity of the girls while simultaneously taking great pains to specify exactly what was done to their genitals. I do not repeat these statements here as I do not want to give the sexualized voyeurism another platform.

Reid's ethnographic style itself performs a certain kind of epistemic and cultural work. Throughout his description Reid attends to the unfolding of the events and ascribes regularity to them:

First a man sat down on the ground.... One of the girls then sat down in front of him.... Each girl was then given some moist guinea-cornflour (ZONGKO) from a spoon, which she took between her teeth and then spat on to the ground, first outside her right foot, then outside her left foot, then between her feet, meanwhile holding her heels together.

By attending to qualities of order, precision, and esoteric knowledge and combining them with descriptions of the procedures that preceded and followed cutting—the preparation of the shea butter, the process of healing—Reid strives to give a ritualized account of a practice imbued with cultural symbolism.

In contrast he devotes only a single paragraph to the second cutting he witnessed, unimpressed as he was with the circumciser and with the event:

On the 10th of August, 1930, I witnessed the operation again. On this occasion the operation was performed, under a tree, on a single girl about 15 years of age. The girl was actually menstruating at the time. The operator was a man of about 50 years of age. He performed the operation in a most unskilled manner. He literally "hacked away" the tissues and did an unnecessary amount of 'trimming' while the raw surfaces were still bleeding.

This paragraph is all that Reid had to say about the second performance of cutting he witnessed. He did not write about the precise unfolding of the event, the presence or absence of helpers or onlookers, or the immediate aftermath of the event. Rather than reconciling the two different events by accounting for the fluid character of ritualized activity associated with cutting, he denounces the second as a poorly executed medical event, an unskilled operation.

Reid was no anthropologist, but his attention to the ideal-typic ritual inscribed with rules and regularity has been a hallmark of anthropological accounts (Kanogo 2005: 79; Pratt 1986). That he and others were compelled to respond in the ethnographic style, rather than to merely answer the questions posed to them, says something about their politics. The excess of cultural information and description of ritualized activity performed a certain kind of political position, one that endowed cutting with a cultural valence rather than depicting it as a cruel act devoid of meaning. The ethnographic style and the surplus of cultural description were put in service of showing that cutting was a legitimate cultural practice. At the same time Reid's inclination to closely describe one event but not grant the other such cultural valence is also indicative of his ambivalence—stripped of ritualized activity, the operation appeared to him as brutal. Reid's conclusions make it clear that he was torn about what he saw. The operation appeared both symbolically

rich and purposeless: he wrote that he was unable to find out "why this operation is done," as "no one can give any reason whatever except to say that it has
been performed for countless generations." This apparent purposelessness led
him to evaluate the operation in medical terms as mutilation: "Apparently
girls allow themselves to be so mutilated . . . to avoid the sneers of old women."

The centrality of colonial emphasis on "reasons" for cutting cannot be
overestimated. Their absence—or, rather, the inability to discern them—led
Reid and others to claim that cutting was purposeless and therefore mutilation. In the governmental framework that granted customs a limited and
codified authority, understanding reasons for cutting was tantamount to
granting it legitimacy. Reid and other men who wrote reports did not know
enough to contextualize the regional practices of cutting and their meanings,
and they would wait a full year before acquiring an interpretive framework.

Understanding Reasons: The "Sensible Officials" and the Work of Cultural Explanations

When in June 1931 the secretary for the Native Affairs Office in Accra for-
warded a pamphlet titled "Female Circumcision and Status of Women in
Tanganyika Territory" to Tamale, the colonial officers posted to the
Northern Territories breathed a sigh of relief. "A most interesting document,"
remarked the chief commissioner in Tamale in handwritten notes on the
cover sheet.[15] "Read with much interest. Thank you, for letting me on such
an eminently sensible [report?]," wrote the Navrongo commissioner. The
Tanganyika pamphlet that provoked such enthusiasm provided the regional
officials with contextualized cultural explanations and plausible reasons for
cutting, albeit at the opposite end of the continent.

The pamphlet was written by P. E. Mitchell, Tanganyika's secretary of
native affairs, on the basis of "18 years of close contact with native society
in Tanganyika" (7).[16] Mitchell is known for his debate with Bronislav
Malinowski and long-standing objections to anthropological theorizing—
Mitchell wanted anthropologists to merely answer questions of interest to
colonial officials rather than ask their own. Yet Mitchell's governance was
imbued with the anthropological sensibility of the time—he learned
Chichewa and Swahili in his early years of colonial service and later invited
Malinowski's student Gordon Brown to conduct research that sought to
determine whether the people were "well governed and content" (quoted in
Mills 2008: 53).

Mitchell's pamphlet was received in the Northern Territories as a powerful retort to Atholl's committee. Mitchell advocated against legislative and other direct interventions against circumcision and proposed a path of "knowledge, sympathy, and . . . [word missing] patience towards Christianity and Europe" (7). Mitchell urged caution on efforts to eliminate circumcision, outlining not only the effects this would have on "tribal institutions" but also questioning whether "European society [was] ready and willing to absorb the African, when he became civilised in this sense" (1). For officials in the Northern Territories, the main import of his pamphlet was that it explained the purpose of cutting that had been elusive to them. "Clitoridectomy causes no mutilation," he wrote, and is a part of "deeper" "initiation ceremonies" that proceed in three stages: "The parting from the old, childish, valueless life, an intermediate period . . . , [and] the final ceremony of admission into the tribe" (2). Given the significance of cutting for tribal membership, he wrote, "It is thought by the natives to be indispensable, and that attacks on it are regarded by them as attacks on the whole of the initiation ceremonies" (3). These cornerstones of tribal social organization needed to be preserved, he said, because "to substitute an alien legal and social system . . . is a thing to be carefully avoided" as the "working system . . . has met the needs of the people" (3, 4). Any change should occur "with sympathetic help and guidance from his [the African's European] teachers" (4).

Mitchell also weighed in on the woman question, arguing against the position of British feminists and humanitarians. He refuted notions that an African woman "has no rights," writing "there is no scrap of truth" in that statement and giving examples of women-initiated litigation in native courts that was decided in the women's favor, the "tribal custom" that regulates the rights of women in polygamous marriages, and women's rights to farm yields (4). He also castigated missionaries who saw Africans as immoral because of their polygamous marriages and not infrequent divorces, writing, "it is necessary to dismiss from the mind the European idea of marriage as a sacrament, and as a sacrament binding two individual persons" (6). "Bantu women are generally happy," he wrote, and are better off than "the working-class women of England" (7). Notably, he knew that he was primarily addressing himself to a masculinist audience, concluding his discussion of women's rights and well-being with a different tone in the report's final sentences. African women needed less, rather than more, freedom, he wrote: "African women at the present day enjoy a degree of freedom which easily degenerates into license, and their need is for more, and not fewer, restraints" (7).

The precise contours of the "eminently sensible" approach that appealed to colonial officers posted to northern Ghana are worth careful scrutiny. Mitchell valued the "tribal system," claimed knowledge of its workings, compared African women's rights favorably to the English while advocating patriarchal control of women's sexuality, and, in another sleight of hand, simultaneously posited African values as equal to European ones. At the same time he conceived of the British as teachers and insisted on the desirability of Christianization, which he equated with Europeanization. For colonial officials in the Northern Territories who were charged with administering indirect rule, the tenets of which were formulated by Lord Lugard based on his experiments with governing Nigeria, preserving the tribal system was sensible in more than one way: it was both appealing and pragmatic. Mitchell's worldview overlapped with theirs, and his knowledge of the cultural context granted him expertise and authority. Their agreement was evident in the supporting remarks and notes written on the cover pages of the accompanying letters that praised Mitchell's views. His contradictory attitudes toward African women resonated among the administrative class, as they were widely seen as "too free (i.e., morally lax) and not free (i.e., exploited)" (Hawkins 2002: 245). The men administering the Northern Territories saw African women's sexuality as a threat to the social order and saw the region as a space where marriage laws and colonial governance could social engineer a patriarchal order that was elusive both in England and in the colonies.

Taxonomies of Governance

Although officers administering the Northern Territories did not have Mitchell's knowledge of the ethnographic context in which they worked, they wrote in the ethnographic style. They specified the terminology for cutting in various languages, provided sociological and demographic data, cultural descriptions, and notes on power and authority in the ritual and about girls' volition, and speculated about the effects of possible colonial interventions, arguing against them. Over time their goal became overtly political: taming London's zeal for condemning and criminalizing cutting.

An analysis of their taxonomies and coordinates of knowledge is telling and significant. They mapped circumcision onto an interlocking grid of sociological and anthropological questions, categories, and sensibilities. This grid is important because it reveals the contours of a colonial reason whose legacies persist in contemporary problematizations of cutting, both anthropological and governmental.

The following is a summary of scores of archival documents; I have retained the original wording, spelling, and punctuation. The regional officials' reports constructed taxonomic knowledge of cutting along the following coordinates of questions and answers:

Which tribes practice circumcision? The answers were partial and contradictory. One document stated that the Dagomba and the Gonja do not practice it but that most others do. The Navrongo officer wrote that it was "practically universal among the bush people of the Northern Province. The exception being the Talansis."[17] The officer in Bawku stated that the Kusasis and Mamprussis do not practice it, but that their neighbors the Yangas and Busangas are encouraging its adoption.[18] The chief commissioner from Tamale, who summarized their accounts for Accra, generalized that cutting was rarely practiced in the southern part of the province, around Tamale, but was common farther north.

At what age is circumcision performed? Among the Dagarti, Grunshie, Issala, Wala, Libi, Wongara, Moshi, and Fulani, the officers said it was performed at four, seven, or fifteen days after birth; among the Kotokoli and Frafra, and across the Navrongo, Zuarungu, and Kusasi districts, at puberty, or when girls are "about 14 years of age."[19] One letter added a preference for circumcision soon after birth, deeming it "less abhorrent" as "the infant is unaware of what is happening to it, the period of suffering is not prolonged, the ritual itself is subject to little publicity, and the danger of malformation and septicemia are considerably reduced."[20]

Are boys circumcised? No.

Where is circumcision performed? In public, underneath trees, next to houses.

When is circumcision performed? If at puberty, after the harvest of the early millet; in Tamale, "in the dry season."[21]

Who performs circumcision? The responses were confident but not in agreement: "always women," "elders," "men."

What kind of ritual is the circumcision associated with? Ceremonial dancing, feast, nothing.

Are there any ill effects? Some treated this question as requiring an objective response. The Tamale-based medical officer answered no, while the acting commissioner of the Northern Province from Navrongo specified: "In the operation 1–2 Fluid ounce *[sic]* of blood are lost; deaths from the operation reported are rare."[22] Others answered the question in relative terms, writing about how the health effects would be experienced and perceived locally. The Tamale chief commissioner wrote: "The operation is considered to be painless and within 10 days there is no visible wound and the girl is not in any way inconvenienced."[23] The Kusasi District commissioner generalized this relativizing sentiment, writing: "I suggest many African customs would be detrimental to a European but are apparently not so to the African."[24]

Who has the decision-making authority? The administrators emphasized that men were not in charge, writing that girls and young women themselves, as well as mothers, made decisions and wanted the ritual.

The purpose of the ritual and the associated beliefs and reasons commanded much attention and disagreement, as nearly all officials tried to offer cultural explanations. Some stuck closely to what they were told by their interlocutors, while others expounded their own interpretations.

Marriageability: "The virgins are then eligible for matrimony," wrote the African Hospital medical officer, as the clitoris obstructs parturition and circumcision facilitates labor.

Cleanliness, purity, custom: "It [the clitoris] is dirty," and circumcision "makes women less promiscuous," "our grandfathers did it," according to the Wa District commissioner, who added, "There is however something to do with SARAH, I think as far the Mahommedans are concerned."[25]

Production of gender: "Girls who have not been excised are generally ridiculed by those who have with such a remark as 'why do you desire to be men.'"[26]

The notion of chastity provoked much disagreement. As quoted earlier, the acting commissioner of the Northern Province wrote that the purpose of cutting was not the reduction of sexual desire but custom, cleanliness, and courage.[27] Dr. Reid agreed, writing that "one has assumed that the purpose is to keep women faithful to their husbands, but this assumption is strongly denied." However, the Wa District commissioner held on to the notion of circumcision as curbing women's sexuality:

> The object of the custom is chastity, the general notion being that desire in women must be curbed in order to lessen their leanings towards promiscuous connection. I have also heard it stated that non-removal of the clitoris would be a hindrance to, and lessen the satisfaction of the sexual act.[28]

The reports offer glimpses of how the colonial officials arrived at the information they presented. For the most part the district chief executives got their information from the chiefs, whom they had installed and with whom they communicated regularly. The acting commissioner for the Northern Province declared himself indebted to the White Fathers' mission in Navrongo and to

Dr. Reid in Zuarungu. The chief commissioner for the Northern Territories was the only one who did not take men's words as representative and who talked to women, consulting with the *magagia* (today *magazia*), who are the leaders of women's groups. Analyzing the prohibition of sati (widow immolation), Lata Mani noted the absence of women as political agents: "The suffering widow remained fundamentally marginal to a debate that was ostensibly about whether she should live or die" (1998: 1). Women, she writes, were "the *ground* for a complex and competing set of struggles over Indian society and definitions of Hindu tradition" (2). In Ghana, women, too, were subjects of debate but were not afforded the status of political subjects. But men, too, spoke because they were impelled to do so and had to answer to the colonial officials, not because they had an actual say in the debate or its outcome.

My main purpose here is not to dispute colonial methods and conclusions or to arbitrate among them, as I am not interested in their truth value but in formations of power-knowledge, as well as the conditions of possibility, sentiments, and forms that animated them. Colonial officials agreed on some matters and disagreed on others. As we shall see, some answers they arrived at can be found in contemporary ethnographies and NGO discourses, but, more important, the questions they answered, and the taxonomies and sensibilities that structured their responses, all persist. Responding to London, regional officials sought to systematize knowledge about cutting, grounding their responses in cultural description, contextualized particulars, and shifts in perspective. The officers knew that the imperial quest for knowledge was itself the terrain of contestation about subsequent policies. Theirs was an effort to tame reformist passions for saving "coloured women in the Crown colonies" by way of carefully calibrated reporting in the ethnographic style.

The Colonial State against Itself: Opposition to Prohibition and Demands for Evidence

Colonial officers stationed in the Northern Territories were opposed to London's interventionist zeal, and their opposition apparently was widely shared among the men administering sub-Saharan Africa. When the demands from London increased and called for campaigns against female circumcision and possible criminalization, the officers stressed the impracticality of such measures.

Regional officers argued that a legal prohibition was simply not feasible. Tribal markings would also need to be outlawed, and that was "impossible to contemplate"—it would mean a "betrayal of the trust placed in Dr. Reid." Also, the legislation could not be enforced; a preferable alternative would be a "propaganda campaign carried out by a Woman Medical Officer who could hold meetings attended by women only and explain to them the uselessness of such a practice."[29] That *feasibility* emerged as the terrain of the debate was itself an imperial marker that bears the imprint of a debate concluded a full century earlier, when in 1829, sati was legally abolished in India after many years of deliberation. As Mani has shown, the concerns about criminalizing sati "had revolved primarily around the political feasibility of abolition rather than the ethics of its toleration" (1998: 15).

The lack of feasibility was a polyvalent discourse. The British did not dedicate human or economic resources to ending cutting, as their ruling apparatus in the Northern Territories was minimal, aimed at crisis management, security, and labor exploitation, not the administration of public health or welfare. The administrators never acknowledged this, writing instead that interventions would fail due to so-called ignorance: "In any case the Zuarungu practice seems brutal and purposeless and I think efforts should be made to discourage it as much as possible, although progress will probably be very slow owing to the ignorance and superstition of the masses."[30] *Slow* was a code word for predictions that ending circumcision, however desirable, was not entirely feasible. The notion of infeasibility allowed the officers posted to the Northern Territories to temper London's reformist passions but was also used to project colonial impotence onto northern subjects, who were figured as ignorant, superstitious, and resistant to change.

In late 1932 the demands from London changed. Rather than asking for information about circumcision or engaging in debate about the best methods of intervention, politicians wanted results. A letter asked for reports "on the steps taken . . . to induce the people of the Northern Province of the Protectorate to discontinue the practice of clitoridectomy and on the measure of success achieved." It was specifically stated that a "bold statement that the Administrative and Medical Officers are doing all that is possible in the matter"[31] would not suffice.

The district commissioners again boycotted the call for interventions by objecting to the notion that they could report specific results. One wrote that "it is yet too early to note any substantial measure of success" from "addressing meetings" or speaking to chiefs, but he stated that he placed his hope in "the gradual introduction of clothing, since nakedness is at the root of the matter."[32] As elsewhere in the empire, morality and its ostensible lack were inscribed in bodily comportment (Boddy 2007). The Wa District commissioner wrote that "no decrease in the practice can be recorded."[33] The Bawku District commissioner wrote that he had spoken to the chief, who had assured him of his opposition to the practice.[34]

The British interest in circumcision waned in 1933, in the wake of the Great Depression, and did not wax again until the end of World War II, when circumcision was outlawed in British-administered colonial Sudan. In 1949 the secretary of state again made inquiries in the colonies, and the acting chief commissioner of the Northern Territories in Tamale was asked to respond. He replied by detailing that "certain tribes" practiced clitoridectomy, wrote that "older women" were responsible for its continuance, and advised against direct interventions: "Propaganda by government officials has had very little effect—if any—and my view is that the custom can be effectively countered only by the increasing education of girls. Penal legislation would serve only to drive the practice still further underground."[35] Like his predecessors, this regional official opposed the prohibition of cutting on the ground that northerners would resist the law. He now had an additional platform to build on: colonial policy had changed and envisioned an expansion of educational opportunities in the Northern Territories, including girls as subjects worthy of education.

Anthropology, Inquiries, and Governance

Colonial inquiries and debates never led to anticutting policies, but we must understand that intervention was embedded in the very character of inquiry itself. If we substitute the term *investigation* for *inquiry*, the force associated with asking for information is more readily apparent. Ghanaians knew to evaluate the questions posed by colonial officials, understanding them as imperatives to end cutting. At least one chief told the district administrator: "This is a very old custom. We can't prohibit it," and, as I mentioned earlier, the Bawku District commissioner wrote that the chief had assured him of his opposition to the practice.[36] The oldest women remembered too. The first formal decree against cutting was issued after independence, by Nkrumah, but the women told me that the injunction to end cutting came "in the Gold Coast era," from "white people."

Anthropologists studying science and governance would readily recognize colonial research as co-constitutive of intervention (Fairhead and Leach 2003). I want to stress that anthropological research is equally constitutive of, and has been constituted by, governance of cutting from its beginnings. This is most clearly evident in hindsight, as Kenyatta's ethnography was itself a political intervention with high stakes. In 1938, eight years after his political testimony before Atholl's committee in London, and after being trained as an anthropologist, Kenyatta published a chapter explaining *irua*, female circumcision, in his book *Facing Mount Kenya* ([1938] 1965). His logic paralleled P. E. Mitchell's, stressing the centrality of circumcision to tribal organization, but Kenyatta offered more forceful arguments for African control of African lives. Kenyatta provided a detailed ethnographic description of the ritual and its symbolic and material entailments, making an argument against the "urge for abolishing a people's social custom by force of law" (127). He elevated circumcision to "the most important custom among the Gikuyu" (128) and wanted his British readers to have "a clear picture of why and how this important socio-biological custom is performed" (129). To that end he wrote about the name of the custom, its function as a moral code and keeper of historical records, described in detail the unfolding of the ritual and attendant ceremonies, the healing process, and the rebirth of the initiates. He also contested claims about the ill effects of the practice on women's reproductive health.

Kenyatta introduced to professional anthropological language what was already the tenet of colonial governance, namely, to put cultural description and explanation of meanings to work as antidotes to imperial reformist zeal. However, Kenyatta also contested the moral and epistemological authority of the British, writing that "the African is [in] the best position to discuss and disclose the psychological background of tribal customs" (148). Despite his anticolonial arguments, Kenyatta used a structure of address that positioned the imperial center as authoritative. Much like the British officers ruling the Northern Territories, he addressed himself to British administrators and publics whose convictions he hoped to unsettle.

Proximity, Distance, and Sensibility

That colonialism was not a monolithic entity is by now well established (Comaroff and Comaroff 1991). Regional officials at the borders of the empire in the Northern Territories were at odds with the politicians and bureaucrats at its seat; so were, I will soon show, the French Catholic church and the British rulers. The oppositional logic of regional officers posted to what is today northern Ghana was shaped by a certain sympathetic affect and the white man's burden of protecting the natives from *other* white men and women. Administrators posted to the Northern Territories were hailed as colonial servants and tasked with advancing the interests of the empire, but they saw themselves as equally serving Ghanaians. This is not to say that they saw Ghanaians as equals—their reports are infused with contempt, clinical detachment, and curious fascination; the differences they formulated were on a continuum that ranges from relativism to overt civilizational racism. But all are subtended by an interest in shielding Ghanaians from the inflammatory discourses and punitive rationality emanating from London. The force of the administrators' agreement with the report from Tanganyika that argued for preserving and valuing native social organization is particularly revealing of the colonial sentiments that shaped opposition to the imperial center's desires.

In contrast the officials writing from London with worries about the "intense physical suffering" of cut girls positioned themselves as motivated by feminist interests and humanitarian compassion. The imperial compassion toward the suffering of girls and women, as well as concerns about their reproductive potential, were both deeply felt and self-interested, as Boddy (2007) has shown, and inseparable from their concerns about reproducing the laboring classes in the colonies. British feminists defined African women's interests as they imagined them, projecting their own notions of freedom, oppression, agency, gender, sexuality, bodies, and pleasures onto African women. They imagined a direct line between the colonizer and the colonized but did not foster connections.

In contrast the regional officials constructed themselves as different kinds of moral subjects—those who mediated between rulers and the ruled. They saw themselves as protecting northern groups from imperial incursions, rather than protecting the empire from the ostensible moral depravities of native customs. As self-declared spokesmen for the interests of the colonial subjects, the protectionist (and, to be clear, patronizing) British men posted to the colonies wrote back to the imperial center and did so in the interest of preserving what they conceptualized as an indigenous way of life—one that, as I will demonstrate, they actually brought into being. Their positioning as British subjects whose own civilized status was not in question and as men who could equate tribal interests with those of local men meant that they took few social risks by being open to the potential meanings of circumcision for the organization of social life.

Sympathetic affect was behind both imperial and oppositional logic. Atholl's patronizing, sensationalist sympathy toward the suffering of native women was coupled with the desire to mobilize the force of sovereign violence. It is thus reminiscent of contemporary mobilizations of feminist humanitarian sentiments that legitimize war or proxy rule in the name of saving women (Grewal 1999, 2014). However, sympathetic affect also enabled a critique from within and the oppositional posture assumed by regional colonial officials. The officials posted to the Northern Territories used proximity, geographic and affective, and the ethnographic style to counter the enthusiasm for legal prohibition and to contest London-driven interventions. These regional officials exercised power that saw itself as primarily benign.

In the discussion that follows, I place this self-imaginary of colonial power in the same analytical frame as the historiography of labor exploitation and underdevelopment in northern Ghana to raise larger questions about the logics of colonial rule and its ongoing permutations. I want to show that the disposition of regional officials was subtended by an entire apparatus built on preserving tradition (Grischow 2006: 81) as a primary mode of governance. As indirect rule morphed into official policy, preserving a codified alterity became the dominant form of rule in the Northern Territories. Historians of northern Ghana have shown that this colonial logic served as a convenient backdrop for labor exploitation, whether intended or not. Keeping these two efforts to preserve tradition in the same frame—the overtly stated critique of imperial interventionism and the simultaneous tacit practice of exploitation backed by the imperial sword—sheds light on the long history of what Miriam Ticktin calls "armed love" (2011: 5), which gave shape to forms of knowledge, affect, and rule whose traces are still visible.

ARMED LOVE: HISTORIES OF RULE

Slavery: Setting the Arithmetic

The colonial conquest of what is today northern Ghana followed a century and a half of violence and dispossession brought on by intensified slave raiding. Although this region has been globally connected for centuries through trade and migration, it was the slave trade that integrated the region into the world-historical system that persists today. Northern Ghana became a source of slaves for the transatlantic slave trade in the seventeenth century and a predominant source of Ghanaian slaves in the nineteenth (Holsey 2008). "At the height of the slave trade," writes Holsey, "European companies stationed on the coast of Ghana came to view the hinterland as a vast pool of potential slaves" while granting coastal residents immunity from enslavement (45). According to conservative estimates, 500,000 northern Ghanaians were enslaved (Der 1998). That's an enormous number: at the beginning of the twentieth century, the population of the entire country was 1.5 million.

In the North the noncentralized groups from the savannah, formerly known as stateless, including those living in what is today the Upper East Region, were particularly vulnerable to slave raiding by surrounding states. They were raided by their established neighbor-states to the south, Gonja and Dagbon, which had to pay an annual tribute in slaves to the Asante: "Between the 1770s and the 1870s, Gonja and Dagbon each delivered somewhere between one thousand and two thousand slaves per year to their Asante overlords" (Allman and Parker 2005: 30). The noncentralized groups lacked the military means to defend themselves; although they were acclaimed as warriors famous for their poison arrows and were later recruited into the British imperial army (Osseo-Assare 2008), these groups lacked guns, horses, and other means of destruction. Toward the end of the nineteenth century, they were also regularly raided by their northern neighbors from the Sahel as well as by Zabarma warriors.

Although the transatlantic slave trade came to a fitful conclusion in the first half of the nineteenth century, the internal slave trade lived on, both in receiving countries such as the United States and in sending countries such as Ghana. In Ghana domestic slavery burgeoned after the demise of the Atlantic slave trade, only to be outlawed during colonial rule. By the 1880s about fifteen thousand people were traded annually in the Salaga market, which became the largest West African market in slaves (Dumett and Johnson 1988). But although the British legitimated colonial occupation by claiming that it was a means for ending the slave trade, the trade continued, and "there was no concerted effort to end it until after 1911" (Miers 2003: 36).

Northerners captured in the second half of the nineteenth century and taken to southern Ghana remained there, becoming incorporated into southern families but under the sign of a lack (Holsey 2008). Unlike free people, slaves were incorporated into kinship as "captive kin" and continued to be marginalized (Miers and Kopytoff 1979: 26). Such was the extent of the trade in northern slaves that the term *odonko*, an Akan word that originally referred to a "bought person" (Holsey 2008: 40), became synonymous with *northerner* and came to connote "servility, primitiveness and abject barbarity" (Parker 2006: 356). The history of disavowed kinship shapes Ghana's north-south relations today; the southern denial of northern interrelatedness is a legacy of slavery.

To legitimize the enslavement of northern groups, Europeans and coastal Fanti and Asante portrayed them as "uncivilized barbarians who were fit only to be exploited as slaves" (Allman and Parker 2005: 31). Northerners were understood as abject cannibals and feral, animalistic subjects with a wild nature and a tiger-like physiognomy. The Asante king Asantehene adopted the colonial distinctions between humanity and animality, proclaiming in 1841 that the "small tribes in the interior fight with each other . . . are stupid, and little better than beasts" (Allman and Parker 2005: 31). Contemporary notions of the unruliness and backwardness of northern Ghana stem in part from this history (Holsey 2008: 46).[37] These representations are sustained by national discourses that depict the North as the *sole* source of slaves in Ghana and thus displace the brutality of slavery onto "savage" northern Ghana; as Holsey astutely argues, southern Ghanaians do so in order to protect themselves from stigmatization by the global order (Holsey 2008: 81).

At the same time that slavery discursively constructed northern Ghana as remote, slavery also materialized it as such. To protect themselves from raiders, some vulnerable groups relocated to the hills and other distant areas, thus "altering their relationship to the landscape" and "producing their remoteness" (Holsey 2008: 44; see also Ferme 2001). Historians suggest that contemporary inhabitants of the Upper East Region are a mixture of various refugee groups and others who migrated during the slave trade and its aftermath (Allman and Parker 2005: 31). My research has also found that some inhabitants of the Bolga and Bongo districts trace their genealogies to various movements in the nineteenth century, when they were subject to intensified raiding. The slave trade thus not only robbed this and other regions of their inhabitants but also altered where some people live, how they identify themselves, and who they affiliate with.

Colonial Rule: Minimal Investment and Extraction of Labor

Although the British were some of the foremost profiteers from slavery, after they formally abolished it, they justified colonial occupation by claiming that it was a means for ending the inter-African and Arab slave trades, mobilizing humanitarian concerns to that end. Fortes and Mayer uncritically endorsed this claim, writing that colonialism brought "peace and more security" to the Tallensi (1966: 5), thus disavowing the decades of war and displacement that resulted from British pacification (Allman and Parker 2005: 31).

Colonial rule did not bring freedom but instead an initial period of local warfare followed by military occupation, installment of indirect rule, and forced and coerced labor. The British annexed the areas north of Asante and formally proclaimed the "Northern Territories" their protectorate in 1901. They had little interest in the region as such and did not foresee profiting from it financially (Sutton 1989). Rather, the British were guided by larger geopolitical interests—they wanted to secure a base in the middle of the French-dominated region of Africa to the north and west and the German colony of Togoland to the east (Benning 1975). To create the northern borders of the protectorate, colonial powers drew arbitrary lines of demarcation that cut across existing social, economic, and political affiliations—the border between contemporary Ghana and Burkina Faso is a nearly straight line that follows the eleventh parallel. But the new polity also crowded together former enemies; these groups viewed each other not as kin but as strangers and had belonged to the same polity only when subordinated.[38]

The Northern Territories were not governed as part of the colony proper but as a hinterland, or, in official terms, a protectorate ruled by a distinct rationality of minimal investment. After the death of the administrator Henry Ponting Northcott, who had spent time in the North, no one was seen as capable of governing it. As Lentz writes, "Neither the Colonial Office nor the Governor of the Gold Coast had a clear idea of what to do with this new appendage of the Gold Coast Colony, except that its administration should cost as little as possible" (Lntz 2006: 33). This imperative meant that colonial governance in Ghana, and elsewhere in Africa, was bifurcated (Mamdani 1996). As Roger Thomas explains, "It commonly featured different administrative policies pursued toward different areas *within* a particular territory. In West Africa, the boundary was usually drawn between the coast, which had a long history of direct contact with Europe, and the hinterland areas" (1974: 427). Since the annexation of the Northern Territories resulted from the British desire for securing territory, not from an interest in administering it, the definition of the region as a protectorate (as opposed to the Gold Coast and Asante colonies) allowed the British to claim it without incurring greater governing responsibilities. Instead they "pursued a minimalist project" (Lentz 2006: 9).

The governance of the Northern Territories was largely structured around labor expropriation, law and order, and territorial control, rather than investments in infrastructure, economy, public health, or education. As Hawkins puts it, the British were more interested in the welfare of cattle than of people (2002: 28). They treated the region as a labor reserve for southern gold mines, public works projects, and the colonial police and army. *Odonko* now became the term for northern laborers in the South (Dumett and Johnson 1988: 100) who became central to the country's most important export economies, gold and cocoa. British officials demanded that northern chiefs—themselves installed by colonial administrators—procure labor for public works. The chiefs were initially suspicious that the men would be taken as slaves, but over time the chiefs themselves resorted to coercion of families; for a time colonial officials paid the chiefs for each man they sent south. Government officials also at times joined hands with private companies for purposes of what they euphemistically referred to as recruiting northern men to work in southern mines. Together with migrants from neighboring countries, northern men comprised 73 percent of the most vulnerable members of the mining labor force, namely, the underground miners (R. Thomas 1973: 80). Conditions were dangerous, workers were flogged and beaten, and many took sick and died. "The workers," writes Hawkins, "resented the deplorable conditions in the mines and the brutal treatment to which they were subjected" (2002: 65). Initially, desertion was a common problem for colonial officials and recruiters, as half the men captured in the Upper East fled on their way south. British policy debates testify to the coercive character of this labor regime: officials contemplated replicating South African policies, such as Pass Laws (R. Thomas 1973: 80), which were the precursors of the apartheid regime and were designed to confine the laborers and control their movement.

Foucault's analysis of governance in what he calls a "historical type of society" offers a surprisingly apt description of colonial rule of the Northern Territories and its peoples:

> Perhaps this juridical form must be referred to a historical type of society in which power was exercised mainly as a means of deduction (*prélèvement*), a subtraction mechanism, a right to appropriate a portion of the wealth, a tax of products, goods, and services, labor and blood, levied on the subjects. Power in this instance was essentially a right of seizure: of things, time, bodies, and ultimately life itself; it culminated in the privilege to seize hold of life in order to suppress it. (Foucault 1990: 136)

Foucault did not intend this description of the juridical form of power to have colonialism as its target; his target was a Western European past that he referred to as "the classical age," after which "the West has undergone a very profound transformation of these mechanisms of power" (136). Yet, with the exception of the last clause in the paragraph quoted—"in order to suppress it"—Foucault's description maps onto colonial rule in the Northern Territories, reminding us of the bifurcations of rule in Western Europe and colonial hinterlands. The colonial regime was not biopolitical, but neither was it deliberately "necropolitical" (Mbembe 1992): the British were not aiming to suppress the lives of Ghanaians—as was the case in slavery, killing was not a goal but a by-product (Hartman 2007). It is clear that colonial rule did not promote social welfare—the British benefited from migrant labor so long as it was readily available, and while workers' deaths were incidental, so was their welfare.

Rethinking the application of Foucault's definition of juridical power draws attention to the pitfalls of analyses that periodize power on a linear timeline, be they historical or contemporary. While David Scott argues that the colonial exercise of power was marked by a shift from "extractive-effects on colonial bodies" to "governing-effects on colonial conduct" (D. Scott 1995: 204), there is no singular or historically unified form of colonial governmentality. Colonial rule of the Northern Territories saw no such radical shift; rather, the governance of conduct was inscribed in policies aimed at safeguarding extraction.

Historians say that one cannot even speak of meaningful rule in the Northern Territories, as governance looked like crisis management (Allman and Parker 2005: 73). This region underwent a pernicious version of colonialism wherein the difference between the promise of citizenship and governance by subjection and minimal care was most pronounced. In practice this meant that colonial government invested little in the North. Although northerners were forced to pay taxes and serve in the army during both world wars, the region received minimal resources for roads, no railway, and little infrastructure for health care. Sporadic "schemes to promote cash crops and commercial animal husbandry were introduced in the north from time to time" (Sutton 1989: 642).[39]

Not all colonial officials agreed with minimal investment. While the central colonial administration begrudged the North its governmental expenditures, administrators posted to the Northern Territories lobbied for greater resources for the region (Benning 1975). Sutton explains:

> There was, however, a distinction between the attitudes of Gold Coast government and officials in the south, and those of local officials in the north. [The latter] were enthusiastic and encouraging about agricultural programs. Such local officials seem to have initiated many of the experimental schemes, badgering the central government for money and personnel. There was a continual conflict over the allocation of resources between officials in the north, who felt that the north must develop a local capital-generating economy ..., and Colony officials, who saw the Gold Coast as a whole, with the north

forming only a minor part in economic terms, except for the supply of labor. (1989: 642)

The Gold Coast officials' view of the Northern Territories as undeserving of resources prevailed. They justified this policy publicly by mobilizing patronizing discourses of preserving native traditions. Many scholars agree that British economic policy "starved the protectorate of investment" (Pellow 2011: 136) in the name of preserving tradition.[40] Another way of putting this is that colonial governance was organized around a particular form of indirect rule that was anti-interventionist *in name*. The British codified traditions they deemed useful to state interests and enacted economic and social policies aimed at halting social transformations that were antithetical to colonial ideology and interests.[41] They thus remade the region as traditional in an effort to slow down social transformations that threatened colonial rule. They installed chiefs as custodians of land and fostered communal ownership under their authority; chiefs were to serve as intermediaries for the colonial administrators and the populace (Hawkins 2002: 123). Equally important, they built only a few schools and capped the numbers of students, initially promoting education only to sons of chiefs so as to train a new generation of English-speaking administrators and later restricting education to practical training and "what the market would bear" (R. Thomas 1974: 429). To keep caps on education, the British reined in the Catholic Church's sphere of influence, limiting the missionaries' projects and the number of schools and hospitals in the Northern Territories to a handful (Der 2001). Missionaries, who arrived in 1906, did not have much influence on colonial governance here and were not welcomed by the British because of the national and confessional differences between the colonial officials and the missionaries—while the British colonizers were mostly Anglicans, the missionaries were French and French Canadian Catholics.

The putatively anti-interventionist colonial rule allowed the British to shape the cartographies of social transformation. The installation and codification of chieftaincy and the drawing of borders and boundaries, both national and regional, modified the structures of authority over land, law, resources, and social relations. Centers of commerce, knowledge, and administration shifted as the British designated new district and regional capitals. They thus redefined who counted as a legitimate authority, who possessed rights to land and resources, and how these rights were to be exercised.

These colonial policies were bolstered by a newly romanticized image of the North. The British no longer conceived of northerners as abject savages but as tribes whose traditions were a virtue, a source of strength that enabled them to "[withstand] the break-up of culture, along with the social conflicts and psychic burdens of modern existence" (Kramer 1993: 44). The "sensible" colonial officials I mentioned earlier were charged with understanding tradition and using this knowledge to support their rule. Some took it upon themselves to write ethnographies of tribal customs, about which they were, on the whole, ambivalent: they reveled in certain cultural difference and ingenuity, from different forms of speech to healing methods, but were repulsed by nudity, frequent divorce, polygamy, and ancestor worship (Cardinall [1920] 2012; Northcott [1899] 2011). Their lens was trained on cultural difference, but, as Jean and John Comaroff write of missionaries as well, the British focused on what they conceived as "the lamentable distance from savagery and civilization" (1991: 174). Even the affirmative accounts, such as Cardinall's praise for the region's men who had fought for the British in World War I, entailed the trope of overcoming what he obliquely termed "the numbing influence of their old surroundings":

> These people of whom I write showed their indomitable courage during the recent war, immortalising their own name and that of their regiment in Togoland, the Cameroons, and East Africa. . . . It was their manliness, their intelligence, their desire to learn that made them seize the opportunity, urged them to discard wholesale all the numbing influence of their old surroundings and practices and established for ever the innate bravery of their race. ([1920]2012: ix)

Over time colonial administrators began to look at customs as a technology for preserving social order, and they reorganized their values and attitudes toward Africans accordingly. In his introduction to Cardinall's book, C. H. Armitage, the chief commissioner of the Northern Territories, writes:

> Even those African native customs that appear to us both degrading and repulsive have in them the germ of some mistaken duty to parents and superiors: of reverence to ancestors, or to an unknowing Being who exercises supreme power for good or ill over the lives and destinies of the devotees. (Cardinall [1920] 2012: iv)

By pointing out the function of native customs as supporting social and ancestral hierarchies, Armitage argues that although mistaken, customs should be seen as the foundation for social order. Anthropologists of the time, from Fortes to Kenyatta, agreed but toned down the moralizing judgment.

THE AFTERLIVES: MATERIALITY, GOVERNANCE, SENSIBILITY

One might salute the colonial efforts to minimize European influence, as education and literacy in English, after all, served to colonize consciousness and minds (Comaroff and Comaroff 1991; wa Thiong'o 1994). However, an upshot of the colonial bifurcated governance was that by its end in 1957, northern Ghana had a total of nine schools in contrast to the more than three hundred in the South. The first secondary school in northern Ghana opened only in 1951 in Tamale (Pellow 2011: 136), and by independence in 1957 only one person from the region had a university degree (R. Thomas 1974: 427). By undereducating the North, the British cemented the region's status as a reserve of menial labor that became, and still largely is, the country's proletariat (Hart 1973).

Given the dearth of historical records, it is impossible to trace precise, much less linear, connections from the longer history of slavery to colonialism and to the present. However, the lives of northern Ghanaians can also be said to be "imperiled and devalued by a racial calculus and a political arithmetic that were entrenched centuries ago" (Hartman 2007: 6). Here, the afterlife of bifurcated colonial governance also entails "skewed life chances, limited access to health and education, premature death . . . and impoverishment" (6). Except for a small class of northern elites and middle-class people like Mrs. Mahama, the director of GAWW, northerners migrate to the South, where they are employed primarily as low-cost labor and are subject to narratives of abjection and hierarchies of social and political citizenship. The story of slavery and colonialism, here and elsewhere, is also a story of disavowed kinship that structures Ghana's north-south relations and denies northerners their national identity in both symbolic and material ways. Yet no singular "political arithmetic" establishes the hierarchy whereby northern Ghanaians are devalued or suffer from what Hartman calls "incidental death . . . when life has no normative value" (2007: 31). In fact, as I will show in the chapters that follow, governmental projects try to *prevent* such incidental deaths while at the same justifying them.

The creation of the colonial protectorate that engendered the Northern Territories as a unified geographical unit in need of a distinct form of governance also lives on. Although northern Ghanaians do not necessarily share cultural or historical affinities, they share a century of experience of governance, by which I mean policies and their accompanying cultural underpinnings. Contemporary development policies, government and donor plans, and NGO projects consider the three northern regions in a single breath, and migrants living in the South often define themselves and are defined as northerners. These taxonomies are imbued with the legacy of being marked as the nation's Other and undeserving of the benefits of citizenship. Anthropology has not done justice to the lived and embodied effects of the category "the North." Although anthropologists have written about this region since the 1930s, the disciplinary unit of analysis has not been northern Ghana as such. Instead anthropologists have seen the ethnic group as a relevant unit of analysis, although its significance as an indigenous category is both questioned and legitimated (Fortes and Mayer 1966; Lentz and Nugent 2000). Both concepts, the ethnic group and the North, were shaped by colonial governmentality, but only the former has an anthropological imprimatur. I suggest that, like the notion of chiefs, the notion of Ghana's North is a colonial construct that has become a historical reality and is here to stay. This is particularly visible in anticutting discourses and campaigns that have the North and northerners as their subjects, although only half the people living in the region practiced cutting historically.

Power-Knowledge and Sensibility

The afterlife of the colonial paradigm is evident in the work of contemporary modernizers and their critics, as I will show in the chapters that follow. At times dramatic and at times subtle, imperial processes "saturate the subsoil of people's lives" (Stoler 2008: 192). The self-declared sensible responses of the colonial administrators, the NGOs' sensitizing campaigns (to educate those considered ignorant), and ethnographic sensibility all are structured by assemblages of affect, proximity, knowledge, subjectivity, and reason. By tracing what constitutes sensibility in domains of rule as well as in analysis and critique, and by analyzing the relationship between sensibility and affective distance, I will explore the political potential of taking the cultivation of the senses seriously, not only as an object of analysis but also as an anthropological and feminist praxis.

The colonial grid of knowledge, sentiment, positioning, and deliberation continues to structure how female genital cutting is made legible and how it becomes an object of regulation. Building on James Ferguson's suggestion that development is anthropology's twin and as such has helped to constitute the discipline (1997), I suggest that contemporary governmental concerns about cutting are better represented as a triad of colonial, activist, and anthropological reason with overlapping questions, taxonomies, and sensibilities. The questions the British colonial apparatus debated in the 1930s about the who, where, when, and why of cutting and about the woman question—the African woman's control of her sexuality and her social status—continue to be asked today, both by NGOs trying to end cutting and by scholars trying to understand it. Answers to these questions are demanded, insistently and passionately. We shall see that NGOs and scholars alike spend much time on inquiries regarding the prevalence of and reasons for cutting. The context in which these purported facts are discussed is crucial to the character of governmental rule: while cultural description serves as an oppositional discourse for anthropologists, GAWW and others who govern hold discussion upon discussion and workshop after workshop about the *reasons* for cutting, only to declare them irrational, patriarchal, and uncivilized. The ethnographic style of the regional officers and their interests in taming imperial spirits therefore bear less resemblance to contemporary interventionists than to anthropologists and Africanists.

Pitting education against legislation continues to serve as the context for debate about the appropriate character of interventions, as does the notion of the "underground" persistence of circumcision. But while regional colonial officials used this notion to forestall legislative zeal, in contemporary Ghana GAWW and others ascribe facticity to the "underground" and use it for opposite ends, to advocate for greater surveillance and punishment. This and other governance discourses are at times uncritically adopted and affirmed by anthropologists. Carolyn Fluehr-Lobban, for example, writes that the 1946 colonial law against female circumcision in the Sudan "had the effect of simply writing its practice underground" (2013: 96), thus conflating the continuation of the practice with its supposedly underground performance—a claim contradicted by scholars who discuss having been invited to witness circumcision (Gruenbaum 2001; Hale 1994).

Knowledge, sensibility, and positioning are still structured along colonial lines of investment. Mary Louise Pratt writes that anthropology inherited its tropes from the imperialism and colonialism against which it has defined itself (1986). But anthropology borrows more than tropes and categories from the colonial paradigm: it also borrows its questions and audiences, and it constructs its sensibility in the same manner as colonial officials posted to the occupied territories. This afterlife is worth thinking about critically and generatively. London-based feminists and humanitarians foregrounded African women's interests, as the British women understood them from a distance. Regional governors and district chief executives in the Gold Coast emphasized the social functions of circumcision and anticipated negative outcomes of imperial reforms. They wrote from proximity to the social groups in question but often reduced these groups' interests to (projected) men's interests. Ghanaian women did not get to represent themselves or be represented.

Anthropologists who offer cultural description in service of relativism share the ethnographic style of regional colonial administrators. Rather than simply dismissing that imperial debris, I am interested in its "distribution of the sensible" (Rancière 2013) in this form of rhetorical structure of arguments against colonial interventions. What colonial officials deemed sensible accounts were born out of proximity and openness but also the inequality resulting from occupation. That those in power would presume and demand intimate knowledge of the Other is itself an exercise of power, yet the resulting knowledge repositioned regional administrators away from the imperial center and in opposition to its will to dominate. I want to suggest that anthropology has inherited this entire matrix. Many writing about cutting align themselves with the interests of Africans but are interpellated by the imperial centers and answer to them. This is why I attempt to write otherwise and to allow questions about cutting to emerge from African engagements with its endings, conceptualized as effects of a world-historical project.

The struggle between the British feminist politicians and the regional colonial officials in the 1930s is emblematic—though by no means a mirror image—of the contemporary disjuncture between anthropology and feminism. The most obvious heirs of Atholl and Rathbone are contemporary Western campaigners and global feminists, and they have been recognized as such and subject to much criticism. I am interested in another, less obvious colonial afterlife that I suggest is evident in contemporary feminist theory and left-of-center scholarship critical of global feminism. This scholarship would not recognize itself as an heir of colonial feminism, but I suggest that it has inherited two of its features, namely, the construction of feminist analysis and politics from a social and affective distance and the certainty of the parameters of feminist critique. Feminist theorists place distance in the service of critique of governance, not interventionist social engineering, but it still has its costs. Critique from a distance reifies its object and imagines it as far more stable than any given social constellation could possibly be. Feminist theory from a distance, be it geographic, class based, or affective, also fosters too much agreement among the speakers. I suggest that for both analytical and political purposes, we need dissensus, not consensus (see Rancière 2010; Povinelli 2015).

I therefore ask which distributions of proximity and sensibility are fruitful analytico-politically, and I suggest that they can be found in a third position, at the interstices of anthropology and feminist analysis rather than theory or critique from a distance. Feminist ethnographers are positioned as close to people whose lives are at stake, and they pay particular attention to the concerns of these people, as they themselves formulate them. As I will show, in my case this includes cut women and advocates against cutting, as well as others involved in and affected by anticutting campaigns. Moving beyond the notion of the "Exotic Other Female" (Engle 1991: 1526) means recognizing that a cut woman—often imagined in the singular, as a uniform subject—is not "one" and not radically different: a woman who holds on to cutting. Rather, differently positioned women take a variety of political positions toward cutting/ anticutting campaigns, and the larger governance of their lives.

I want to suggest that feminist anthropology comes *near* without speaking or feeling *for* the ethnographic subjects. It does not presume either identification or fundamental alterity, nor does it erase difference in subjectivity and positioning. In doing so, it is able to attend to subtle protests and political potentialities that are immanent in any given exercise of power. Illuminating them is my ultimate goal in the chapters that follow. Nonetheless, this analytical project is not a political coup. That women are no longer simply the muted ground of a discourse (Mani 1998: 2) but are speaking subjects means that their political marginalization is reconfigured, not resolved. Cut women and activists have been talked *about* and silenced, but today they are also impelled to speak by anthropologists like me, as well as by NGOs that use participatory methods in their campaign and governments of the global North that co-opt the voices and figures of "native informants." Thus listening, recognition, voice, and speech entail both governmental operations and possibilities for uncovering some of their damage.

In Accra, They Say

This is not a cultural practice!

This is not an indigenous practice; it's the foreigners who do it.

Watch out and make sure they don't cut off yours!

There are no campaigns against FGM in Ghana.

You want to learn about the this thing—female genital mutilation. Ha, ha, ha. How is your research going? Ha, ha, ha.

2

———

Making Harmful
Traditional Practices

June 2002, Bolgatanga District, Upper East Region. "Bismillah." Elizabeth turns the ignition in her green pickup and shoots me a quick glance from the corner of her eye, discretely gauging my reaction. Elizabeth is a devout Catholic who prays for hours every dawn, but for her, God is a She, and Bismillah a good invocation for a safe journey. She and her sisters embraced Christianity decades ago, in their youth, and were now trying to convince their traditionalist father, an almost ninety-year-old retired police officer, to do so as well. Elizabeth's last name bears traces of Islam, as does my first name. Were some of her ancestors Muslim? I do not ask her, and she does not ask about my name either. Her prayer, I have since learned, is as much a reflection of her family history as a nod to mine.

I met Elizabeth several weeks earlier on a flight from Frankfurt to Accra; we sat next to each other and struck up a conversation. Initially embarrassed to tell her my precise research question—yet another (quasi) Western woman asking about female genital cutting—I described my broader interests in NGOs working on Ghanaian women's rights. She was a director of such an NGO in Bolga, she told me. I planned to travel to Bolga, I then said, since I wanted to look at regional efforts to end female genital cutting. Elizabeth did not blink when I specified my interest—like other "gender workers" (Manuh 2007) from the region, she focused on economic development, domestic violence, and "harmful traditions" with material consequences but collaborated on anticutting campaigns when the opportunity arose. She was eager for me to come to Bolga, as "most people stay in Accra" and never learn about the North. "You just come and stay with me," she offered, and I did. Elizabeth welcomed me into her house, a neotraditional structure she built when she returned to her father's village after a life of exile, education, and marriage on several continents. She introduced me to her friends and helped me connect with Dr. Adjei, whose NGO, Rural Help Integrated, would become one of my main fieldwork sites.

On this day she was taking me on a day trip to Tengzugu in the Tongo hills, one of the region's main tourist attractions; in subsequent years I would take my visitors there as well. Elizabeth takes a shortcut, driving down a dirt road that takes us past the small hamlets she represents in the district assembly. She offers a ride to a woman carrying a load of firewood collected on the fringes of the forest, asking how she is and where she is going. As a successful NGO director, consultant, and ambivalent politician, Elizabeth generates and sustains social relations wherever she goes, from villages to coffee shops, the World Bank, or an airplane. The woman initially refuses help, saying she does not have far to go, but then climbs into the bed. Elizabeth shakes her head and comments, "They are so used to this hard work, they just do it."

As we begin the ascent to the hills, Elizabeth asks me whether I know about Fortes, the famous British anthropologist who first came to the region in 1930s. With pride in her voice she tells me he liked it so much he had a wife here. Colonial-era anthropology has an ambivalent legacy, but local intellectuals fondly remember Fortes and Rattray, who brought the region some visibility and wrote historical accounts of its life and people that still hold a place in cultural memory. To readers of anthropology, the Tongo hills are the home of the people Fortes, following colonial practice, called the Tallensi. Fortes did not intend to classify people living here as a separate, self-contained ethnic group, and he explicitly warned against doing so (1936), but authors are not in control of the reception of their work, and "the Tallensi" have been institutionalized in anthropological thought as an ur-ethnicity with a stateless society. To Elizabeth, Tongo is simply a neighboring town, home of her sister's in-laws and people no different from her own. Most of the inhabitants of the Bolgatanga, Bongo, and Tallensi-Nabdam districts are called Frafra today; the name is another relic of colonial hubris, yet the term has become locally meaningful through governmental force and repeated usage. *Fara-fara,* loosely translated, means "well done" and is used as a greeting; greeted profusely, the British thought they were being offered ethnic identifiers and began to refer to the people, as well as their language, as Frafra. This name has stuck, although Ghanaian linguists have been trying to pare away the colonial nomenclature and now call the language Gurene or Frafra-Gurene.[1]

The Tongo hills and Tallensi rituals are familiar to anthropologists and Africanists because of Fortes, but it was recent scholars who helped turn them into tourist attractions. The historians Jean Allman and John Parker helped establish the ecotourism project we visit in the hills; they were writing a history of the Tongnaab, the powerful shrine frequently visited by southern Ghanaians looking to ameliorate various afflictions. The shrine sits amid an imposing landscape of granite boulders perched on top of one another. It epitomizes the Upper East Region: while it is assumed to be traditional, inhabited by isolated people in a stateless society governed only by spirits and gods, it has in fact long been cosmopolitan, both "global and historical," as Allman and Parker put it (2005: 3). I would add that the region is also a reflection on Africanists, insofar as it has been discursively constructed and materialized by scholars past and present.

The men in charge of receiving tourists know Elizabeth and give us a warm welcome. We first visit the chief's house, a hundred rooms stitched together into a single compound of three hundred people. Next we are taken to tall rocks, where we are told about the histories of hiding from slave raiders and battles with colonial occupiers. We are also told about festivals that are presented as meaningful despite having been commoditized for tourist consumption. As we climb the rocks, from which we can see the green valleys, with Burkina Faso to the north and the White Volta to the south, Elizabeth tells the guides that I am a researcher who will be "studying FGM." One of the men, a teacher, turns to me and asks, "What do you think about FGM?" "What is there to think about?" Elizabeth interjects. "It is an outmoded practice whose time has passed."

By the time I left Bolgatanga, I had decided to make it the main vantage point for my research. I had initially planned to conduct most of my research in Accra, hoping to contribute to the anthropology of urban Africa. I had planned to study the national advocacy of the Ghana Association for Women's Welfare (GAWW) and the community-based anticutting campaigns of the NGO Muslim Family Counseling Services (MFCS) in the Nima neighborhood, as well as the relationships of these NGOs to donors and the Ghanaian government. I quickly learned that I would not be able to study the community-based projects that were my main interest: while

MFCS leaders were not only welcoming but eager to attract a "white Muslim" researcher, they had run out of funding and had largely ceased operations; their offices were deserted. Meanwhile, in the Upper East Region, efforts to end cutting were alive, intense, and complex. There was much talk about FGM everywhere, although the practice of yabega ŋma, Gurene for "cutting of the initiates," or commonly, ŋma la, "cutting," was waning in at least some parts of the region.

Those who governed the region had come to see cutting as an "outmoded practice whose time has passed," as Elizabeth put it. Statements like this invoked both the ending of the practice and the imperative to end it: cutting was said to exist in the present but was regarded as not of the present. In the words of the Bolganaba, the chief of Bolgatanga, this meant that "the obsolete customs, cultures, and traditions must give way to modern times" in the name of development and social progress. The notion of cutting as an anachronism renders in a popular idiom what is officially known as a discourse about "harmful traditional practices." How did this codification of harm come about? And how was it possible for it to become an unquestioned consensus in Ghanaian public culture? Elizabeth's and Bolganaba's words speak to more than the issue of cutting; for those who govern Ghana, the "harmful traditions" that are said to subjugate women and children and destroy rural livelihoods are the primary frame of reference for governance.

Theorists of development have critically analyzed the primacy of linear and teleological notions of time and space in modernization theories (Ferguson 2006; Fabian 1983; Povinelli 2011b; Escobar 1995; Pigg 1997) and revealed their colonial origins, including the articulation of racism as the basis of colonial rule (Gupta 1998; Hodgson 2001; D. Moore 2005). My goal is not to critique the notion that traditional practices are inimical to development—other scholars have written extensively and persuasively on this topic—but to examine the work this notion performs in contemporary Ghana and to show how it has morphed, how it lives on and sustains its hold on governance, and what it costs those who govern and are governed by it.

In this chapter I focus on how anticutting campaigns mediate and embody the governance of northern Ghana, which constructs harmful traditions as the main cause of the region's continued scarcity and political marginalization. I examine the discourse of harmful traditions and analyze its genealogy and contemporary articulations. I want to show that the codification of harmful traditions is embedded in the larger frameworks of modernization and development, which have shifted over time. I suggest that anticutting campaigns employ this notion to mediate the fraught North-South relationship and the place of the North in the Ghanaian polity. GAWW and other organizations conceptualize cutting as a practice that is in the present but also out of it, and in the nation but not proper to it, thus characterizing northern Ghana as a counterpoint to southern civilization and modernity. The public acceptability of NGOs' characterizations of FGM as a harmful tradition is a result of both the prevailing understanding of Ghana as a country with "inhibiting cultural baggage" and the unloading of this baggage on northern Ghana and its rural populations.[2] As I will show, the national discourse of harmful traditions is the primary mode of problematizing northern poverty; it draws on neoliberal technologies of recognizing scarcity while shifting the responsibility for it to northern Ghanaians and their traditions.

In Chapter 1, we saw that northern Ghana has long been governed in reference to tradition. Today, rather than being codified, managed, and selectively valued, cultural practices are codified and devalued. The upshot is that they serve as the basis for problematizing, and intervening in, seemingly everything: subjectivity, family, society, economy, climate change.

A Diplomatic Solution

GAWW introduced the notion of "harmful traditional practices" in 1984 to make it possible to campaign against cutting without having to name it as such. Rather than concentrating public attention on the potentially contentious question of cutting, GAWW sought to cultivate acceptance by carefully managing the framing of its projects. The NGO's application to form an association did not mention cutting, and the choice of its bland name, Ghana Association for Women's Welfare, suggested that there was nothing objectionable or radical about the organization. Similarly, GAWW hoped that the notion of harmful traditional practices would forestall any objections to anticutting campaigns by appealing to public aspirations of national development and modernization.

GAWW's strategy to avoid any explicit naming of cutting came from its mother organization, the Inter-African Committee on Traditional Practices Affecting the Health of Women and Children (IAC). The idea was conceived even earlier, by IAC's precursors, the NGO Working Group on Traditional Practices Affecting the Health of Women and Children. The terminology was envisioned as a way of preempting opposition by African diplomats and governments and of making the campaign against cutting more palatable. So it is important to understand this naming strategy as a joint Afro-European and global construct, as it involved participation of diplomats and activists from around the world.

In 1977 the NGO Working Group on Traditional Practices was formed in Geneva. Despite the name, everybody knew that, as Dorkenoo and Elworthy put it, "the Working Group concerns itself exclusively with excision and its grave consequences for women's health" (1992: 20); some described the group's name as "a euphemism, notably for the practice of female genital mutilation" (Sanderson 1995: 23). The terminology appealed to diplomats and UN organizations and traveled widely. In 1979 the World Health Organization's Regional Office for the Eastern Mediterranean organized a watershed event in Khartoum, a weeklong seminar entitled "Traditional Practices Affecting the Health of Women and Children: Female Circumcision, Childhood Marriage, Nutritional Taboos, etc." (World Health Organization 1979). A Moroccan diplomat named Halima Embarek Warzazi details how the terminology "came to the rescue" of UN bodies that wanted to address "female circumcision" without alienating African diplomats. In 1983, when the group proposed to "authorize two experts" to conduct a study on female circumcision, not everyone was on board:

> A number of representatives of African countries where the practice was current were unenthusiastic about the Sub-Commission's proposal. The representative of Senegal came to the rescue by changing the title of the proposal and calling for a vote on a resolution requesting a study of traditional practices affecting the health of women and children.

The resolution passed after "the question of female excision" was "watered down in the title of the study."[3]

The Inter-African Committee, GAWW's umbrella group, inherited an acute awareness of the politics of naming, especially the implied threat of feminist neocolonialism. Given their contemporary militancy and their emphasis on a platform called Zero Tolerance to FGM, it might be hard to imagine that, in their early years, the IAC believed "in a 'softly, softly' approach to the abolition of female circumcision" (Dorkenoo and Elworthy 1992: 21).

Good Customs, Bad Customs: Cultural Triage and Its Cost

Although GAWW's notion of harmful traditional practices (often abbreviated as HTPs) aimed to prevent dissent, danger lurked nevertheless, for postcolonial Ghana had struggled to find a middle road between two demands that are seen as conflicting in the framework of development: modernizing the country and respecting Ghanaian culture and particularity. As Meyer astutely describes, the Ghanaian state is invested in promoting national pride and national heritage, such as festivals and "the myths, rituals, songs and dances of Ghana's ethnic groups" (1998: 316). Culture is mapped onto the past, and the desire to reclaim it is represented by the Adinkra symbol Sankofa—one of the Asante symbols that stands for the nation at large—that signals that the past guides the future. As Meyer writes, Sankofa "is understood as a call to retain valuable 'traditional' elements rather than allow Ghanaian culture to be swallowed up by Western values" (316).

To make advocacy against cutting not only palatable but desirable in this context, GAWW savvily promoted what we might think of as the work of "cultural triage." Rather than focusing solely on ending cutting, GAWW represented its work as that of sorting out good from bad traditions and of promoting the former while eradicating the latter.[4] The NGO's objectives, stated in its application to be recognized by the government as a nonprofit organization, specify this in detail:

a) To continue the work of the Dakar seminar of February, 1984 on Traditional Practices Affecting the Health of Women and Children in Africa.

b) To identify traditional practices in Ghana that affect the health of Women and Children.

c) To assess such traditional practices that have or may have positive or negative effects on the health of women and children in Ghana.

d) To focus national attention on these practices.

e) To educate the public especially women on the effects of such practices with the aim of eradicating the harmful ones and encouraging those which have healthy effects.

From the NGO's inception its leaders recognized the importance of public perception and worked assiduously to craft an innocuous and nonthreatening image by relying on existing IAC frameworks as well as the rhetorical skills that Ghanaians take pride in. GAWW regularly invokes cultural triage in its documents and at public events; to this day the NGO states that its interest is in promoting beneficial practices, such as breast-feeding, as much as eliminating harmful ones. In practice its sole focus is ending cutting. Much as secularism was a more palatable alternative to the threatening notion of atheism (Asad 2003), the vernacular modernity that GAWW proposes is not a radical concept but an assimilationist view that accommodates codified particularity within a dominant teleological development framework.

In addition to performing cultural triage, GAWW conceptualized cutting as a practice that was in the nation but that did not originate there and did not belong to it. To gain government and public support for its advocacy, GAWW wanted the public to see cutting as a "national issue" whose cessation was of vital interest to national development. This was an argument that had to be made repeatedly. Dr. Adjei recalls that NGOs had to continually fight for state recognition:

> In Ghana FGM is not a National issue despite the fact that a law has been passed outlawing the practice. After all, it is prevalent only in "the northern regions" of the country. This geographical area of Ghana is periodically plagued by life threatening epidemics such as Cerebro Spinal Meningitis, Cholera, Measles and Yellow fever. Scarce resources are directed at containing these epidemics and not much Governmental support is given to eradication of FGM.[5]

For Dr. Adjei the neglect of efforts to end cutting was an extension of the larger neglect of the region.

GAWW's interest was not in improving public health in northern Ghana but in getting government support for anticutting campaigns. GAWW knew that the danger of associating cutting with Ghana was that shadows of abjection and shame would be cast onto the nation-state. The organization sought to prevent that by portraying cutting as foreign to Ghana, both in its origins and in terms of the people who practiced it. Turning cutting into a national issue meant simultaneously constructing it as Ghanaian and non-Ghanaian—as existing in the nation-state but not belonging to it. It helped GAWW's cause that cutting was practiced by groups already considered marginal. Although it had been practiced by some southern groups (Oware Knudsen 1994), cutting is largely northern and rural and is thought of as foreign and Muslim. Unlike Akan symbolism, kente cloth, or the institution of queen mothers, the cultural practices of northern Ghanaians are neither venerated nor co-opted by the state. Thus it was easier to declare cutting harmful, but at the same time it was more difficult to get the state to pay attention to it.

The framing of cutting as a harmful traditional practice was welcomed by Ghana's ruling bodies and eventually was enshrined in the Constitution and the legislation against cutting. GAWW members were actively involved in the design of the new, democratic Constitution, which was approved in 1992, and they take pride in their advocacy for Article 26, which bans "dehumanising and injurious" customs. Article 26 states:

1) Every person is entitled to enjoy, practise, profess, maintain and promote any culture, language, tradition or religion subject to the provisions of this Constitution.

2) All customary practices which dehumanise or are injurious to the physical and mental well-being of a person are prohibited.

In addition to setting limits on customary practices and banning the injurious and dehumanizing ones, the Constitution required chiefs to modernize customary law. Rather than leaving modernization up to NGOs, chiefs were charged with evaluating "traditional customs and usages with a view to eliminating those customs and usages that are outmoded and socially harmful."[6] The spirit of constitutional reforms, and Article 26 in particular, laid the groundwork for subsequent legislation that criminalized cutting, which was passed two years after the Constitution.

Bringing cutting into the national consciousness came at a steep cost for northern Ghanaians, in that it redrew the boundaries of political belonging and governmental care. In public culture cutting is mapped onto the North and carries the added baggage of savagery and barbarity. Regional NGO and government workers find themselves in a difficult situation, having to distance themselves from cutting and cutting from the region. Their solution is to provide alternate cartographies of the origins of the practice. When Fati Paul, who was a GAWW member, an official of the National Council on Women and Development, and from the Northern Region (where most Muslims refrain from cutting), gave a report at the 1990 IAC conference in Addis Ababa, she said: "Although the indigenous people of the North do not practice FC, about 25% of the population who are migrants from neighbouring regions of Ghana and other countries such as Togo and Burkina Faso, are found to be practicing FC in the region."[7] I have often heard similar statements from many who claim that cutting "is not a cultural practice" indigenous to the region but a foreign one.

Disassociating cutting from indigeneity meant redefining what and who counts as Ghanaian. In the absence of historical evidence about origins of the practice, different NGO and government workers place cutting at a distance from the groups and places to which they belong. For Christian reformers, declaring cutting nonindigenous means asserting that it was introduced to Ghana by Muslims. As I will discuss below, in the rendition of Mrs. Mahama, the GAWW director, not just any Muslims but evil ones—Arab slave traders—were responsible. Others claim that cutting was brought to Ghana by nonindigenous minorities and is therefore "not a true tradition" of northern Ghana. For Muslim reformers who belong to groups that have not practiced cutting, it means declaring that only foreign Muslims engaged in the practice. Meanwhile Muslim reformers from groups that practiced cutting separate it from Islam and claim that cutting is not Muslim at all but African or "traditional" in origin. These explanations are tied to the officials' own affiliations and identities, which are threatened by theories of nonindigeneity. Securing their own claims to citizenship therefore comes at the expense of those around them. In other words, expunging harmful traditions from Ghana has reduced the parameters for belonging and redistribution of care. Northern Ghana and groups that practiced cutting now receive more attention but less care.

FEELING LIKE AN NGO: HOW TO EMPATHIZE WITH THE IRRATIONAL?

It is May 2004 and GAWW has convened a two-day workshop, FGM Education for Nurses, in Tamale. Tamale is the capital of the Northern Region, and the nurses participating in the workshop have arrived from the far corners of the Northern and Upper West regions, from rural clinics and urban health centers. All twenty-five nurses are women, and nearly all hail from northern Ghana, though not necessarily from the regions where they are posted. They are proud to have been selected and see the workshop as an important occasion for professional development.

Mrs. Mahama, who is leading the workshop, has a difficult task ahead of her: she must reconcile two conflicting goals. She wants to teach the nurses to empathize with cut women and not to blame them or shame them for being cut. But she also wants to teach them to see cutting as a harmful traditional practice that is unreasonable, abject, cruel, both dehumanizing and inhumane, and to see the daughters of cut women as threatened by their mothers. Throughout the workshop Mrs. Mahama will find herself oscillating between these goals, at times stating calmly that nurses should try to listen and understand cut women and, at others, encouraging righteous

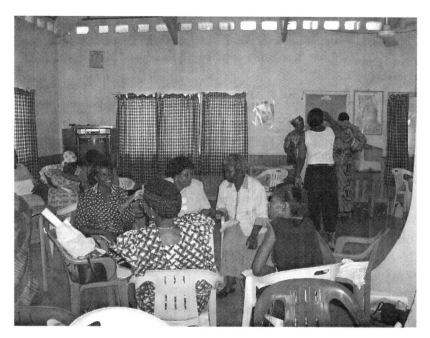

FIGURE 2. Nurses socialize during a workshop.

indignation. The workshop is a condensed space that reveals how anticutting campaigns want to distinguish the object of shame from the people who practice it but ultimately collapse the two.

Nurses have long been at the forefront of interventions against cutting. Mrs. Emma Banga, a nursing professor and the longtime president of the Ghana Registered Nurses Association, was one of the first active board members of GAWW, and Mrs. Mahama is herself a nurse. Elsewhere in the world, nurses and doctors such as the Ghanaian expatriate Efua Dorkenoo and the Egyptian doctor Nahid Toubia founded their own NGOs to end cutting. In her book, Dorkenoo recounts her first experience with cutting as a nursing student in the United Kingdom:

> Twenty-two years ago, while studying obstetrics in the UK as a part of my training to become a nurse, I was suddenly thrown into a situation for which I was not prepared. An African woman had been admitted to the labour ward: she was about to deliver and had undergone the radical form of female genital mutilation as described above. She came from a community where it was an accepted norm to infibulate all girls. What was left of her natural external genitals was a mass of scar tissue with only a small opening, hardly enough to admit the little finger. Without splitting the vulvar scars, there

was no space for the baby to be delivered. This threw the midwives and obstetricians into panic as they were not familiar with this practice and none of them knew how to deliver her so the baby was born by Caeserian [sic] section. (1994: 2)

An encounter with an actual cut woman facing a health-care system unable to care for her is cited as a motivating factor for Dorkenoo's subsequent advocacy. However, the NGO she founded in London did not make health care for cut women a priority, nor have other anticutting groups or governments in the global North or in Africa done so.[8]

At the GAWW workshop only one session is to be devoted to health issues and none to health care for cut women. The purpose of the workshop is not to enhance the nurses' clinical practice in reference to cutting but to train them to be modernizing agents who will help end cutting. This involves teaching the nurses to think and feel differently and asking them to substitute care for cut women with a concern for their children and the surveillance of their bodies. The upshot is that cut women are to be talked about, worried about, researched, and legislated against but not cared for.

Making Modern Subjects: Naming Harms

Workshops are one of the prime sites of public culture where Ghanaians are continually reminded of modernization theories and the need to end harmful traditions. All manner of development workshops reconstruct modernization theories time and again and invite their participants to understand themselves as modernizing subjects. The paradigm of harmful traditional practices is always under construction, and the work of specifying, dissecting, and situating harmful practices with respect to northern Ghanaians is never complete.

NGOs analyze social problems by first solidifying the interpretative framework for those problems. This is why more than half, if not two-thirds, of each NGO event I attended in the Upper East Region was devoted to the enumeration and classification of "harmful traditions" and the overlapping "women's issues." Although workshop participants are familiar with these taxonomies, NGOs and donors repeat them time and again in participatory exercises. In keeping with this, GAWW representatives spend the first day of the workshop re-laying the "tracks" (Pigg 2005: 45) of modernization theory, which couples development to the abandonment of tradition. Before the nurses can be taught about FGM, they are reminded of the larger discourse within which concerns about FGM are nested. The following detailed ethnography of the GAWW workshop reveals how this discourse operates in a context in which northern Ghanaians are compelled to participate in their own subjectification. The notion of FGM as a harmful traditional practice hinges on the construction of a larger discourse about northern Ghana, and rural populations in particular, as ruled by harmful traditions. Nurses are trained to see themselves as knowledgeable of these traditions but free from their grasp and able to free others as well. As Pigg puts it, the authority of health workers "rests on knowing villagers without aligning themselves closely with them" (Pigg 1997: 276).

"What are some of the harmful traditional practices in our area?" Mrs. Mahama asks the participants in one of the first exercises of the day. As the nurses begin to volunteer answers—teenage pregnancies, forced feeding, tribal marks—Mrs. Mahama writes them on a large flip chart, inviting further reflection about the harmful effects of each. The flip chart begins with an organized format:

HTP	Effects
Teenage pregnancy	Prostitution, broken homes, malnutrition, school dropouts, difficult labor
Forced feeding	child gets choked, infections, loss of sense of smell, malnutrition, retarded growth
Tribal marks	Tetanus, anemia, septicemia/sepsis, keloids
Breaking the lobes	Abscesses, infection, pain, hunger for the child, marasmus of the breast after delivery

The topics of conversation exceed the list, as Mrs. Mahama and the nurses offer numerous illustrative remarks and stories. And as issue after issue is broached, nurses are mobilized into a crescendo of indignation, turning more and more enthusiastic. Each item on the chart occasions clarification and illustration: "Some even go to a soothsayer," one nurse offers, introducing *some* as a word for referring to those not present. Because the subjects she refers to consult soothsayers and engage in divination, they are marked as non-Christian and non-Muslim people who live in rural areas. "Some force-feed with maggot water," another nurse adds, raising the shock quotient. The nurses who speak up locate the practices at some distance from themselves: it is not *we* who are subjected to tradition but *they*.

Mrs. Mahama is quick to introduce death as the ultimate harm. "There was a case two years ago in the Upper West where an old lady did the [tribal] marks. She cut too deep on the baby's stomach and all the intestines fell out. The child got infected and died, even though they took it to the hospital." "So then the baby died, the people stop," one nurse replies provocatively, and the other participants take the bait, responding: "They say the baby didn't come to stay." "They won't stop." "It's a sign of royalty." Many of the assembled nurses have visible tribal marks on their cheeks, but they are not supposed to recognize themselves in the discussion. The formal emphasis on *them*—the rural and traditional subjects whose practices are being scrutinized—ensures the safe distance necessary to denounce practices rooted in "superstition."

The naming and specification of harms is a collectivity-building process, forging a common ground among nurses in opposition to the people they are meant to care for. "They also expel the colostrum," one nurse says. "Why?" "The child will get frequent stools." Mrs. Mahama adds: "In our area, they put ants in the calabash with the colostrum, and if they don't swim out, the child can't drink milk." "Others do it and wait for the ants," a nurse rejoins. "If ants come, the milk is sweet." Mrs. Mahama: "A woman from Sandema came to the clinic in Accra; all her babies had died. She had flat nipples and said her milk was not sweet. She gave the babies formula with water and all the babies died." Thus modernizers see harmful traditions as belonging to uneducated northern populations who trust in ancestral spirits. Their ostensible proximity to nature and use of animals—maggots, ants, and chickens— for purposes of divination marks them as only liminally human.

As the nurses compile more examples of harmful traditional practices, Mrs. Mahama stops organizing them on the flip chart. Words flow: bathing of postnatal mothers, widowhood rites, kalgoteem (an herbal medicine), wife inheritance, child betrothal and early marriage, beating of virgins, and woman-woman marriage. When someone mentions "widowhood rites," Mrs. Mahama slows everyone down and intervenes to say, "It isn't the rites that are bad, but some of them are dehumanizing." In keeping with GAWW's practice of cultural triage, she emphasizes that cultural rites or rituals have some beneficial aspects. After this qualification she goes on to explain that something is wrong with many widowhood rites, the purpose of which is to ascertain whether a wife is responsible for her husband's death: "In many tribes in Ghana, no man dies a natural death. The woman is the one who killed the man. Even if he was a drunkard, she is blamed." This prompts the nurses to name the most objectionable features of widowhood rites they have heard about.

"You lie with your dead husband."

"You must go backwards."

"They give you a smeared calabash to eat out of."

"Sisters-in-law put pepper in [a] widow's eyes."

"You must wear the same cloth and can't bathe; you get skin infections."

"You don't lie on a mat, you lie on dirt."

"And if an ant bites you, you are a witch!"

The voices reach a crescendo.

Suddenly, one voice rises above the rest, as a nurse exclaims that she, too, had suffered, shouting, "I ran away from the rites!" Her exclamation is met with silence. Even though the nurse then explains that she was subjected to widowhood rites against her will, and that she has since escaped from them by finding Jesus, her connection to tradition is too uncomfortable, too intimate. By including herself as a subject of tradition, she has violated the central feature of the exercise: it is not supposed to be about an experience shared by *us* but about the hypothetical *them* and their harmful traditions. The nurses are to name "harmful traditional practices in our area," which suggests an intimate knowledge of the practices discussed, but they need to be careful not to recognize themselves in them. GAWW's purpose is to construct the nurses as knowledgeable about harmful traditions but not as subject to them; they should understand themselves as modern subjects who oppose harmful traditions and who are not in their grip.

GAWW wants the nurses to become so secure in their distance from cut women that they can be empathetic reformers. When one of the nurses begins to complain about women who "won't go to the hospital" and see "TBAs" (traditional birth attendants) instead of professional midwives, Mrs. Mahama exhorts her and others not to blame rural women for being cut or for their health-seeking behavior: "Most women do not attribute their suffering to FGM, so we must teach them. Don't blame them—she didn't know. Don't say, 'Look at how you're bleeding'—tell them not to do it to their daughters."

As a former nurse Mrs. Mahama knew that doctors and nurses regularly talk down to and berate their rural and poor patients—whether for failing to access health care in a timely fashion, taking medicine improperly, or for otherwise being bad patients. Mrs. Mahama wanted the nurses to see themselves as reformers who discipline cut women, not by scolding them but by educating them. The nurses should be understanding and empathetic, she insisted, otherwise rural women "will not listen." This goal proved difficult to reconcile with the exercises that focused on harmful traditions and cast rural women as abject.

We Have Never Been Modern: The Modernity Exam

The exercise in creating modern subjects gets more complicated later in the day, when an invited guest speaker, a government official with the title of deputy community development officer for the Northern Region, gives a lecture on modernity and tradition. Like GAWW, the development officer divides the world of northern Ghana into urban-complex and rural-primitive binaries. However, he believes that the nurses carry a residue of tradition inside them and should expunge it, lest they be complicit in FGM. To join the fight against FGM, he says, they should change all their values. He explains in a sociological disquisition on the concept of social values that Ghana is "a society with culture," by which he means that Ghanaians hold traditional values that are ultimately damaging:

> Values are the underlying things that influence our decision-making. How do we know that we have shared values? You have a shared value if you are able to convince the other person of your opinion. No matter where we are in society, we share some common interests, no matter how primitive or complex the society is. Some are not comfortable with "primitive." But they are underdeveloped. Aha. In rural areas, they do simple, simple things. Urban areas are more complex.

To demonstrate that the nurses uphold traditional values and are therefore ultimately responsible for upholding FGM, he distributes a test with four questions:

1a) Have you ever heard of FGM?
1b) Should it be continued?
2a) Have you ever heard of teenage marriage?
2b) Should it be continued?
3a) Have you heard of chieftaincy?
3b) Should it be continued?
4a) Have you heard of traditional medicine?
4b) Should it be continued?

After giving the nurses time to write down answers, he explains the purpose of the test:

> This exercise is to tell you how traditional you are and how modern you are. These are just four out of fifteen questions. These questions normally have scores. We don't have time to do an analysis to see how traditional you are, how backward you think, and how modern you are. The exam lets you know: Am I thinking like a modern man? Am I thinking like a yesterday person?

The nurses' answers are a window into the Ghanaian vernacular modernity that accommodates some traditions: they are opposed to FGM and teenage marriage, value chieftaincy, and have mixed opinions about traditional medicine. For the development officer this incomplete modernity is one of the reasons why FGM continues; his notion of development and modernity leaves no room for anything "cultural":

> Culture is still very active, still predominant in our society. This was aptly demonstrated with the question about chieftaincy. People here should be fed up with chieftaincy, but no! In other societies, people forget about chiefs. But here people kill one another because of chiefs. We must look at practices that are negative to development.

His remarks are met with amused laughter, as the nurses do not see themselves as upholding harmful traditions. While the officer wants them to question the authority of chieftaincy and abandon all traditions, the nurses embrace the more pervasive state model of vernacular modernity that makes room for practices codified as traditional. GAWW's hospitable model of cultural triage, which distinguishes harmful from beneficial cultural practices, resonates with them.

The development officer concludes his presentation by emphasizing that "FGM continues because people like us are not committed to fight against it," and he asks the nurses to tell him how they will personally strive to end FGM. This exercise will be repeated in more detail the following day, at the very end of the workshop, which, following common practice, ends with pledges of commitment. As the nurses mention such strategies as forming girls into groups and educating them, advising parents in clinics, educating young men, and organizing community forums, they are also tasked with working on themselves. By educating and converting their "unfortunate brothers and sisters," they are told, they can produce themselves as suitably modern.

The last exercise of the day brings into full view the tension between producing nurses as empathetic caregivers who understand the struggles of the women they are trying to reach and concerned reformist citizens. On the program is a discussion of a story, "Tradition, Tradition. A Story of Mother Earth," written by Efua Dorkenoo and published in the Students' Manual for Nurses and Midwives by the World Health Organization. Encouraged by the WHO manual to initiate a liberal dialogue about the story, Mrs. Mahama arranges the chairs in a circle and asks the nurses to read the story out loud, one paragraph at a time. The story is set in a fictional kingdom called the Land of Myrrh, which is populated by "proud people of great cultural heritage" and women who are ambitious, astute, elegant, and self-possessed. However, all the women have only one leg, because it is both traditional and fashionable for women to get one of their legs cut off. Mother Earth is sent to check up on the kingdom because "there had been a very bad drought, people were hungry, and naturally the Great Creator was concerned." Confused about the one-legged women, she tries to find out "the reasons" for this phenomenon. However, she deems the reasons unsatisfactory, as she does not believe that women with two legs would become prostitutes or sexually insatiable, unable to bear children, or have their remaining leg grow into a tree. Furthermore, because she has a direct connection to the Great Creator, Mother Earth knows that the Great Creator does not demand that a leg be cut off. Finally, an old woman gives Mother Earth a satisfactory answer: the practice started when an old ruler was threatened by gender equality and, afraid that he would lose a dancing competition to a woman, passed a decree that women should have one of their legs cut off. When Mother Earth solicits the views of people in the kingdom, they tell her that they suffer from the practice but are afraid to change it. They had tried once, when "the food situation in this drought stricken land was getting worse and worse" and when women "walking on crutches . . . found it difficult to work the land and to travel far and wide to find richer pastures and foliage for the animals." Prompted by a crisis of drought and scarcity, people began to question the tradition by exposing and challenging the myths given as reasons. But the ruler thwarted their plans, and "little girls continue to be mutilated to this day." The story ends with a call to children: "But come along, children. We have a game of survival to play, and for this we need both our legs. So come along!"

Dorkenoo's story validates the mutilated women while demonizing the practice and is thus reflective of her own position as a diasporic Ghanaian woman from London, as well as of GAWW's advocacy. The story portrays female genital cutting as absurd and unreasonable, and the reasons people give—are impelled to give—are presented as myths that need to be exposed as such. In this view, nothing about cutting is beneficial; it threatens survival by disabling women who are already suffering from drought and scarcity. Dorkenoo's solution is to end cutting by spreading the idea that women would be better able to handle the extra labor necessary to survive drought. The moral of the story is that if women and children learn to question so-called irrational myths and subsequently halt the practice of mutilation, their suffering will abate, and they will be able to persevere through scarcity.

After the reading was over, Mrs. Mahama attempted to lead a discussion using techniques outlined in the WHO manual that entail a liberal pedagogy of "learning to question"; the discussion should reproduce the nonjudgmental form of questioning exemplified by Mother Earth. Mrs. Mahama tried to guide the nurses through a process of self-reflection so that they could achieve an empathetic understanding of the rural Others. But neither the story's characterization of cutting nor Mrs. Mahama's pedagogy lent themselves easily to empathy. Mrs. Mahama began by explaining the importance of empathy and reflection: "She [Mother Earth] starts with questions, so we should also start questioning tradition. She was not judgmental, didn't condemn them. If you're judgmental, they cut off. Mother Earth listened with empathy, she reflected on the answers. What was the outcome?"

"They gave her the answers," a nurse ventured.

"People started reflecting themselves!" Mrs. Mahama corrected the nurse. "It motivated some of them to take action."

This part of the exercise proved to be a performative contradiction. Mrs. Mahama asked a question, received an answer that did not align with the WHO manual, and then quickly stated the answer that did.

MRS. MAHAMA: Whom does the Mother Earth represent?

A NURSE: Those who are against FGM.

MRS. MAHAMA: Mother Earth represents all of us! We should all start questioning traditions that are not in our interest, that are outmoded.

Mrs. Mahama constructed a tightly woven discursive space in which some statements were welcome and others were not. The nurses were supposed to recognize themselves in the agential and attentive figure of Mother Earth, who empathizes with the cut women while demonstrating that cutting is driven by irrational myths. But the nurses had difficulty recognizing themselves in the figure of Mother Earth, and, after the morning exercises of naming and constructing abject harms, the nurses could not embrace the imperative to empathize. The only nurse who saw herself in the story was the woman who had earlier claimed she was a subject of tradition. She identified not with Mother Earth but with the limbless and mutilated women: "I didn't do the widowhood rites! And I was sanctioned, I am the outcast! Jesus has freed me from these things. They gave my birthright, my inheritance, to my sister."

"She's a rebel, but how many can do this?" Mrs. Mahama interrupted, in an attempt to move the discussion.

But the nurse raised her voice: "They forced me to be naked for the funeral rites."

Mrs. Mahama interjected again: "Women don't want to be outcasts, so they submit—"

The nurse cut her off: "I didn't finish! I was pregnant. My sister was also pregnant. I had to wash the corpse. But the mother-in-law said I shouldn't have done this."

Mrs. Mahama interrupted the nurse and told a story of a Bolga teacher who submitted to family pressure and got cut. Then Mrs. Mahama asked, "What lessons have we learned?" One nurse volunteered: "People are afraid to talk about it—you become an outcast if you question." The nurse who never finished her story started shouting: "I am an outcast and I am liberated. Jesus is my husband!" Mrs. Mahama ignored her and offered the correct interpretation of the lesson: "This story tells us: traditions are difficult to change. You need patience and people who will start questioning."

The nurse was silenced because confessional statements did not belong in the space of the workshop. Mrs. Mahama is a devout Christian who preaches in her church; in other contexts she would have welcomed the nurse's narrative of suffering from tradition and subsequent liberation through Christ. But Mrs. Mahama did not find this narrative appropriate in an NGO workshop where the nurses were supposed to recognize themselves as concerned and empathetic citizens with political agency, not as suffering subjects of a suffocating tradition. While in some West African contexts NGOs promote confessional technologies such as personal testimonies of illness (Nguyen 2010), these forms of subjectification are not always called for.

Nurses were supposed to identify with those who remedy suffering, not with those who embody it. The nurse's affect was excessive, uncontrolled, and uncontained and thereby marked as irrational. The affect that GAWW desired was one of righteous indignation. Concerned citizens are supposed to feel intensely, but these feelings must be carefully channeled toward proper objects.

On the first day of the workshop, the nurses were asked to think about FGM as one of many outmoded and harmful traditional practices that impede development, subjugate women, and therefore have no place in modern Ghana. They were also asked to situate themselves with respect to these traditions as reformers and to work on themselves to become modern subjects and join the campaign against FGM. If the purpose of the first day was to consolidate the classification of harmful traditional practices and interpellate the nurses as modernizing subjects and concerned liberal citizens, the second day was designed to map and specify FGM, situating it further outside liberal tolerance (Brown et al. 2006) and within the realm of "repugnance and abhorrence" (Povinelli 2002: 85).

Mapping FGM: Reanimating Colonial Taxonomies

The GAWW workshop is a useful vantage point from which to view the construction of FGM as a discursive concept in its own right. FGM is not a descriptor of practices of cutting; it is not the English term for a practice called yabega ŋma in Gurene. FGM is a construct grounded in colonial taxonomies (described in chapter 1) that are more developed today. These taxonomies are evident in questions Mrs. Mahama posed and answers she provided:

> Why call it FGM? It is mutilation and WHO has a definition we all use now.
> How did FGM come about? It came to West Africa through the Arab slave trade.
> Where is it done?

Mrs. Mahama displays a world map and a map of Africa on transparencies and writes the following text on flip charts:

> How prevalent is it? 120–140 million women have had FGM, most of them from Africa, and every year, two million girls are taken through.

She adds, "In Ghana, we don't have much statistics to go by; you can give us data."

> What are the Ghanaian tribes that do it? Kassena, Nankane, Walas, Builsas, Dagabas, Kusasis, Busangas, Lobis, Fra-Fras, Kotokoli, Fulanis, Wangaras, Moshis, Sisalas; also settlers in Accra and in the Brong Ahafo and Northern Regions.
>
> What are the reasons for FGM? 1. Tradition. Some don't even know why they do it, it was just handed down to them; 2. Cultural and social pressure, insults; 3. Initiation rite in the Upper East.
>
> At what age is it practiced? From birth to death; in some places they will do it even on dead bodies.
>
> What types of FGM are there? Types I, II, III, and IV.

The questions and answers are from the WHO manual, and Mrs. Mahama supplements them with some regional inflections, explaining Ghanaian particularities. The underlying taxonomy is global and is supposed to be transplantable to any African country.

A common anthropological objection to Mrs. Mahama's grid would be that it is at least partially inaccurate, exaggerated, and collapses a multitude of practices of cutting into one phenomenon—FGM—that it then disaggregates into types. These objections would be correct, but my interest here is not the inaccuracy of the answers but the questions that organize this grid of global knowledge about FGM. As we have seen, these questions were first posed by British colonial officials and continue to be asked today. Understanding FGM means mapping it onto the interlocked historical, demographic, anthropological, and epidemiological matrix structured by these questions. The making and remaking of this FGM grid is a normative practice pervasive in both scholarly and governmental cultures of expertise about cutting. Many a chapter or article on cutting begins with this taxonomy, and its absence produces confusion. Anthropologists provide it in the name of contextualizing cutting, while scholars from other disciplines thus perform knowledge about cultural dimensions of cutting. The question remains why the taxonomy established during colonialism continues to serve as the ground for contextualizing cutting. What do we lose by taking the colonial taxonomy as our orientation to what needs to be said and known about cutting? One answer is that staying tethered to this grid prevents us from understanding how we unwittingly participate in the perpetuation of governing taxonomies and operations of power-knowledge that proceeded from imperial centers and demanded answers from the colonies.

Mrs. Mahama's grid would be familiar to NGO workers and civil servants from northern Ghana. She places cutting outside the nation-state: it is not an original Ghanaian practice but one introduced by Muslim migrants who continue to spread it through ongoing migration, she says. The map extends beyond Ghana. That mutilation is recognized as a global problem categorized by types and practiced in a variety of countries helps deflect responsibility from the nation. The grid is motivated by anthropological questions about tribes and reasons but populated by modernizing responses; all the proffered reasons are deemed unreasonable. The grid also aims to produce feelings, but those are largely off the page.

In the space of the workshop the mapping exercise produces Mrs. Mahama as an expert with factual knowledge and the nurses as learners, surveillance workers, and properly moved citizens disturbed by cutting. The exercise engenders various affects in the nurses. They laugh to avert discomfort as they help Mrs. Mahama name the "tribes that do it"; there is something shameful about the enunciation of tribal names. The nurses are shocked and pained when Mrs. Mahama tells them that "the old ladies will do it even before the baby comes [at delivery]," and "on the dead bodies." The nurses are also eager to learn and begin asking more and more questions. They are confused about the types of FGM.

To explain the four types of FGM, Mrs. Mahama pulls out the IAC-produced anatomical model and the nurses assemble it on a table. They mingle around it, confused and curious at the same time.

"Please, sister, what is practiced in Ghana?," one of the nurses asks. Mrs. Mahama points out the model for clitoridectomy but then quickly moves to explain infibulation, or, as she puts it, "the most radical form of FGM." Infibulation is virtually nonexistent in Ghana, but it has the strongest shock value, and globally it has come to stand for the dangers of FGM. The anatomical model shows what infibulation looks like, but Mrs. Mahama's words more affectively materialize its horrors. As she tells the nurses about the thorns with which girls are ostensibly infibulated and immobilized, the "old ladies' dirty nails" that "snip it [the clitoris] off," and girls in Ethiopia who are left in the bush to be attacked by wolves that "get the smell of blood," the grammar of oral disapproval expands. "Tsk, tsk, tsk" and groans emanate from the nurses' visibly disturbed faces.

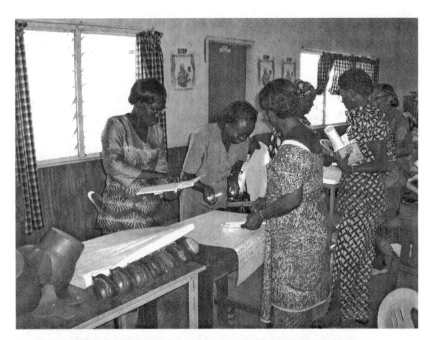

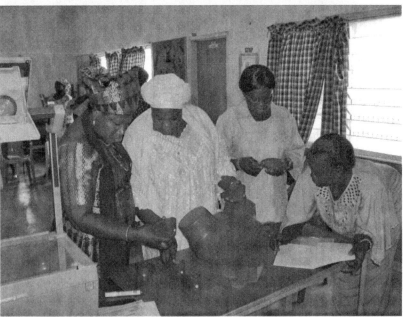

FIGURE 3 (*Top*). The anatomical models: hemorrhage and "FGM types."

FIGURE 4 (*Bottom*). Nurses examine the anatomical models.

Knowledge for Surveillance: Redistributing Care

The mapping exercise aims to inculcate facts and feelings but also to redistribute the nurses' attention, care, and concern toward different objects. Rather than thinking of themselves solely as health workers who offer care to cut women, the nurses are asked to care about the taxonomic grid itself. It has become difficult to accrue data on rates of cutting on the basis of interviews, Mrs. Mahama says, referencing the "denial paper" that highlights cut women's unwillingness to tell the truth to researchers (see chapter 3). She says that the nurses are therefore best positioned to conduct research on cutting. "You can give us data," she encourages, explaining a process of secretive surveillance of cut women and their children who come to clinics. "If you do good examination, you can jokingly say you want to look [at the girls' genitals]. When you want to find out [whether a child was cut], you record it, but don't make the mother uncomfortable. After some three months, you'll have the data."

Mrs. Mahama knows that it is not likely that the nurses will take her up on this suggestion this time, but she mentions it to plant the seed for subsequent projects. The mapping exercise is an effort not only to share knowledge but also to construct knowledge as an object of concern: the FGM map itself needs the nurses' labor and care. The GAWW workshop thus resituates the nurses in relationship to their patients and advocacy against cutting. The nurses should see that the ultimate value of their labor lies in producing epidemiological knowledge about the prevalence of cutting.

GAWW is so certain in its convictions that Mrs. Mahama and Edna, a GAWW affiliate who runs some of the workshop sessions, make no effort to hide this redistribution of care. Unlike WHO officials and members of the U.S. Congress, who, as I will discuss later, motivate the search for knowledge by stating that epidemiological data on prevalence will result in better care for cut women and children, GAWW makes no such pretenses. Rather, as Edna suggests, the nurses' offer of care should enable them to trick mothers into having their babies and older children examined: "Nurses in Wa told us they pleaded with the women to tell them [whether their children were cut] so that they could counsel them how to take care of the baby: 'You're a special person to us, we want to take care of you.'" Gathering data requires simulated affect: the nurses' affable jokes and performance of care should pave a smooth path to knowledge.

In the workshop's only discussion of health and cutting, the focus is not on health care for cut women and children but on portraying the potential health consequences in the worst light possible. To that end Mrs. Mahama assembles medical knowledge and affective storytelling. While her slides display a sterile map of immediate, intermediate, and delivery consequences—categories derived from the WHO classification—Mrs. Mahama supplements it with shocking stories, offhand remarks about cut women's lack of humanity, and exaggerated statistics. In contrast to the WHO, which carefully calibrates the admixture of sober fact and horrific detail (Hodžić 2013), GAWW is not driven by liberal anxieties that require that FGM be treated with cultural sensitivity. The NGO feels no need to perform nuance, given the widespread public conviction that cutting is harmful, barbaric, and non-Ghanaian.

> [On the slide] Complications: Immediate
> Pain, haemorrhage, shock, urinary retention, infection, septicemia, tetanus, delayed healing, fractures.
>
> MRS. MAHAMA: The clitoris is slippery. They put ash or sand on it to be able to cut it. The circumciser spits at it first. Some use cow dung.
>
> [On the slide] Complications: Intermediate
> Dysmenorrhea, cysts and abscesses, keloids, damaged urethra.
>
> MRS. MAHAMA: Most of them get dysmenorrhea, there is always tension there. Most women get the abscesses—you see them walking like this [she walks with legs wide open]. Most of them develop keloids. Most often they lose their babies, so they try to deliver more, and it hurts always. What is suffering to a man, to enjoy his sex? . . . Then infertility—because of PID [pelvic inflammatory disease], UTIs [urinary tract infections]. Some of them, most of them have kidney failures and stone formation. Some even have anal incontinence. Some develop false vaginas. The man pushes anywhere at all and creates other holes.
>
> [On the slide] Delivery Complications
> Delayed second stage, tears, ruptured uterus, bleeding, macerated stillbirth, prolonged and obstructed labor, fistulas
>
> MRS. MAHAMA: According to Dr. Adjei, the baby was hanging [from the woman's body] for three days before they brought her. The baby started decomposing. This woman in Bolga kept the fistula for 17 years.[9] The

women won't go to the hospital because of shame. They have four times more stillbirths than nonexcised women. My own cousin lied to the doctor and said she delivered three times, but it was nine times. As for FGM, most women are frigid. There are psychological effects. They say they are not complete, they feel like they are incomplete women. Many feel depression. I used to have the story by one Waris Dirie, a very beautiful Somali woman. It was a best-seller. She's in this campaign against FGM, and she talked about the psychological trauma she went through.

I had first heard Mrs. Mahama claim that "most of them die" on my first trip to Ghana in 2002, when I attended a GAWW meeting about a proposed amendment to Ghana's legislation against cutting. Point C of the memorandum accompanying the amendment read:

Furthermore, it has been established that the practice in all its forms causes untold hardships and medical complications often leading to the death of the victims. It is therefore being proposed that the name of the offence should be changed from "Female Circumcision" to "Female Genital Mutilation" (FGM) to reflect it is [sic] actual nature.

My attention was drawn not to the main subject of the paragraph but to the phrase "causes untold hardships and medical complications *often leading to the death of the victims.*" No one discussed this claim; I was newly arrived in Ghana and the only person startled by it, and I asked how it would be received by the attorney general. A government worker responded with another exaggerated claim: "FGM leads to death often enough. We know that two out of ten women will die."

In subsequent years I attended numerous events at which Mrs. Mahama claimed that "most of them die," "most of them lose their babies," "most of them develop keloids"; in all these cases I saw nurses, teachers, and government officials nod in affirmation. For GAWW members and others, "most of them die" was precise enough, as nobody takes this statement literally; rather, it is interpreted as an indication of the potentially serious health problems caused by cutting. These claims are not meant to reflect evidentiary facts but serve as metaphors for the gravity of invoked consequences.

As she is talking to the nurses, Mrs. Mahama supplements the biomedical metaphors of harms with a mobilization of affect. Since the nurses may not find cutting itself repugnant enough, Mrs. Mahama depicts it as crossing numerous boundaries. The mixing of dirt, bodily fluids, and animal waste in the form of ash, spit, and cow dung violate the body and pollute the social order. These impurities are a public threat, and their invocation is meant to depict cutting and the people who practice it as abject and impure, raising doubts about their humanity. FGM is constructed as not only violent and harmful but also abject and inhuman.

Mrs. Mahama's efforts appear successful, for the nurses are disgusted and repelled. Some fight back tears; some are incredulous about the foolishness and selfishness of men. The nurses are indignant about lies that rural women tell doctors. To heighten their affective responses, Mrs. Mahama brings out a photo album with "fresh pictures" from Wa, where a circumciser was arrested with the help of GAWW. Mrs. Mahama distributes the photographs of the cut children and comments on their victimhood.

Afterward she screens an old IAC documentary, *Beliefs and Misbeliefs*. Filmed partly in Nigeria, the film portrays cutting at a safe distance; Muslim Nigerians who settled in Ghana are often viewed as unwelcome slum-dwelling migrants, and GAWW often attributes cutting to them. Given the poor sound quality of the film—"It's an old tape, more than ten years, but we don't have the money to buy another one," says Edna—the narration is unintelligible, but Mrs. Mahama offers only minimal explanation along the way, as the point is to visualize the horrors of FGM.

The film begins with a close-up of bodily scarification and cutting, and the nurses become distressed. They gasp as the knives are being sharpened and cry out loud as the film proceeds to show the act of cutting. They shout:

"The hands are bloody!"
"We can't watch this!"
"They cut it like meat!"

The purpose of the screening is not to foster understanding but indignation and horror, and Mrs. Mahama invites the nurses to join in an affective and moral commentary as they watch the film. She directs their attention to the mother of the cut child, inviting the nurses to judge her: "Look at the mother! She is happy!" The nurses know these words call for a response, and some comment on the mother's ignorance. Mrs. Mahama comments on the cut girls: "They're happy, dancing. They've become women. As if they're drugged!" The official from the Ministry of Health, otherwise quiet, joins in: "They wanted it, they didn't cry. These are the people who migrated to Ghana!" Since the feelings of disgust are too much to bear, they have to be displaced onto the nation's Others, so this official, like many others, ties cutting to migrants or, as others call them, settlers and foreigners. This discourse has traction; as a regional director of the Commission on Human Rights and Administrative Justice, a government agency, told me, everyone knows that FGM is "disgusting."

The film put an end to attempts to foster empathy toward cut women, replacing it with revulsion, moral judgment, and the symbolic revocation of citizenship. There is little room for understanding and caregiving when cutting and the people who practice it are depicted as repulsive foreigners. GAWW's inability to reconcile the imperative of compassion with its construction of FGM exemplifies the larger double bind of problematizations of cutting: although NGOs attempt to bracket value judgments when talking to rural men and women, they are, as I discuss later in this chapter and in chapter 5, perfectly aware of their subordinate status and the constant scrutiny that attends it.

At the end of the workshop, the nurses thank GAWW. "I have elected myself to talk on the behalf of the group," says one nurse to smiling approvals from others. "Thanks to the facilitators from Accra. We've been hearing about it, but we haven't had proper insight into it. By the grace of God, we can help save our sisters." For GAWW this means that the workshop has been successful.

TRADITION AS A PARADIGM FOR GOVERNANCE

In chapter 1, I described how colonial rule of the Northern Territories was predicated on preserving specific understandings of tradition and treating it as a foundation of social and political orders that legitimized minimal investment in the region. Ghana's decolonization ushered in a different relationship to both tradition and investment, giving way to talk of national unity and investment in regional education and economies. At independence in 1957 all of Ghana was set on the path of certain types of de-ethnicization; Nkrumah wanted to rid all groups of tribal marks and also expressed disapproval of female circumcision in that context. He also tried to industrialize the northern regions and educate its people so that their employment prospects were not limited to menial labor. Education was made free and compulsory in the three regions that today comprise northern Ghana, and some people benefited from it, forming the first northern intellectual elites with social and political capital (Pellow 2011; Nugent 1995). But the general population remained underserved; the 2000 census showed that three-quarters of the population in the Upper East never attended school, and educational infrastructure remained poor.[10] As late as 2010 the headmaster of Bongo Senior High School warned that the school was at full capacity and would not be able to enroll any new students. Meanwhile the postcolonial drive to industrialize the country came to an abrupt end. The empty shells of a meat-processing factory in Bolga, a tomato-processing factory in Tongo, and a rice-processing factory in Tamale stand as reminders of some of the postindependence investments made by the state.

Additional state attempts to bolster the regional economy were undermined by Cold War politics, military coups, severe regional droughts, and structural adjustment and economic liberalization policies imposed by the International Monetary Fund (IMF). Between independence in 1957 and the acceptance of IMF structural adjustment policies in the mid-1980s, the Ghanaian state had fewer than thirty years of what might pass for sovereignty over its economy and social investment policies (see Pierre 2013).

Anthropologists with long-standing regional interests agree that "deepening poverty" is a feature of postausterity politics (Whitehead 2006; see also Pellow 2011). In addition to causing currency devaluation and inflation, market liberalization has exacerbated regional inequalities (Grant and Nijman 2004), and the poorest districts feel the effects of declining food production and inflation most acutely. An example is the virtual destruction of regional rice production by the removal of Ghanaian government subsidies and reduction of import tariffs; local rice is now more expensive than imported rice, and half a million farmers have been "driven out of business" (Harsch 2008: 4).[11] Not surprisingly, regional rice production has largely collapsed; when NGOs such as the Single Mothers Organization from Zuarungu try to revive production, they do so on a small scale. Nonetheless, donors praised Ghana for its democratization, liberalization, and quick ascendance to middle-income status that turned the country into a "neoliberal poster child" (Piot 2010: 175). This neoliberal progress has stalled since 2011, and funding for many NGOs and government projects has since dried up.

There is now more migration south than ever and its character has changed. Although NGOs and the government portray them as subsistence farmers, people from northern Ghana are itinerant migrants who make up some of the country's internal diaspora. As in north-central Togo (Piot

1999), the makeup of households here is thoroughly shaped by migration, and many people are simultaneously northern and southern (see also Pellow 2015).[12] What began as slavery and was followed by forced labor later morphed into migration to secure livelihoods and employment; the entire twentieth century was a period of southern migration. Migration is both a central strategy of economic survival and a practice of self-actualization for many young men and women (Lobnibe 2010; Hawkins 2002). Women and men in rural Bongo told me about lives spent in southern Ghana, as well as sporadic, seasonal journeys to "Kumasi" (which stands for southern Ghana). I never specifically asked about these histories, but they inevitably came up in conversations and interviews. Many told me that they worked on farms or "washed bowls" (at an eatery), meaning that they were situated at the margins of the informal economy. Indeed, the very concept of an informal economy is based on Keith Hart's studies of the Frafra labor proletariat in Accra (1973).

In recent years the composition of migrant bodies has shifted, as has the public perception of them. Men were recruited as laborers during colonialism, and northern families were hesitantly welcomed after World War II, but more girls and women now migrate independently (Cassiman 2010), often out of sheer desperation. For those girls whose families cannot afford education beyond primary school, migration is a rite of passage into adulthood. "She ran away to earn money for her school fees," many parents told me, referring to their teenage daughters, most of whom never returned. In popular discourses these young women, who work as hawkers and porters, are seen as a national problem and serve as a fulcrum of moral anxieties about social decay (see Smith 2014). Migrant women themselves are acutely aware of regional inequalities: they see the disconnect between their struggles for survival and burgeoning urban infrastructures, including glassy skyscrapers, lavish homes, and conspicuous commodities.

In contrast to the northern migrants who regularly move south, southerners see the North as less desirable. This region of Ghana is bereft of doctors, nurses, and teachers, as many assigned to work there never arrive; officials regularly complain about those who fail to report to their jobs but receive salaries nonetheless, as well as about agricultural extension officers who sit idly in their urban offices. A few years ago the *Ghanaian Times* reported that "of all the doctors newly posted to the Upper East Region in the last four years, only one had reported for duty." The *Times* found that there were more doctors in Ridge Hospital in Accra than the total number of doctors in hospitals and other health facilities in the Northern, Upper East, and Upper

West regions combined.[13] For health care professionals, the labor market is global, and the brain drain that has sapped Ghana of health workers is a national concern.[14] Ghanaian nurses and doctors are in high demand in the global market; they are among the few exceptional labor migrants who are wanted and welcomed to the global North.

Regional Gap and Harsh Culture: Poverty and Neoliberal Recognition

The status of the Upper East Region and northern Ghana as a reserve of labor migrants is continually obscured by governmental and development policies. Rather than reckoning with joblessness and the region's exploitative terms of integration into the national and global economies, these policies construct it as isolated, static, traditional, and agricultural. As in the Lesotho described by James Ferguson, the economic policies applicable to northern Ghana represent it as a "stagnated agricultural peasant economy" (1994: 58). At first glance the region has benefited from the recent emphasis on poverty reduction by the UN Millennium Development Goals. However, governmental attempts to alleviate poverty build on the problematization of harmful traditions as the main cause of the region's troubles. In other words, poverty is explained away by intensely localizing discourses that attribute culpability to the region's inhabitants and their traditional practices. The management of "harsh culture" becomes the primary goal of development workers and "sensitization" its means. Borrowing from Elizabeth Povinelli's analysis of liberal recognition (2002), I suggest that these problematizations entail what we might call neoliberal recognition. This is a form of governmental identity that brings benefits and harms by resubordinating the subject within the very categories that are supposed to liberate it—in this case poverty caused by harmful traditions and attendant concepts.

Prevailing problematizations revive the imperial discourses of culturalism that figure African practices as superstitions and values as pathologies (Pigg 1996; Gupta 1998; Ferguson 1994) and then turn them into explanations of poverty. Here the symbolic violence of racist imagination becomes a theory of poverty that, in consonance with neoliberal reason, shifts responsibility for poverty onto those recognized as "extremely poor," which is an official category for people living far below poverty levels. The contours of this discourse are familiar, and I analyze how it is reanimated, not because it is new but because it endures.

Scarcity has been a mutable but persistent feature of life in the Upper East Region (Allman and Parker 2005; Whitehead 2006). Even though I have experienced food shortages and limits of humanitarian care firsthand, I was unprepared for the chronic scarcity both in urban Bolgatanga and rural Bongo districts, its reverberations across the social body, and its marks on physiological bodies. What to say to a working-class friend, who tells me, "It's been long since I have tasted milk"? Or to another, who cannot afford to buy the malaria medicine for her son and hopes that it is "malaria small" and will clear on its own? How to look away when a rural family has a roaring quarrel about food and resources when a relative's visit lasts for a day longer than anticipated? In Bongo my research assistant, Constance, firmly insisted that we refuse all spontaneous invitations to partake of food because "they do not have enough to feed themselves." Given her family's relative wealth and husband's wage job in town, Afua, my host, was one of the rare women who always had enough to feed the children who came to play with her sons. The early millet was not yet harvested, and the previous year's crop did not last long enough, but they too ate the red millet usually seen as unfit for consumption and used only for pito brewing.

Recent governmental accounts describe northern Ghana as disproportionately poor and suffering from "extreme poverty" and a "regional gap." Resulting antipoverty measures have been epistemologically bolstered by new technologies of marking and measuring gaps—notably, not inequalities; these measures compared the three northern regions with the rest of the country and found that the North is significantly poorer. A report for the World Bank uses economic indicators, showing that average per capita incomes in northern Ghana are "2–4 times lower than elsewhere in the country" (Shepherd et al. 2004). A UNICEF report the highlights disparities in children's health: "In northern Ghana, IMR [infant mortality rate] is twice as high and U5MR [the mortality rate among children younger than five] three times as high as in the capital region" (UNICEF 2008). Public health analyses of the country's Demographic and Health Surveys show that northern Ghanaians suffer from malnutrition to a greater extent than people in the South, and that nearly half of all children younger than five are stunted, or too short for their age (Van de Poel et al. 2007). In the Upper East Region 15 percent of women have acute undernutrition, and nearly half are anemic. Among the children, chronic malnutrition and disease are so prevalent that 36 percent are stunted and nearly 90 percent are anemic (ICF Macro 2010a, 2010b).[15]

It is difficult not to be alarmed when confronted with such statistics, but the indicators of northern poverty have had ambivalent effects: they have generated support for development projects while also placing northern populations under greater scrutiny and reanimating the explanatory framework of cultural pathology. One result is that governmental regimes have winnowed the pool of explanations for northern scarcity and regional inequality down to the notions of "harsh environment" and "patriarchal traditions," or what we might refer to as "harsh culture."[16] Northerners are hungry, officials say, because they hold on to traditional food taboos; their land is infertile because they are hostile to their own environment, burning and overpopulating it. Even when NGOs and the state account for other factors, they culturalize and localize them.

Anticutting NGOs are well aware of the overwhelming scarcity in the Upper East and Upper West regions but either see themselves as unable to remedy it or deflect responsibility by declaring that people are liable for their ills. GAWW in particular casts scarcity as an effect of harmful traditions, primarily "food taboos." GAWW leaders have long been aware of the discrepancy between their narrow focus on "eradicating FGM" and the concerns of the women they try to reach. So have others—it is not a coincidence that in her story "Tradition, Tradition," Efua Dorkenoo narrates the struggles of cut women within a context of drought and scarcity (World Health Organization 2001).

Already in the 1980s, GAWW leaders told the anthropologist Takyiwaa Manuh that they had received feedback that the NGO should work on "alleviating the terrible material and socio-economic conditions under which they [cut women] live" (1989: 131). Disturbed by GAWW's lack of attention to material conditions, Manuh confronted the organization's leaders directly, asking them how they felt about talking to women in Northern Ghana about female circumcision in the face of severe economic hardships. GAWW leaders were aware of this problem and regretted it (Manuh, personal communication, 2003), leading Manuh to believe that GAWW would seek donor support to address issues of scarcity in order "to be more relevant to the communities in which they work" (1989: 139). They never did. Instead, the organization popularized the notion that food taboos imposed on women and children are a leading cause of hunger, malnutrition, and poor health. To legitimize this explanation GAWW relied on scientific expertise, inviting scholars to give presentations at conferences and workshops and sponsoring research on the topic. The researchers stressed that poverty produced food taboos, not the other way around, but GAWW articulated food taboos as the cause of malnutrition and poor health. This explanation became quite popular, and other NGOs and public health officials came to rely on it.

Development policies for northern Ghana see poverty as rooted in over-population and the ostensibly low productivity of farmers and their supposedly inferior and rudimentary farming methods and "poorly functioning markets."[17] The IMF's Ghana: Poverty Reduction Strategy Paper claims that "traditional farming practices" are economically unsound, environmentally harmful, and a threat to sustainability (2006:33). The United Nations' International Fund for Agricultural Development (IFAD) relies on this document—produced by Ghana's government for the IMF—to bolster long-standing Malthusian and modernization theories that posit that the region's main problems are too many people on the one hand and the lack of modern technology on the other.[18] This discourse reanimates long-standing World Bank and IMF axioms (Ferguson 1994) that postulate that poor land use practices cause poverty. This discourse is now given a new life: northerners' reproductive and farming practices serve as explanations for climate change and environmental degradation.[19]

Climate Change

Climate change indeed affects northern Ghana. Drought in Ghana has persisted since the 1970s and has been interspersed with periods of flooding, such as the 2007 northern floods that "devastated the year's crop and left fifty-six people dead and more than 330,000 homeless" (Glazebrook 2011: 763). In the Upper East both farmers and scientists tell stories of extreme weather, insufficient and unpredictable rainwater that results in agricultural decline, reduction in livestock, and disappearing vegetation (Dietz and Millar 1999; Dietz et al. 2004). It is impossible to attribute causality for any single event or short-term historical development to climate change; such events merely highlight that we need to take the farmers' grievances about erratic rains seriously. Rural women also point to the disappearance of grass they need for weaving baskets; they used to be able to gather it around their fields but now have to purchase it or travel south to pick it.

I witnessed concerns about drought the summer I lived in Bongo, when the rain was so scarce that village women performed a rain dance for the first time in a generation. I first heard about it from one of the neighboring elders whom we went to greet, the head of the household that Constance's cousin had married into. The news about the dance spread quickly around the village, and Afua encouraged me to go see it. As a Christian she was not going to participate or watch the dance but was palpably excited about it.

The sky was getting dark as we set out toward the earth shrine, and rain seemed imminent. Constance was disappointed and said she wished they had danced the day before, as now "they will attribute the rain to the dance, but we won't know the truth." She knows something about making rain as her grandmother's brother had the power to make rain or clear the sky. Constance had never witnessed it but knew about the time when the sky darkened as her grandmother was plastering her roof, and her brother cleared the sky for her.

We heard the women's ululating cries from afar and eventually came to a rock where we joined a small group of women and children who were standing and watching the ritual. About twenty yards ahead of us a hundred women dressed in skirts made of twigs and leaves were dancing, asking their female ancestor, their old mother, to make rain. Gathered around a sacred tree and rock were girls, young mothers with babies on their hips and backs, middle-aged women, grandmothers, and great-grandmothers. Several men were seated next to the women, drumming the beat that supports the dance. The women's skirts were similar to those girls wore when they were cut. Some women also had leafy head wraps or tops made of leaves that they had tied around their breasts. "They will only be wearing leaves," my host's uncle, the clan head, had told me earlier that morning, much to the consternation of his son. "Wearing leaves is not proper," the son had said, "some people will go clothed." The old man saw no need to argue, for he knew that he was right.

The women sang rhythmically, mixing in ululation and cries. The old mother has called them to perform the dance for her, they said. Soon the sounds of thunder were followed by the drizzle of an incipient rain. The women continued dancing and ululating, and it started raining hard. We returned home soaked. The women danced again the following week, for the rain was abundant but brief.

The power to make rain cannot be overestimated. Thousands of people converted to Catholicism in 1932 when the White Fathers prayed for rain and the rain came (Hawkins 2002: 142). Some converts later left the church, when they realized that the priests' power was limited and circumstantial. In nearby Tongo the men, not women, made rain, according to Fortes, and the only participants were the powerful men from the Namoo clan of the chiefs (1970: 151). There is no mention of women's ritual activity or power in Fortes; like others of his generation, he underestimated the ritual authority and power of women (see Amadiume 1997). But in Bongo a hundred women sing and dance to make rain among the rocks and trees that are said to possess supreme powers of the land, or Earth (tiŋa).

To the donors, government, and NGOs, northern life itself is the cause of climate change in that it shapes nature in pernicious ways. I often heard that the ecology of the savannah had been mismanaged and abused by local populations, as they burn the bush, put pressures on the land, and cause desertification. In turn, these practices are described as consequences of local "tradition," "ignorance," and "resistance to development." Anthropologists at times uncritically affirm such characterizations. Although, as Laube writes, "it has been shown that the agricultural practices of local farmers are much more adapted to their environment than scientists and administrators would like us to believe," and that climate change is caused by greenhouse gases, the depletion of the southern Ghanaian rainforest, and the construction of Lake Volta, "the main reason for the degradation of the area is certainly the increase in population" (2007: 46–47). Meanwhile his own research shows that the district's population remained constant for decades because of migration south (48).

This conception of climate change fails to account not only for the global North's overwhelming contribution to the problem but also for political decisions that led to technologically induced environmental disasters. For example, the catastrophic flooding that decimated crops and destroyed houses in the Upper East in 2007 was not caused by rain or the "local mismanagement of riverbeds," as is often said, but by Burkina Faso's decision to open its dams in order to reduce upstream flooding (Glazebrook 2011).

One major upshot of dominant blueprints for interventions is that NGOs and the state primarily govern by "sensitizing people," not by redistributing resources. Since ignorance and cultural pathologies are seen as the causes of environmental degradation, poor education, malnutrition, sickness, scarcity, and a host of other problems, sensitization and (informal) education are practiced as solutions. Sensitization is another form of governance by information (Riles 2001); to sensitize, in the language of Ghanaian NGOs and the government, means to educate those considered ignorant. In practice, as I will show shortly, this means informing people about how their own behaviors and practices are harming them.

CRITICAL DISCOURSES

Ghanaian and other social scientists have long critiqued reductionist accounts of poverty and resulting policy platforms. They agree with NGOs that hunger, scarcity, and illness are problems but sharply disagree about their causes, manifestations, and remedies. In 1979 Nii Plange asked in an influential paper whether the "underdevelopment in Northern Ghana" was caused by "natural causes or colonial capitalism" and argued for the latter:

> The "natural" conditions of soil, climate and even population have been used by several anthropologists and historians to "explain" the relatively underdeveloped condition of Northern Ghana during the colonial period and its aftermath. Such explanations take no account of the requirements of the colonial economy for the labour power for mines and cocoa plantations. (1979: 4)

Ghanaian geographers, economists, and political scientists have pointed out a multitude of historical forces that have disenfranchised northern Ghana (Plange 1979; Konadu-Agyemang 2000; Saaka 2001; Songsore 2003). Anthropologists also disrupt the connection between environmental degradation and harsh culture, revealing that population density in West Africa often results in more forests rather than deforestation (Fairhead and Leach 1996). Whitehead shows that poverty has increased in the Upper East region even where land is readily available; she also refutes the overpopulation thesis by showing that the largest households are the most economically secure (2006, 2002).

The question of whether northern Ghana is poor or impoverished, undeveloped or underdeveloped, involves key terms that encapsulate different theories of the causes of poverty: those in the first camp (poor, undeveloped) see poverty as intrinsic, while those in the second camp (impoverished, underdeveloped) implicate capitalism, exploitation, and other world-historical forces. At stake in this disagreement is the understanding of causes of scarcity: Is it an effect of nature or culture? If the latter, is it a product of cultural pathology or political economy? Are the forces that shape it local or global?

I understand scarcity, a term I prefer to poverty, as a world-historical artifact, an effect of the longue durée of history and the shifting global and national political economies. The decline in livelihoods does not have a single cause but results from a compendium of forces that include climate change, austerity-based structural adjustment programs, and the increase in inequality that followed Ghana's economic liberalization. I suggest that scarcity cannot be understood without accounting for the effects of violence and exploitation that beset the region with the Atlantic slave trade, continued during colonial times, were only partially remedied after independence, and are exacerbated under neoliberalism. However, my goal here is not to advance my own theory of scarcity under neoliberalism but to show how differently positioned Ghanaians construct their own etiologies of scarcity.[20] We have seen that NGOs and the government do so in concert with long-standing capitalist and Malthusian discourses that persist despite critiques by scholars and certain activists. Now I want to account for rural women's perspectives and their problematizations of scarcity and governance by sensitization.

You Count, So Be Counted: Abandonment and Sensitization

Although people in the region, scholars, and development institutions agree that "poverty is real" (Apusigah 2005: 8), they do not interpret this statement in the same way, nor do they ascribe it equal valence. Unlike middle-class and urban Ghanaians, rural women and men do not use the languages of development or enlightenment to describe their social position or their scarcity. They do not say, "We are poor," "we are undeveloped," "we are ignorant," "we have not seen the light," or "we are not modern." Nor do they share an understanding of either themselves or Ghana as backward. Rural women do not describe themselves as poor (*nasa*) but refer instead to specific types of suffering: food shortages, lack of blood and weak bodies, and a lack of opportunities to earn money (see chapter 5).[21] They understand poverty in relational terms: those who can claim this status are marginalized women who live in small households with few family members and hence lack social and economic support (see also Whitehead 2002: 582). Poverty is also stigmatized, as wealth correlates with respect; calling oneself poor entails taking considerable social risks. These rural women's most bitter complaint is that their harvests do not yield enough grain and legumes to last them the whole year and that they have no money to purchase food, which has been made prohibitively expensive by staggering inflation.

Everybody suffers from scarcity, my host, Afua, told me, but not in the same way: "There are some women who are looking for money to buy stocks to weave hats; there are also some who are looking for money to send grain to the grinding mill. Yet some others don't even have salt to cook with. In Bongo here we are suffering too much." Agnes, an enterprising woman who brews *pito* (red millet or sorghum beer), sells snacks called *wa'asa*, and farms a groundnut (peanut) field that she started with a loan from IFAD, also wanted me to understand that although she is better off than others, it is "not so much." Agnes is a returned migrant who spent one year

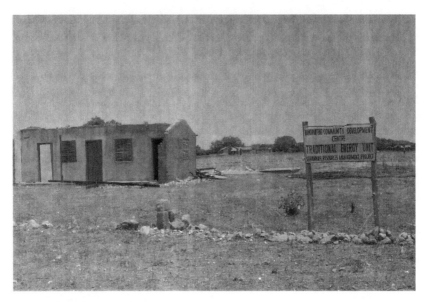

FIGURE 5. Abandoned development.

farming corn in Kumasi before returning to Bongo and starting her pito brewing business. She had hoped that educating her children would provide them with opportunities, and although she did not go to school, she made sure that all five of her children did. But the education they received did not make their lives more secure, and her sons did what the generations before them had also done—they migrated south. One has a job making soap in Accra, she told me, but the other one doesn't have (proper) work, as he pounds *fufu* in a chop bar to make ends meet. Neither is married, as marriage is out of their economic reach.

Much of development activity that takes place in the village is sensitization, although there are some infrastructural and individual empowerment projects as well. At first glance the village is bursting with various NGO and governmental activity. In recent years the government built a school and a social center, an NGO built latrines, and government contractors delivered poles for suspending the wires that would bring electricity to the village. But the school is overcrowded and underfunded, with eight hundred students served by four teachers, the latrines were unwanted and go unused, the social center began falling apart before it ever acquired doors or windows, and the poles that promised electricity never delivered it—during my last visit they were still piled by the side of the road.

Development schemes oriented toward sensitization of the villagers are numerous. In 2002 a UNICEF delegation visited the village, and Mr. Robert, my host and the village assemblyman, chronicled the event in a new notebook, in which he subsequently recorded every NGO, government, and donor visit.[22] On his list were names of representatives from the Voluntary Services Overseas NGO; the Ghana National Association of Teachers; the Bongo District Assembly; a multisectoral government delegation; the District Health Management Team (Community-Based Nutrition and Food Security Project); Ghana Education Service; Catholic Relief Services; Programme for Rural Integrated Development (PRIDE, another NGO); Department of Community Development; the regional office of the government's Nonformal Education Division; the Best Solar Company; Ghana Health Service; the District Water and Sanitation Team; and a Seventh-Day Adventist pastor. My name also found its way onto the list, and some of the chief representatives interpreted my request for research permission as a request to "sensitize women about cutting." As Robert told me more about the various visits, I understood just how sensitization shaped the character of governance here. The projects Robert chronicled consisted of meetings that took the form of information transfer combined with "community sensitization" projects such as durbars (ceremonial gatherings). NGOs and government organizations "sensitized" the villagers about water safety, nutrition, food security, HIV/AIDS, sanitation, and reproductive health.

I knew women were ambivalent about sensitization projects; they were not particularly bothered by them but saw them as irrelevant to their suffering. Rather than rejecting this type of outreach, they welcomed some talks and tolerated others with equanimity. This is also how they evaluated the efforts to end cutting: their shared sentiment—"let them talk"—does not mean "we will not listen" but points to the limits of what talking and listening can achieve (see chapter 5). For these women sensitization is not simply an inadequate response to the problems they faced but beside the point.

The UNICEF delegation, with its white visitors, was a frequent topic of conversation and speculation, evoked in part by my own presence in the village. Villagers became suspicious of UNICEF when they noticed the delegates digging around the water wells: "Were they looking for gold?" I was asked. Many thought that the UNICEF delegation must have sought to profit by exploring the possibility of extraction. The villagers were suspicious that their land would be exploited and they would be cheated of their share.

Rural women saw that money circulated in development and government networks but saw themselves as cut off from this flow and bereft of their fair share of government funds in particular. Many told me that nobody—neither the state nor NGOs—had done anything to address their problems, even though "the government says we are government people," that is, citizens of Ghana for whom the state has responsibility. When I asked Agnes, a well-respected, outspoken woman, what the government could do to help them secure a livelihood, she said, "I don't know, I've never seen their help." Cecilia, who was assisting me with some translations, tried to correct such statements. "What about the rooms they built?" she asked one of her neighbors whose house was destroyed in a recent flood and later rebuilt with donated funds. "What about the weaving you learned?," she asked another woman who had participated in the PRIDE basket-weaving project. "I forgot about it," the woman answered. The forgetting was itself a commentary on the inadequacy of development projects. Their complaints that nobody has helped them were meant to point that they were eventually cut off and abandoned and that antipoverty projects did not make a significant dent in their experiences of scarcity and suffering. If the state could forget them, as Agnes would say, they could also forget the state.

While Cecilia, out of loyalty to the NGO she volunteered for and to her uncle Robert, the local politician, wanted me to have accurate information, the women she questioned made it clear that humanitarian gestures and short-lived projects were inadequate, as they did not guarantee sustenance. The women I got to know recalled how they were mobilized to participate in projects that seemingly understood the magnitude of the scarcity they faced but proved incapable of remedying it. Because development projects are gendered and women are the most frequent participants, this meant that they experienced a series of promises made and broken. The agricultural and basketry projects in Bongo were intended as one-time measures, and others were started but never took off. Some women received fertilizers and seeds but only once. Others were trained in new weaving techniques but were unable to sell their baskets. They showed me their unfinished baskets, which they had stopped weaving because PRIDE, the NGO that had initiated the project, never returned to buy them. (PRIDE had to cancel the project early on because the NGO found it difficult to break into the already crowded market in baskets, where middlemen profit at the expense of weavers.)

Afua told me about another project that she and some of her friends and neighbors participated in: "Some time ago, they formed groups and lent money

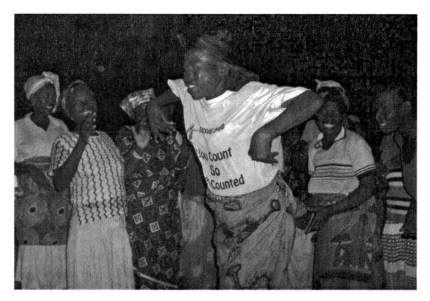

FIGURE 6. The Census: "You count, so be counted."

to the groups. We collected the loans, but it was difficult for us to pay them back. So that arrangement is no more there and we haven't seen anyone coming here to help us." She and some other women had received funding from a short-lived microcredit project but were not convinced that microcredit would be a self-sustaining, ever-expanding growth mechanism. From these women's perspective, it was not sufficient for NGOs to give them a loan once—they needed ongoing, continual support. The continued circulation of investments, loans, and debt that they saw as necessary indeed subtends many world economies, but these women were not able to participate in ongoing circulation.

Nearly everyone complained about living in what Povinelli calls the state of abandonment (2011a), and their indignation was aroused by democratic governance itself. The national census, and the intensified political campaigning in the wake of democratization and the decentralization of governance, gave them a sense of the importance and economic and political materiality of their individual and collective lives. "You Count So Be Counted" admonished the t-shirts they received during the 2000 census—and they did. They learned that the village had more than five thousand inhabitants, far more than previously counted. The upshot was that they began to understand themselves in biopolitical and democratic terms, as a population with rights to resources correlative to their numbers.[23]

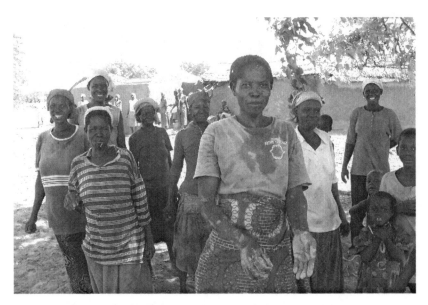

FIGURE 7. "Will you help us?" Women repairing a house invite me to participate.

At one youth meeting a group of teenagers attending high school else-where in the region returned to the village to discuss demands for electricity, and one of their main arguments was their strength in numbers. Because they came from one of the larger villages in the district, they deserved elec-tricity, they said, and wanted to send a warning to the district assembly: "If they deny us, we will not vote in the upcoming elections." This message caught on in the village, and I heard Afua repeating it a few days later, despite her husband's protests.

Aradhana Sharma has argued that people in Uttar Pradesh, India, also used the NGOs' and the state's own technologies to demand more "resources as rights" (Sharma 2008: xxii). This is just what the students and others had in mind. But even as they protested, women in Bongo seemed to think of their citizenship only in terms of a performance of political agency in the form of a threat. While they proclaimed the injustice of their situation, they had little hope that, even if they refused to vote, anything would change, that anyone —except, for some, "perhaps, God"—would alleviate their scarcity.

Since to ask about someone is to care, and since I posed a lot of questions, several women thought that I would be able to provide some solutions to their problems. When I asked my hosts' neighbor Atampoka, a destitute woman who suffered from mental illness, if she thought that anybody would help with her scarcity, she replied: "I think it is God. So now that she is here, I think she is my god."

Cecilia asked her, "You don't think it is the government?" And Atampoka replied: "If the government helps me, I would like it, but if the government does not see me, what can I do? I don't understand English."

Researchers are routinely interpellated as potential benefactors or patrons, as are volunteers, tourists, and others who come through the region. For women like Atampoka, who lack wealthier family members and who live in the context of abandonment by the state—where, as she put it, she was invisible and had no capacity to make herself heard—the desire for a benefactor is greater than usual. Moments like this taught me that the desire for the humanitarian hero, the individual who takes on the task of saving African lives, is not only a Western projection but a joint construction of Ghana and the global North. However, benefactors do not always materialize. I was acutely aware that I, too, might be counted as yet another person who arrived in Bongo, asked women what they wanted, and failed to bring a project later. These women have much in their lives that sustains them, but the open wound—the gaping difference between global opulence and the scarcity they experience—cannot be easily sutured.

CONCLUSION: GOVERNANCE BY TRADITION AND SENSITIZATION

In this chapter I have shown that the discourse of harmful traditions is central to problematizing both cutting and northern poverty. As a result the management of harsh culture is the primary goal of development workers, and sensitization is their means. In this region and elsewhere, much development work is discursive, affective, and social, not infrastructural or economic. NGO governance hinges on educating and sensitizing people, thereby producing new subjects, shaping both those who govern and those who are governed (see also Nguyen 2010). Sensitization projects go hand in hand with neoliberal recognition of northern poverty, which shifts the responsibility for scarcity to northern Ghanaians and their cultural pathologies. Northern Ghana and groups that practiced cutting now receive more attention but less care. I have shown that GAWW taxonomies that make FGM intelligible entail casting it and the people who practice it as repugnant and abject, which leaves little room for understanding them as deserving of respect and care. Becoming sensitized about FGM thus entails becoming desensitized to the lives and perspectives of the actual people said to embody it. NGO workers and civil servants, including the nurses, are told they should identify with the value of national progress and distance themselves from rural women. Cut women, then, should not be understood as casualties of governmental care (Ticktin 2011), since little care is offered, but as subjects and casualties of concern.

As a result of this mode of governance, NGO and government workers find themselves in an unenviable position in their own everyday lives. For example, they have to campaign against slash-and-burn agriculture and the burning of wood to make charcoal, but they, too, depend on some of these practices, which are said to be environmentally destructive. On a drive home from a workshop in Tamale, one NGO worker stopped the car to inquire about the charcoal prices at a roadside stand. It was too expensive and she did not purchase it, but when she returned to the car, she told me about the harmful environmental effects of wood burning for charcoal production. She assumed I shared the opinion that using charcoal is bad, but confronted with the necessity of purchasing it at the lowest possible price, she felt the need to perform her knowledge of the effects of environmental degradation and align herself with this morally charged discourse. She and other regional development workers do not have the option of formulating alternative discourses, since opposing the prevailing view would endanger the only form of expertise they are sanctioned to deploy.

GAWW workers and affiliates also know firsthand that the sensitization projects are limited at best. When I interviewed Olivia, the GAWW coordinator for the Upper East Region, I asked her to comment on the various dimensions of what she referred to as "women's suffering." A well-known teacher, activist, and host of a show called Women in Development on URA Radio, Olivia she said she started speaking up on gender issues when she moved to Bolgatanga from southern Ghana, where, as she put it, she was "born and bred" to migrant parents. Women in Northern Ghana "suffer so much more," she said—they perform more labor, are responsible for feeding the family, but do not have the economic resources to provide for them, and are subjected to stringent social expectations and moral judgments as a result of local traditions. At the end of our conversation I asked her what she believed to be the primary cause of women's suffering. Laughing, she responded: "Economic issues."

Yet she and others who are dissatisfied with sensitization have few options, as donors prefer to fund educational workshops instead of redistributing material resources, and both NGOs and the government depend on donors to approve expenditures and projects. For instance, because Dr. Adjei viewed sensitization as an important but insufficient mechanism for ensuring reproductive health, his NGO, Rural Help Integrated (RHI), used what he called a "holistic" approach, which meant including "income-generating activities." This small project consisted of donating five grinding mills and shea butter–processing machines to villages deemed "particularly needy." I attended the commissioning ceremony for one of the machines, strategically scheduled to coincide with a visit by monitors for the UN Population Fund (UNFPA), which funded the project. On our way to the ceremony, Andrew, the UNFPA representative, questioned Dr. Adjei about the purpose of the mills and was dissatisfied with the answers; to Andrew grinding mills had nothing to do with reproductive health. Had rural women been included in the conversation, they would have vigorously disagreed: grinding mills are coveted because they offer a reprieve from the arduous task of grinding millet by stone. The machines allow women to rest and regain their strength, a benefit that should not be underestimated in areas where women work during most of their waking hours and see this labor as damaging to their health (see chapter 5). The village where I conducted research was included in RHI projects but did not receive a machine or other resources. When virtually all villages suffer from scarcity, but only the extremely needy receive goods, we see the overlap between development work and humanitarian governance that saves lives but does not foster them (Fassin 2012; Redfield 2013).

Earlier I suggested that James Ferguson's poignant analysis of the development imaginary illuminates the nature of contemporary Ghanaian governmentality, and I now want to clarify the limits of this comparison. Northern Ghana is not Lesotho, and development is no longer what it was. The very concept of development has also undergone a profound global shift: development agencies have scaled down their goals and now work toward poverty relief or reduction rather than elimination. The original development dream of modernization entailed a promise of global parity that was never realized; that dream has now been abandoned. As anthropologists are increasingly suggesting, development looks more like humanitarian emergency relief and vice versa (Gabiam 2012; Mathers 2010; Ticktin 2014). Many critics of development now experience what Wendy Brown calls a "melancholic situation" (2003): waxing nostalgic for something (global parity) that could never be embraced, given modernization's attendant ideologies of capitalism and Africa's lack.

Many Say

They won't tell you the truth—they will tell you what you want to hear.

3

―――――――

When Cutting Did and Did Not End

Bolgatanga, May 2004. GAWW has come to town and arranged for local students to march in celebration of the Zero Tolerance for Female Genital Mutilation day, which has been newly inaugurated by the Inter-African Committee on Harmful Traditional Practices Affecting the Health of Women and Children (IAC). After being corralled and organized into lines, students in their early teens walk down the main streets to the beat of drums. They wear their brown-orange school uniforms and GAWW t-shirts that depict a bleeding circumcised baby girl. Shopkeepers, their customers, and passersby—some curious, others bemused—watch the marchers. I am accompanying one of the teachers who organized the event, and on Commercial Street we overhear two shopkeepers discussing their confusion about the point of the march. The posters are in English and denounce "FGM"; the women understand the acronym but are curious about why the students are marching—cutting has ended in Bolgatanga, so why protest? "Are they still doing it?" one asks. Since cutting is no longer in their consciousness, the governmental concern about it seems out of place. Not so for NGO workers and civil servants. The teacher with whom I am walking hears the women and remarks to me that cutting has not ended and that "they still do it on the outskirts."

Cutting is ending in Ghana, however unevenly and incompletely, but in public discourse the ending of the practices is largely disavowed. The state, the media, and most NGOs claim that rural communities continue to practice cutting "underground" and "resist" anticutting campaigns. What is more, some assert that the practice of cutting is not just "intractable," but on the increase; they contend that groups that say otherwise are "hiding the truth." Ghana is one of the many countries where cutting is on the wane, but the discourse about its intractability and underground proliferation prevails. Following the example of GAWW and the national media, regional NGO and government officials reinforce the underground discourse in their public statements, contending that cutting continues, as the teacher put it, "on the outskirts." However, some regional NGO workers and civil servants have fine-grained understandings of where cutting did and did not end, and they put those to use in their practice (chapter 4).

As I discuss in this chapter, cutting began to ebb in Ghana before interventions by NGOs, and it plummeted in their aftermath, to the point of near-disappearance in parts of the country. But rather than emphasizing the questions "Exactly when and where did cutting end?" and "What percentage of Ghanaian women practice it today?" I suggest that it is more important to ask when cutting could have ended and did not, for whom it ended, and what is left in its wake. In this chapter I explore these questions to critically respond to the dominant narrative of underground resistance. My focus is on Ghanaians' problematizations of the ending of cutting, and I attend equally to those who uphold and contest the discourse of underground resistance. To that end I contrast official governmental discourses that propagate moral panics about cutting with the narratives of cut women and circumcisers that emphasize its ending. They recognize that they are seen as resistant to NGO interventions and try to disrupt this image.

In this chapter I also show that the nostalgic discourse about the loss of patriarchal values is the only public discourse that attests to the ending of cutting. As we shall see, officials bemoan the demise of cutting and the disappearance of the traditional patriarchal values they believe it upheld, thus inadvertently testifying to the demise of cutting. This nostalgia for cutting is notably expressed only by those never subject to it—while the uncut women and male officials might miss cutting, cut women do not. Nor do circumcisers. They feel a loss but miss not cutting itself but the relationship to gods, as well as their benevolence and protection, which cutting secured. In the aftermath of the enactment of anticutting legislation, the circumcisers position themselves as nonsovereign subjects of history who are owed care but are "abandoned," in Povinelli's terms (2011). Rather than desiring the return of cutting, they want the state to enter into the kind of reciprocal relationship they had with the gods, one of taking and giving, mutual attention, care, and accountability.

UNDERGROUND RESISTANCE: CUTTING IS ENDING, BUT FGM LIVES ON

Despite indications of long-standing decline, and the more recent and dramatic near-disappearance of cutting in Bolgatanga and Bongo, the discourse about "the intractability of FGM" is stronger than ever, and GAWW has been one of its main proponents. The NGO points to arrests of circumcisers, media reports about cases of cutting, and pictures of cut children Mrs. Mahama took when traveling to the Upper West Region and visiting families with cut children. They circulate these in meetings and workshops as evidence that cutting is an ongoing problem and that, as they say, northerners "still do it" and "do it underground." Dr. Adjei has been one of the few voices of opposition to this discourse. But while he proudly states that there have been no cases of cutting in Bolgatanga since he started his NGO's outreach, he keeps to this modest claim and, moreover, rarely speaks to the media. So the position of GAWW, an Accra-based NGO focused on national public advocacy, carries the day.

As I showed in chapter 1, the notion of an underground proliferation of cutting did not originate with GAWW but stems from colonial debates about potential criminalization of cutting. Regional colonial administrators used this claim to oppose the legislative measures desired by London and to argue that criminalization would not be feasible. Today NGOs use the notion of underground resistance differently; they argue for stricter law enforcement and greater punishment, constructing northern Ghanaians as undeserving of benevolent governance (see chapters 6 and 7).

What exactly does *underground* mean?[1] In interviews, public statements, and conversations officials say that cutting continues "on the outskirts," or "in the periphery," or when one goes "deep into the villages." Such "remote communities," they say, avoid surveillance by sending girls and circumcisers across the border to Burkina Faso. Border areas are accused of taking advantage of their location to circumvent law and order. In actuality, if people crossed the border for purposes of cutting (as one circumciser told me he did in the past, before he stopped cutting), they did not do so to circumvent the law or to perform some act of underground resistance but because cross-border movement is part and parcel of everyday life. For instance, I learned from market traders in Bongo that they included Yelwongo, a town in Burkina, in their list of rotating market days. (They identified Yelwongo,

Bongo, and Bolgatanga as the markets they visit every three days.) Although the border between Ghana and Burkina Faso is policed, regulated, and managed, people maintain rights to land and water on both sides (Lentz 2003), and cross-border trade is licit, illicit, and everything in between (Chalfin 2001). Regional NGO workers know this, and for them "the outskirts" is also a metaphorical territory that is farthest from urbanity and civilization, which are understood as the counterpoints to cutting.

Even when families do not send girls "to Burkina," the story goes, local circumcisers perform cutting at night or farther away from the village, by "the river." GAWW members and some civil servants also claim that many groups now "do it to babies because babies cannot complain." Practicing cutting underground, then, means that a deliberate and nefarious alteration of the practice has occurred in order to evade governmental scrutiny. This popular discourse thus frames northern Ghanaians as not only unruly but cruel, willing to harm and silence their children in order to retain their tradition. The political consequence of such claims has global reach—this discourse has been taken up the U.S. State Department's *Human Rights Report* for Ghana, which erroneously states that only children are cut in Ghana. (Such reports are widely used to adjudicate asylum claims.)

The underground discourse got a boost in 2003, when word spread that Fefe Dari, a woman from the Upper West Region, had been arrested for having circumcised three infants and young children. GAWW and other organizations portrayed this case as proof of an emerging mass movement of cutting babies. To make this claim they skillfully set aside what they knew about the different contexts of cutting: while in some groups, such as most of those in the Upper East, cutting initiated (pre)pubescent girls into womanhood, in some of those in the Upper West (including where Dari was from), cutting was historically performed on young children and infants (Oware Knudsen 1994). GAWW was well aware that cutting an infant in the Upper West did not reflect the existence of an underground resistance movement, but the narrative was familiar and useful.

Assertions about underground resistance are nested within larger notions of northern Ghana as a site of unruliness and disorder. Discourses from the state, NGOs, and the public rarely acknowledge that social change occurs in the North. According to the prevailing view, northern Ghana is rife with harmful traditions because local people stubbornly hold onto them and are resistant to the values of development, modernity, and rule of law. Statements about unruliness and backwardness are coupled and frame both public and governmental understandings of the North: they are dominant in everyday conversations and in the media (see Holsey 2008: 81), as well as in Ghanaian NGO workshops, government reports, legislation, and legal judgments.

The notion of resistance allows NGOs and the state to transfer responsibility for all manner of deprivation to northern Ghanaians themselves. To resist is to refuse development and thus to be responsible for scarcity and privation. Contrary to its positive anthropological valence, "resistance" functions in a different hierarchy of values in Ghanaian public culture, where it bolsters ideas about disorder at the margins of the state, justifying socioeconomic inequalities as well as exclusions from the benefits of citizenship. The issue of cutting, which figures in both global and Ghanaian political cultures as the epitome of a premodern disorder, brings this discourse into sharp relief. Ethnic groups that practice cutting are understood as especially unruly and ungovernable, and cutting is conceived of as both a bodily and social pathology.

Claims about underground performances of cutting hold the status of public truth. Officials repeat them at workshops, on the radio, and in newspapers in ways that betray both fascination and excitement. These claims gain strength as they travel, in part because the border-crossing discourse mobilizes increasing anxieties about threats to sovereignty and national boundaries. The border is figured as a site of transgression used for personal gain and against public interest; this discourse is evident in long-standing governmental concerns about corruption and smuggling (Chalfin 2010).

Public concerns about border crossings are unusual in that they are deeply felt and motivate action. An NGO director from Accra, for instance, someone who was not otherwise involved in interventions against cutting and not in need of any additional work, was moved to propose a cross-border, transnational project. She spoke passionately about a concept paper she wrote for a joint education and surveillance project with Burkina Faso; the paper proposed that customs and police officers and border guards collaborate to prevent the cross-border traffic in girls for purposes of cutting.

What Counts as Evidence: How Science of Resistance Travels

Accra, October 2003. Since the office of the U.S. Agency for International Development (USAID) in Accra was said to have funded several projects against cutting, I arranged a meeting with Lynn, the agency's reproductive health officer. Lynn was exceedingly forthcoming as she had noticed my e-mail address from the University of California, Berkeley, with which she identifies as an alumna; she is a graduate of the School of Public Health. In advance of our meeting, she had prepared a CD for me that included copies of documents and reports about FGM projects and interventions in Ghana and was ready to tell me more about them. The documents addressed the FGM Eradication Experiment by the Navrongo Health Research Center, the UN Population Fund (UNFPA) workshop to disseminate Dr. Adjei's research findings, the U.S. Embassy's official report on FGM in Ghana, a donor-mapping report, and several others. But Lynn was most excited about the results of the Navrongo study that measured rates of cutting over time in the Kassena-Nankana District: "Have you heard about the denial paper?" she asked. I had not. Over time I would learn that this article, which argues that cut women cannot be trusted, received global attention, whereas contemporaneous analyses that corroborated the ending of cutting did not.

Donors funding Ghanaian interventions against cutting have been one of the main parties interested in finding out whether cutting is ending and, if so, how it is ending. In recent decades documenting which interventions were working became an aspirational norm and *evidence* a key term for attracting funding and justifying projects (Hodžić 2013). To many in Ghana the Navrongo Health Research Center (locally called simply Navrongo), located in Upper East's Kassena-Nankana District, was the research hub most ideally suited to answer these questions. The center understands "accurate measurement of the circumcision status" (Jackson et al. 2003: 200) to be necessary for evaluating and testing interventions, and it conceives of its own role as crucial to supporting rationalized governance. Otherwise known as a "population observatory," the research center employs demographers, other social scientists, and trained fieldworkers who speak regional languages and administer the Navrongo Demographic Surveillance System. This is a survey-based population-monitoring system "that has registered individuals present in the district, demographic events, population characteristics, and social relationships" (Jackson et al.: 202). Navrongo researchers have published scores of articles on cutting alone (see Ako and Akweongo 2009; Oduro et al. 2006), but Lynn's enthusiasm for the Navrongo paper was less a reflection of her well-deserved trust in the center than her predilection for what is interesting—a simple tally of cutting rates is less interesting than discovery of a problem.

So what did the "denial paper" find? Navrongo researchers (Jackson et al. 2003) interviewed nearly twenty-four hundred women in 1995 and 2000, asking them, among other things, whether they were cut. The paper outlines the discrepancies the researchers noticed in some of the responses to this question. More specifically, 13 percent of women changed their responses between 1995 and 2000; the paper labels these women as "deniers ... who reported in 1995 that they were circumcised and reported in 2000 that they were not" (203). The younger the woman, the more likely she was to change her response about being cut. As to why these women did so, the paper suggests that the law banning cutting gained recognition in the intervening five years, after a circumciser from the district was arrested and imprisoned. In addition, younger women face the greatest pressure *not* to get cut, the researchers write, as the "social acceptability of the practice declines" (208). The paper concludes that "questions must be raised about the validity of self-reported data" and that the inability to secure conclusive evidence about the demise of cutting might serve as proof that cutting was indeed *not* ending: "Denial of being circumcised in women's self-reports may spuriously inflate estimates of the impact of [NGO] interventions" (208). In other words, rural women were said to resist both researchers and NGOs, and the impossibility of ascertaining a complete truth was read as an indication of mendacity.

By framing cut women as untrustworthy and unreliable, this article bolsters the prevailing discourse of northern ungovernability and resistance by endowing it with a scientific aura. The specter of deniers conjured by the researchers contributed to the idea that cutting was untamed and ungovernable and that cut women could not be trusted to tell the truth. Left out of the subsequent reception of the article was that the percentage of women whose statements did not match their earlier interviews was, at 13 percent, rather small; 87 percent made consistent statements. Since the paper emphasizes the findings about deniers, its message is that cut women's statements about the demise of cutting cannot be trusted. Lynn was not alone in her excitement about this interpretation; in subsequent years I heard references to the "denial paper" from various UN officials working on anticutting campaigns from Washington, D.C., to New York City and Geneva.

If the administration of clinical trials requires patients to be "treatment naïve" (Petryna 2007: 28), it seems to follow that the research center requires its respondents to be "research naive." But while the Navrongo researchers held recent legislation and NGO advocacy responsible for the loss of naïveté, northern Ghanaians have long been seen as not naive enough. The colonial ethnographer A. W. Cardinall wrote in his book *The Natives of the Northern Territories of the Gold Coast* that "the desire to please the white man, to anticipate his wishes, makes it difficult to find out the true practices and the reason therefore" ([1920] 2012: ix). In fact, he continued, he was once told explicitly, "I will say anything the white man wishes." Cardinall's remarks suggest that people knew that answering to those who rule them is a politically charged act. Today few Ghanaians draw strict lines between research and interventions. Asking a question, after all, is an indigenous way of teaching, research is just another component of development projects (Elyachar 2006), and evasion is a useful weapon no matter who is asking the questions.

The discovery that, in the wake of NGO and state interventions, a small number of women, young women in particular, feel pressured to state that they are not cut is important, and this is a phenomenon I also witnessed firsthand. Several young women who were locally known to be cut told me that they were not—their own cutting was not something they were willing to discuss with a researcher. Consider the following situation. I sat down with A., who shall remain nameless to avoid the semblance of ethnographic intimacy, transparency, and verisimilitude that pseudonyms provide (see Visweswaran 1994). A. was said to be one of the last women cut in Bongo, but A. told me she was uncut and that she could talk to me only about other women's experiences. A.'s mother-in-law, who stood nearby, shook her head and motioned upward, suggesting that I keep on asking. She herself was cut and saw nothing wrong with it—like other older women, the mother-in-law was lighthearted about both cutting and its endings—but the situation was more difficult for younger women, and A. had her own stance:

> Silence can be a plan
> rigorously executed
>
> the blueprint to a life
>
> It is a presence
> it has a history   a form
>
> Do not confuse it
> with any kind of absence
>   (Adrienne Rich,
>   "Cartographies of Silence")

I borrow these words from Rich because cutting is silence for some women. We need to attend to silence, not because it diminishes the possibility of knowing the complete truth about the rates of cutting but because it illuminates the consequences of the demise of cutting for the last generations of cut women and sheds light on the affective components of governmental campaigns. Today cut women are shamed and not only by their peers, as the Navrongo researchers suggest (Jackson et al. 2003), but by NGOs, campaigners, and interviewers. "During that time," I was told by a woman talking about the past in Bongo, "they used to laugh at them [the uncut women], but now they rather laugh at those of us [who were] cut." I saw the traces of this shaming when Angela, a public health nurse in Bawku, proudly told me that she scolded cut girls when she gave a talk at their school. She asked them: "Don't I see that you have shaved your heads?," her way of saying that she knew that they were recently cut. In response the girls bowed their heads in submission, discomfort, and shame. I was also inadvertently implicated in such shaming, as ethnographic research also furnishes an opportunity for moral pedagogy. From watching how NGO workers interview rural women and men, and working with translators, I have seen how easily an interview turns into a moral lesson. "Now that you know that cutting is bad, would you do it again?," a translator with whom I worked for a few days in Bawku asked one young woman after we were finished with the interview. "No, no, no," she replied.

The Limits of Reason

Ghanaian demographic and epidemiological research on rates of cutting has been concentrated in the Upper East Region, because of the Navrongo research center's location in the Kassena-Nankana District and Dr. Adjei's research in regional hospitals, villages, and towns. Persistent, long-term community-based campaigns against cutting have taken place in exactly those select pockets of the country where the research has taken place—the Kassena-Nankana, Bolgatanga, and Bongo districts of the Upper East Region—and with the involvement of the same actors. Both Dr. Adjei and the research center sponsored campaigns against cutting and conducted research, at times combining the two.

While deeming cut women unreliable interview subjects, researchers turned to hospital observations in delivery units as a preferred method of ascertaining how many women were cut. Soon after the publication of the denial paper, a trove of epidemiological data on rates of cutting showed that cutting was indeed waning, albeit unevenly across the region.

The research center itself reviewed the data from the Navrongo hospital and established that 29 percent of women who delivered between 1996 and

2003 were cut. The researchers also affirmed the waning of cutting over time: rates of cutting dropped from 61.5 percent among women aged forty and older to 14.4 percent among women aged twenty and younger (Oduro et al. 2006). Dr. Adjei's research with more than six thousand women who delivered in three regional hospitals between December 2001 and June 2003 shows just how much the numbers vary across the region.[2] Bolgatanga had the fewest cut women (8.8 percent) and was followed by Navrongo (18.5 percent). In contrast, the majority of women who delivered in Bawku (81.5 percent) were cut.[3] His aggregated results also show striking differences between younger and older women: while 49 percent of women aged thirty-six to forty-nine were cut, the rate dropped to 29 percent among those twelve to nineteen years old. This disparity between older women and girls and teenagers suggests that the incidence of cutting has been cut nearly in half in the last thirty years. So while cutting was dwindling during the twentieth century, more recently the decrease has been rather dramatic, especially in those districts that have experienced the most campaigns and scientific scrutiny.

Contradicting their earlier emphasis on deniers, Navrongo researchers now concluded that "practice has shown a significant decline in the district in recent years due to the prevailing campaigns and intervention studies" (Oduro et al. 2006: 87). The analyses of delivery data by Dr. Adjei and the research center stand as important correctives to official discourses about the intractability of cutting but should not be fetishized. Statistics are constructed and embedded in the context of their production, but something else is at stake here as well. In the context of reigning discourses, knowledge could not trump the popular conceptions of cutting as intractable and Upper East women as unreliable. While Navrongo's "denial paper" resonated widely and traveled globally, the center's subsequent paper did not, and is virtually unknown. Dr. Adjei's findings about the waning of cutting were recognized by only a few Ghanaian media outlets.

In addition, at a time when women were no longer trusted to speak the truth about cutting, this research displaced the search for evidence onto their bodies; instead of the women themselves, experts like nurses, midwives, and physicians were considered epistemic authorities who now read cut bodies as objects and did so objectively. The transition from the authority of experience to authority of expertise is also notable with respect to other suspect, putatively untrustworthy groups such as asylum seekers; their own testimony is viewed with circumspection, and physicians and others, including anthropologists, are often called upon to provide expert opinion (Fassin 2012; Ticktin 2011; Redfield 2013).

Resistance and Surveillance

Something about cutting or rather, the way it is constructed in scholarly and governmental discourses, seems to imply resistance. If there is one site where anthropological accounts of cutting are congenial to governmental discourses, it is in the notion that interventions will likely be met with resistance (see Hodžić 2010). Time and again, anthropologists assert that NGO interventions are likely to fail. Whether this belief is true or not—and this is not an unimportant question—we need to recognize that its public acceptance can be damaging.

The discourse of underground resistance incites increased public health surveillance and harsh legislation. Because rural women are said to be untrustworthy, GAWW teaches northern nurses to examine the genitals of infant girls brought in for medical care (chapter 2). Even more striking are consequences for lawmakers and law enforcers, who read the ostensible lack of reports about instances of cutting as resistance to the law, which eventually led to longer sentences and harsher punishment (see chapters 6 and 7). We shall see that notions of "resistant people" and "harsh culture" are applied to justify "harsh sentences" and regulation of northern groups.

To be clear, Ghana is not the only place where cutting is ending, FGM lives on, and the notion of underground resistance is mobilized for purposes of surveillance and criminalization. In the European Union, United States, Canada, and Australia, African and Muslim immigrants are placed under scrutiny by social services, teachers, medical authorities, and the legal system. German feminists stopped collaborating after one NGO proposed to have the genitals of all immigrant children inspected by medical practitioners. In the EU epidemiological statistics about the prevalence of cutting are constructed in ways that maximize the numbers of at-risk girls.[4]

Such is the grip of the notion of "resistance" that it has motivated new practices of surveillance spanning different continents. In one example, an Ethiopian family residing in Germany was prevented from traveling to Ethiopia because German Social Service agents were worried that the daughter would be cut during the trip. To verify the claim a German Embassy representative interviewed the grandparents in Addis Ababa and approved the trip after he was assured that they opposed cutting. In response to similar incidents, Somalis living in Sweden have taken the state to court and have received monetary compensation.

In the United States the discourse of underground performance of cutting is recent but powerful and is used to mobilize calls for tough "zero tolerance for FGM" legislation. Central to this campaign is the mobilization of another version of the "native informant": an African immigrant activist who claims that African immigrants subject their daughters to cutting. Jaha Dukureh is an immigrant who was born in Guinea and runs an NGO in Atlanta whose purpose is to spread national awareness of the dangers of cutting. A self-described victim of cutting, Dukureh has been touted as the most prominent voice raising awareness of the ostensibly rampant underground performance of cutting on U.S. soil. Articles about Dukureh carry such headlines as "The Shocking Rise of Female Genital Mutilation in the United States," "Alarming Trend: The U.S. Female Genital Mutilation Crisis," and "America's Underground Female Genital Mutilation Crisis."[5] Dukureh and the journalists who write about her point to cut immigrant girls as evidence that cutting is practiced and on the rise in the United States but do not explain that those girls were cut before they arrived in America. This is exactly what Swedish authorities faced—in their many attempts to prosecute parents of cut girls, they kept finding that the girls were cut before emigrating and thus before they were subject to Swedish law (Johnsdotter 2009).

In the United States the discourse of underground resistance extends beyond the issue of cutting and is mapped onto married African American men who are said to engage in "down-low" (secretive) homosexual activity and therefore are blamed for increasing HIV/AIDS rates (Snorton 2014). As Snorton shows, the down-low discourse about the spread of HIV/AIDS places black sexuality in a "glass closet" marked by "hypervisibility and confinement, spectacle, and speculation" (4). It too relies on "native informants"—here, African American women and men—as the public voices that propagate the discourse. Like the down low, the discourse about the underground performance of cutting links blackness with duplicity and legitimizes concerns about a vulnerable population that is ostensibly harmed by its own members by relying on the authority of native informants. If a whole population is to be distrusted, some of its members must be elevated to the status of exceedingly trustworthy subjects who will bear witness to the duplicity of others; such is the status of select "native informants" like Dukureh or Hirsi Ali (see also Mahmood 2008). The similarities between discourses of underground resistance and the down low testify to challenges in critically confronting the governance of subjects figured as suspect not-quite-citizens in the so-called postracial age. This is a challenge for anthropology as well: Joanne Passaro's analysis of anthropological receptions of her work on homelessness in the United States also reveals that, as she writes, "some 'natives' could not be trusted to speak for themselves"—neither the general public nor Passaro's anthropological audiences trusted homeless black men (1997: 155).

AT THE BORDER: THE ENDINGS OF CUTTING
IN THE BONGO DISTRICT

I first heard about the underground perseverance of cutting from GAWW's director, Mrs. Mahama, who told me that the practice persists in border areas such as Bongo. I took her at her word and, wanting to understand more about the women who found themselves at the center of NGO attention, decided to spend a part of my time in the rural Bongo District. Once there I learned that cutting was ending and that a whole generation of young women was uncut. The women I got to know dated the endings of cutting differently. Some, like the wound dresser, said that cutting was common "during the Gold Coast era" (that is, during colonial rule) but that it ceased after independence: "Under Nkrumah they didn't cut the [facial] marks or the clitoris." Others referred to their family histories, and many women with grown children said that they were cut but their daughters were not. Cutting, it seems, waned during the course of several decades. In this village the last cutting of women occurred in about 2000.

Ethnography can illuminate only the traces of these trajectories and must leave their contours as nontransparent as they are to Ghanaians themselves. Only in the Bawku District was I told that cutting continued and noticed it myself: while I knew only a few young women from Bongo and Bolgatanga who were cut, in rural Bawku I met many cut women who were in their late teens. I also learned from the data I collected at the local courts and the Tamale prison that most of the circumcisers who had been arrested were tried by the Bawku Circuit Court. Bawku is also where Esther, the gender desk officer (a district-level government official charged with promoting gender equity), continued to receive reports of cutting. A less obvious ethnographic detail is nonetheless telling. In conversations with groups of villagers, I was typically asked about my own views of cutting. I was uncomfortable with the ascription of authority that the question often entailed, but it was also a way for the villagers to learn more about me. While I was in Bongo people asked me whether I agreed with the NGOs and whether I thought that cutting was truly harmful. In Bawku people asked whether I thought girls *should* continue to get cut; Bawku was the only place where I was asked this question. I would have liked to conduct more research in Bawku but was limited to day visits, primarily because of political violence that had destabilized everyday life in the district.

In Bongo I witnessed the immediate and extended aftermath of the demise of cutting. Agnes, a middle-aged pito brewer, was seventeen when she was cut, one year before she got married in the 1970s. She and her friends decided to get cut on their own, as was common in her generation, and then informed their parents: "We asked our parents and they gave us the path. They understood us and agreed that we should cut." The parental consent was expected, since cutting was then normative and nearly universal. Everybody wanted to get cut, Agnes said, even the girls whose ancestral spirits opposed cutting; some in the latter group asked to get cut, but the circumcisers refused them. Their desire for cutting was shaped by duress, she emphasized:

> In those days, people insulted you if you didn't cut. They would tell you have fear in you. They would tell you not to jump their *wane* [pumpkin] plant. If you didn't cut, it's not proper for you to marry, and they said if you cut, you're a woman, but if you don't cut, you're a man.

Agnes mentions insults—regarding cowardice, threats to reproduction (of plants and women), and gender. But I learned from her and other women that uncut girls, who were rare in Agnes's generation, were not *actually* insulted—instead they were told that they *would* be insulted if they remained uncut. The threat of insults was itself a form of social sanction meant to impel girls to get cut. Thus, rather than being punished, uncut girls were compelled to get cut. Insults functioned as the law of cutting, to incite girls toward culturally desired practices. That law should compel and discipline, rather than punish, speaks to larger cultural logics of law, as I will show in chapters 6 and 7.

Cutting, Agnes said, ended in Bongo in the 1980s, and she pointed out that her oldest daughter, who was then thirty, was uncut. Now that cutting has ceased, she continued, women do not suffer from its consequences, but life is still difficult. Afua, my host, had been cut more recently, in the mid

1990s, and in unusual circumstances. She had no acquaintance with cutting when she was growing up in southern Ghana. When she was fifteen, she was sent to Bongo to live with her aunt and soon after was given in marriage to Robert, the local politician and development worker. No one expected her to get cut, but she did not feel like she belonged in Bongo, she told me; being uncut also precluded her from participating in some conversations. One of her sisters was cut at this time, which planted a seed in Afua's mind, but it took what Jennifer Johnson-Hanks calls a "vital conjuncture" (2002), the death of an infant, to move her to action. She and Robert had tried to conceive for several years, and she eventually became pregnant, but the child did not survive. Soon thereafter she went to her aunt's house to get cut and heal under her aunt's care. In retrospect she does not characterize this as a decision but as a whim. "It was only for fun," she told me, and for respect: "This person has done the cutting—they respect the person more than the one who hasn't done it." Respect was important to Afua, who presented herself as someone who upheld cultural norms, whether by valuing elders or receiving guests. Did ideas about improving reproduction motivate her, given that some attributed cutting to improved reproductive potential? If so, she did not mention it, talking instead about her desire to fully belong.

Faith is of the same age and class as Afua, but she is not cut. Like Afua, she is the wife of a local politician and owns a small business. But while Afua grew up unaware of the existence of cutting, Faith grew up intending to get cut but never followed through. When I first met her, she was selling *coco* at the market; she had learned to make the porridge when she lived in a Hausa-speaking neighborhood in Kumasi with her husband. They returned to Bongo to try to make a living, but although her husband was successful, making ends meet still was difficult. As a girl Faith had imagined that she would get cut and was told she needed to "go for cutting" before marriage. However, her marriage was hastily arranged—her brother needed four cows to arrange his own—and as a result she married uncut. She soon found herself in a double bind, as her mother wanted her to temporarily return to the natal home and get cut, but her husband did not want her to get cut at all. She eventually agreed with him, and once they moved to Kumasi, away from her natal family, the matter was settled.

Cecilia, Afua's niece, is not cut nor are her peers. Ten years younger than Afua, and a high school student when I first met her, Cecilia was a volunteer and peer counselor on sexuality, cutting, and HIV/AIDS for the Programme

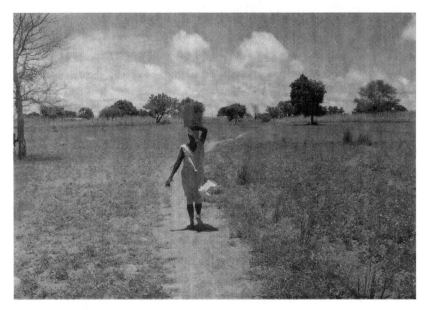

FIGURE 8. "Come visit me."

for Rural Integrated Development (PRIDE), the organization cofounded by her uncle Robert. One of Cecilia's duties was to advocate against cutting, but she found this task unnecessary, since young girls were not disposed to get cut. When I asked one of Cecilia's peers why she did not get cut, she asked, "Why would I?" Cutting, she said, "was not on our minds."

Cut Women's Perspectives on the Discourse of Resistance

The notion of underground resistance to ending cutting also structures cut women's accounts of the ending of cutting and their responses to NGO interventions. Women and men in the Bongo District responded to this discourse by emphasizing their compliance with NGOs while articulating an alternative historical account that situates cutting, as well as their experiences of marginality, within a shared national framework. In chapter 5, I explore this response in detail, showing how rural women refuse the governmental "institutionalization of meaning" (Mbembe 1992: 2) rather than NGO efforts to end cutting. Here I wish to highlight that rural women and men are well aware of the charges of cultural pathology and unruliness, and they try to defuse them. Therefore they do not merely say that cutting has ended but invest themselves in the truth of this claim.

Some portray cutting as belonging to a bygone era: "We used to cut in the 'olden' days." When was that? Three, five, ten, twenty, or forty years ago, I am told. Others stress that they "have nothing to hide." Many address the resistance discourse and accusations of unruliness implicitly, but an elderly wound dresser who used to tend to cut girls told me that she could now "speak the truth" since cutting *has* ended. Their temporal detachment from the practice and their insistence on the truthfulness of their statements about the ending of cutting reveal that they are aware of their official status as untrustworthy subjects.

They also want to be viewed as being responsive to NGO interventions, since they believe that a performance of compliance is a prerequisite for attracting additional NGO projects and their elusive benefits. Consequently, the people in Bongo did not merely inform me that cutting had stopped but also assured me time and again that they have heard the NGO message. These assurances index both their relationship to NGOs as well as their understanding of my research. My inquiry did not appear to be much different from the NGO campaigns that instructed Bongo women about the negative consequences of cutting. Ethnographers and NGOs both ask questions and do so in similar ways; in fact, Ghanaian NGO campaigns often share the formal characteristics of ethnography. For instance, PRIDE did not tell rural women that cutting is harmful or insisted that they stop it. Instead, NGO instruction is structured by participatory questions that appear to be open ended: NGOs pose quasi-Socratic questions about the women's views. At the same time NGO workers ultimately make it clear that their inquiries are meant to elicit correct answers. Rural women thus often presented themselves to me the way they presented themselves to NGOs—as willing to speak and as having listened and heard.

This constellation poses an ethnographic challenge, as anthropologists are no longer, and have never been, the only people who intently listen to "the local" people and ask them questions. The standard techniques of disassociating ourselves from reformists or bureaucrats do not suffice in a context in which knowledge and governance have long been intertwined (see also Hawkins 2002). Rural women were aware that their utterances were often measured for explicit governmental purposes. In this sense Navrongo researchers were right to raise questions about the limits of social science research, but this does not mean that rural women were lying. Rather than understanding the social as newly tainted by the governmental, we need to acknowledge their long-standing social entanglements. Rural women's accounts of the ends of cutting are mediated by layers of governmental interventions, and I suggest that no truth about cutting exists outside the truth regime in which NGOs, the state, scholars, and rural women all partake. Furthermore, understanding that rural women experience giving an account of themselves as a governmental technique of surveillance is important not only because it points to the contingencies of ethnography but also because it helps us understand how life is lived in the wake of efforts to end cutting and other governmental interventions.

WHERE ARE THE VIRGINS?
NOSTALGIA FOR A PATRIARCHY THAT NEVER WAS

Sometimes when they are hotly debating the virtues of the African female, I ask myself: "But who am I? Where did I come from?"

AMA ATA AIDOO
Our Sister Killjoy

Katie, a Canadian lawyer with whom I was staying in Accra for a few days, rushed to the small verandah of her house in Labadi and called me inside: "You must come, they are arguing about FGM! It's a real fight." The parties to the argument were Josephine, Elizabeth's sister and a formidable gender activist, and a Burkinabe man who was Katie's boss. They were discussing the demise of public morality and agreed on many counts but were at loggerheads when the conversation turned to the problem of girls' unruly sexuality. Josephine insisted that FGM was a worthwhile practice because it safeguarded girls' virginity, while the Burkinabe man begged to differ. Katie was astonished, wondering, "What is going on here?"

Katie did not expect a woman known for her lifelong activism to defend cutting. Josephine's words were informed by discourse that I refer to as the "virginity hypothesis"—the claim that, as an anthropologist writing for the UNFPA puts it, "in the past, cutting checked sexual promiscuity, pre-marital sex and unwanted pregnancies" (Awedoba 2008: 106). Josephine, a feminist and an ardent Christian who enjoys being provocative, does not like to be pigeonholed and today would not endorse cutting if asked about it. She is concerned about girls' sexual morality and believes that the purpose of cutting was to safeguard virginity and "to show that you're a virgin," but she says that she has no nostalgia for cutting:

Some people feel that [uncut] girls are not able to control their sexual feelings. But I'm not in that group. I am in the group that says, "Even if we've lost something, we can still find another way of letting the girls appreciate themselves more than, you know, going to do a thing like that." You know?

Whence, then, Josephine's support for cutting on that evening in Accra? My sense is that Josephine was thinking through arguments made at the workshop she had attended earlier that month, to which I will turn shortly. However, the virginity hypothesis and the nostalgia for cutting are much larger phenomena than a single NGO workshop. In addition to keeping alive the discourse of underground resistance, which stresses the intractability of cutting, public figures in the Upper East Region embrace another official discourse that acknowledges the ending of cutting, but this one is tinged with regret. They invoke cutting with wistfulness and long for the days when it was still performed, as they claim that it preserved girls' virginity and sexual morality. I suggest that they are nostalgic not only or even primarily for the practice itself but for the patriarchal social order that they believe it protected. The ending of cutting, it seems, can be acknowledged only in negative terms, as a demise of the social order. As a result cutting remains marked by official concern—whether because it is said to be intractable or because it is said that its disappearance has undermined public morality.

The virginity hypothesis is part and parcel of public masculinist discourses about social problems that critically evaluate the present by bemoaning the loss of morality and the decay of social order and cultural norms and that displace these problems onto young women in particular. Ghanaian media, government, and NGOs, as well as male elders—both rural and urban, ordinary and powerful—often discuss what they cast as the morally problematic behavior of youth and women—hence the many discourses about idle youth, teenage pregnancies, street hawking, loose girls, and fallen women. Women's behavior thus is cast both as a cause and a symptom of trouble in contemporary Ghana. In recent years the figure of the *kayaye,* a young northern girl who migrates to work on the streets and markets of Accra, has become emblematic of these concerns, on the part of both the government and elderly rural men. But some feminist NGOs occasionally join the conservative chorus; they, too, are preoccupied with the loss of sexual morality and girls' failures to exemplify virginal virtues.

"The Magic of Their Differences":
The Patriarchal Cunning of Recognition

The workshop Josephine attended in Bolgatanga was organized by Elizabeth. Although focused on voter education, it inadvertently promoted the virginity hypothesis and restored sexuality to the normative patriarchal order. The project's goal was to ensure and enhance the participation of women and people with disabilities in political decision making, both as voters and as candidates for office in the upcoming national elections. Twenty NGO and government representatives were invited to the leafy garden terrace of the Royal Hotel to become trainers within the so-called TOT (training of trainers) framework—participants were to learn skills that they would pass on to citizens in their home districts. During the next three days they were supposed to learn how to hold candidates accountable for their promises, how to communicate political demands effectively, and how to measure whether politicians are addressing them.

Despite the stated focus, the workshop began with the usual enumeration of northern harmful traditions, and the first day was consumed by discussions of FGM, forced marriages, betrothals, and witchcraft accusations. The problematization that posits culture and patriarchy as the main source of the region's ills is a staple of northern NGO events and a ritualized act in its own right that repeatedly lays the tracks for making modern subjects. Like initiation rituals themselves, this ritualized act teaches participants the obvious and already known (Piot 1999: 100). Whereas after cutting, mothers would teach their daughters how to keep the yard tidy and wash their bowls, even though they already possessed such knowledge, NGO discussions of harmful traditions also repeat the already known. In workshop spaces the already known that is nonetheless taught is the civilizing discourse that builds on colonial and anthropological taxonomies and categories.

Elizabeth had something entirely different in mind. She had recently returned from South Africa, where she was trained in a so-called positive approach to development called Appreciative Inquiry and became, as she put it, a convert. Appreciative Inquiry was initially developed in the United States as a management technique, and it evolved to combine various elements of the American spirit—positive thinking, self-help, growth, possibility, and the dream of continuous self-improvement—with postcolonial awareness and a desire to affirm Africa. Elizabeth was one of the people who used Appreciative Inquiry to design InterAction Leadership, a British

Council program that promotes the core values of "a positive revolution in change":

> The Interaction leadership programme is enabling men and women to engage the challenges that Africa faces by honouring success and learning from what has worked and is working in Africa. By *recognising* Africa's contributions to the world, *the deficit view of the continent can be challenged,* and hope for the future can grow. The Interaction leadership programme is designed by Africa and UK partners working with the principle articulated by the New Partnership for Africa's Development—*Africa for Africa, through collaboration.* Interaction brings people together across the continent from North to South and from East to West to network, *to share and celebrate the magic of their differences.* Through such exchanges, participants can challenge assumptions about themselves, their environment, and their continent. The programme encourages people to work in a way that *appreciates indigenous knowledge and differences* and to encourage their contribution to bringing transformation to the continent. (emphasis added)[6]

Refusing to perpetuate the "deficit view of the continent"—the perspective that postcolonial scholars and anthropologists have long criticized—the people behind this project want to acknowledge Africa's contribution and pan-African collaboration but within the paradigm of liberal recognition that codifies difference and indigeneity. In contrast to the colonial rule of northern Ghana that preserved tradition, and contemporary governance that sees northern traditions as harmful, the AI approach is primarily recuperative. Its purpose is to mobilize culture and indigenous knowledge for transformation, which puts it in step with certain approaches to neoliberal governance itself (Elyachar 2002).

Elizabeth wanted to bring Appreciative Inquiry home. On the second day of the workshop she asked the participants to challenge their understandings of "local harmful traditional practices" by reflecting on them from a positive perspective. "Finding out positive things is difficult for everyone, but it's interesting," she said and used FGM as an example:

> The outcome is bad, but the ritual process is good. Your grandmother will give you a talk, teach you life skills—how to be a good woman, what it means to be a wife, how to wash your calabashes, how to be bold, how to dance. The suitors will watch.

Elizabeth's description of cutting as a publicly celebrated ritual that involves dancing and observation by suitors, and that pedagogically transmits gendered values across multiple generations, represents the prevailing governmental imaginary. Rather than reflecting historically existing cultural forms, this imaginary uses anthropological theories of coming-of-age rituals that have only limited resemblance to regional practices of cutting but that have morphed into governmental knowledge. Grandmothers were rarely involved in cutting—the ritual focus was on healing rather public celebrations—and the making of a good woman was a process that far exceeded domesticity and cutting alike, whereas being a good woman meant respecting oneself and others and sustaining relationships.

Elizabeth's articulation of the value of cutting as a production of gendered subjectivity that is both properly domesticated and "bold" is one of the strategic essentialisms she often used to make gender activism palatable to male public figures. I once saw her scold herself when she realized that such essentialisms may not be necessary. Invited to give a speech at a fund-raiser for a girls' school she attended, she appealed to the men in the audience, telling them that well-educated girls will make good wives and mothers. After noticing that the largest donations came from women, Elizabeth laughed at herself, saying she needed to change her thinking, meaning that she did not need to appeal to masculinist expectations. But she did not change her practice, as her NGO also upholds the discourse of family values as the foundation for Ghanaian stability and order while challenging only rural and non-Christian patriarchal formations seen as rooted in tradition and custom.

Workshop participants had difficulty emulating Elizabeth's appreciative approach, which required putting cutting in context and condemning the physical effect of the practice but not its purpose or value. NGO workers are used to "cultural triage" that separates good and bad customs but not to sorting out the good and the bad *within* a single practice. After workshop participants broke into smaller groups, they were given the task of identifying "cultural norms and values that can promote the cause of PWDs [people with disability] and women," and Elizabeth pleaded for a positive outlook: "Please remember the concept of appreciative inquiry—let's stay positive to counteract the negative."

But how to stay positive? I sat at a table with a group from Bawku. For a long time no one said a word. Other groups were equally perplexed by the task, I noticed when I looked at neighboring tables and saw confusion on people's faces. Our group finally figured a way out. Since Elizabeth had mentioned "good things" about cutting, participants tried to find something good about it as well.

"Cultural practices used to ensure women's virginity, and now, there is nothing to keep women safe and faithful."

"They won't say you're carrying a man's organ."

"And it [FGM] is not bad when you're not married."

It shortly became clear that all the groups had flipped the habitual discourse of harmful traditions on its head. Rather than decrying how traditions inhibited development and progress, they now cast them as promoting good patriarchal values. Although they articulated the "African family" as one that controlled and exploited the sexuality and labor of girls and women, the workshop participants now figured exploitation as positive: FGM was good because it kept girls virgins; widowhood rites were good because they confirmed women's faithfulness; girls were considered valuable property their fathers could marry off; polygamy was good because it ensured "numbers in terms of children and family size"; uneducated girls are valuable house help for their rich relatives, a relationship that "helps knit the African family together and redistributes wealth"; girls are more of an asset than boys because girls are younger than boys when they start working ("at age five she can fetch water") and because girls can be converted into currency through dowry. The participants' discomfort in making these statements was mixed with confusion and disbelief but also relief. The air was thick with anticipation, and even though something wasn't quite right, everyone went along. Men and women, NGO workers and civil servants, Christians and Muslims all temporarily aligned themselves with the most conservative public discourses about gender and the family. These discourses hold the waning of cutting responsible for a weakening of social mores regarding sexual and marital relations. As such the end of cutting is not seen as just one of many social transformations but as *the* cause of the deterioration of a core social institution that had safeguarded tradition—the patriarchal, heterosexual family system.

Elizabeth was dismayed. She had not anticipated this outcome and tried to rein it in by moving to the middle of the terrace and speaking forcefully: "We need to realize that responsibilities don't go with rights. Girls may have a lot of positive responsibilities but do not have the matching rights. And we need to see how those positive responsibilities can be moved from the home into the community." But it was too late to change the tenor of the meeting, and Elizabeth knew that the damage was done. The attempt to reevaluate culture brought about a crisis in knowledge and value. The discursive ties between northern culture and patriarchy are so firmly established that the only response to the request to value culture was to assert the value of patriarchy and to see it in everything.

Moments like this have traction. The virginity hypothesis may not reflect a historical fact, but it has moved from theory to reality by way of such moments. I learned as much when I asked cut women in Bongo about virginity and sexual self-control. No one had ever mentioned these associations with cutting on their own or volunteered them as motivation for getting cut, and some, like Agnes, had told me explicitly that it was not true that uncut women now chased men—that happened only, she said, "if a girl already wants to follow men." But when I asked about this again in 2009, several women told me, "Yes, cutting allowed us to control ourselves better."

Governmental Histories

The notion of cutting as a means for controlling women's sexuality does not have a solely Ghanaian provenance but emerged as a Ghanaian-British construction: the virginity hypothesis was first articulated in colonial debates of the 1930s. Historians and anthropologists alike have shown that colonial law overemphasized the centrality of marriage and virginity and did not reflect African values or conjugal practices (see Hawkins 2002; Tambiah et al. 1989). As Hawkins writes, "The Victorian ideology of marriage perceived sexuality not as a condition coincidental with marriage, but rather one to be repressed within it" (2002: 34).

Even early on, the virginity hypothesis was a polyvalent discourse that could be used for opposing political ends. As I demonstrated in chapter 1, while British feminists wanted to end cutting so as to liberate African women's sexuality, a desire that hinged on British notions of what African women needed liberation from, at least some colonial officials were happy with having women's sexuality curbed. Recall that they were enthusiastic about Mitchell's relativizing report because he refuted the claim that cutting minimized women's rights, insisting instead that African women have sexual rights and rights to sustenance in marriage and that women were indeed too sexual and required restraint.

Many Ghanaian anticutting campaigners and sometimes scholars present the virginity hypothesis as an indigenous explanation of the purpose of cutting. Take GAWW, for instance. In her contribution to the report on the 1984 Dakar seminar that inaugurated the IAC, Marjorie Bulley, cofounder of GAWW, wrote: "Some Ghanaian tribes engage in female circumcision at varying ages. Its purposes are to provide proof of virginity and to preserve chastity."[7] Bulley's claim was not based in any intimate knowledge of groups that practiced cutting; in the 1980s GAWW leaders knew little about cutting as it was lived or practiced. Bulley was basing her claim on a common tendency to identify a single origin of cutting, often in Egypt, and the description of the original purpose of cutting as control of women's sexuality. A population studies report from the University of Ghana thus states, "The commonest explanation of FGM is that, though carried out by women, it was devised by men to control women's rampant sexual desire" (2000: 5), positing women's rampant desire as the supposed origin of the need for control. Ghanaian feminist scholars agreed with such statements; as Takyiwah Manuh wrote, "for women working in the GAWW for instance, female circumcision is *correctly* perceived as an instrument to enhance male pleasure, even at severe cost to the physical and mental health of women" (1989: 148; emphasis added). At this time GAWW and Manuh understood cutting as shaping a mutually exclusive notion of pleasure—men gained from women's loss. GAWW articulated concerns about women's sexual pleasure obliquely, by displacing it on men as the proper subjects of satisfaction. That men were said to have mistaken women's pain for pleasure, as Manuh also reports, reveals the understanding, prevalent in the 1980s, that men were the agents of cutting and that cutting was performed for their benefit.

In recent decades GAWW and other anticutting campaigners have supplemented discussions of sexuality with more proximate reasons and meanings for cutting, which they regularly discuss and codify. The virginity hypothesis is one of many such reasons that confounds easy distinctions between local and governmental conceptions, as control of sexuality and virginity was colonial in origin but articulated as having a local etiology. Scholars and public officials alike have adopted governmental understandings of cutting, reconstructed them as local truths, and repurposed them for both feminist and conservative ends. Not everyone agrees. Dr. Adjei was incensed about repeated assertions of the virginity hypothesis because his research with high school students showed that cut girls were more sexually active than uncut girls, as well as more likely to drop out of school.

The hold of the dominant discourse is such that anthropologists giving an account of cutting and its endings must frame their discussion in terms of the virginity hypothesis. In the discussion of cutting in his report for UNFPA, *Cultural Sensitivity and Programming,* Albert Awedoba, an anthropologist at the University of Ghana and a specialist on the Kassena-Nankana District, reveals his struggle with this discourse. Awedoba adopts two voices in the report: the voice of the people which he knows well, and the voice of a public official. The public voice asserts the official mantra: cutting controlled girls' sexuality, kept them from having premarital sex, and prevented teenage pregnancies (Awedoba 2008: 106). But in writing from the perspective of the Kassena-Nankana peoples, Awedoba refutes the virginity hypothesis: "Practicing communities rarely argue that circumcision reduces the libido and sexual desires of married women" (77). The shift between the two voices is evident in the terminology: the official voice speaks of FGM and the other of circumcision. From the perspective of those Awedoba knows best, cutting was not intended to ensure virginity or chastity by eliminating desire but "signaled that a woman was ready for marriage and suitors then began to woo her formally" (78).

My own ethnographic perspective partially coincides with Awedoba's, but rather than resolving his dilemma, I want to contextualize and reframe it. Cut women in Bolgatanga and Bongo also told me that cutting was usually the beginning of sexual relations, not a means of discouraging them. There was little need for efforts to keep girls away from men until cutting, as the normative age for cutting was the onset of puberty, and before that hardly any girls had sexual encounters. Cutting was not a prerequisite for marriage ("a certifiably chaste girl is ready for marriage") but one of possible beginnings for courtship and marriage: suitors initiated the period of courtship after girls were cut.[8] They sent girls gifts of food during the healing and recovery period, and most girls were married a year or two after cutting.

The main context in which cut women brought up their sexual experience was in their explanation of gifts or payment to the circumciser. "The knowledge of men," I was told, was what determined the expected amount of payment. *Yapeliga* was the cutting of girls who did not "know men," and *yasablega* referred to the cutting of those who did. But "knowledge of men" or "meeting men" does not necessarily refer to virginity. These are not the same semantic categories. "Knowing men" reflects on experience, while "virginity" intertwines it with ontological and moral claims about bodily purity and virtue. For the circumciser Atanga, childbirth was the relevant factor for determining how dangerous the procedure was and how high his payment would be: "If the girl had already given birth, she gave me a goat, but if she had not given birth yet, she gave fowls." His purpose was not to ascertain whether a girl was a virgin but to perform cutting with the proper blessings of the gods. Because the performance of cutting on girls who had "met men" or given birth to children was more dangerous, the payment was higher. Indeed, Afua was the only woman I met who had the *yasablega* performed.

I find myself in a situation similar to Awedoba's: even though I give credence to neither the virginity hypothesis nor the discourse that attributes the demise of the social order to the ending of cutting, I cannot *not* account for their popularity. The popularity of the virginity hypothesis means something, and I would venture that it reflects the larger moralizing discourses about social change and Westernization (from urbanization, shifts in kinship formations, delayed marriage, and migration of girls to the South) that are expressed in reference to sexuality (see also Smith 2014). Family and sexuality have long been at the center of moral panics, and the genealogies of these concerns are anthropological as much as governmental. The virginity hypothesis is informed by rising moral panics about sexuality that are shaped by the recent ascendance of religious morality and fears about the spread of HIV/AIDS.[9] The latter are institutionalized in abstinence-only campaigns, "virgin clubs" for girls organized by volunteer groups such as the Christian Mothers Associations, and in virulent opposition to public assertions of queer and homosexual identity and concomitant claims for public recognition.

As I noted earlier, the affective tone expressed here is sentimental: some Ghanaians find something attractive about the imaginary of a patriarchal past at a time when the pursuit of gender equality has become a dominant governmental project. The nostalgic voice allows public officials to articulate something redemptive in patriarchy, even if that means being sympathetic toward practices that they otherwise despise and denounce. They thus enter a patriarchal bargain: declaring "patriarchy was a good thing, for it safeguarded social order" is worth the cost of saying "FGM had something good about it, for it protected families."

Sexuality, Cutting, and the "Status of Women"

The question of cutting as an effect of the status of women in African societies, and of African women's sexuality in particular, has been debated since imperialism. Despite the historical record, which shows that colonialism diminished the rights of women and entrenched patriarchy by redistributing property and authority to men (Lindsey 2007; Manuh 2007; Macharia 2012), the prevailing public imagery is that the West African precolonial past was patriarchal. In the epigraph to this section, Sissy, the character in the prose poem *Our Sister Killjoy* by the Ghanaian author Ama Ata Aidoo, takes to task the way African intellectuals contribute to this image. Sissy cannot recognize herself in the picture of a virtuous, servile African woman; she contrasts women at home with British women, "the dolls the colonisers brought along":

> No, My Darling: it seems as if so much of the softness and meekness you and all the brothers expect of me and all the sisters is that which is really western. Some kind of hashed-up Victorian notions, hm? Allah, me and my big mouth!!
>
> See, at home the woman knew her position and all that. Of course, this has been true of the woman everywhere—most of the time. But wasn't her position among our people a little more complicated than that of the dolls the colonisers brought along with them who fainted at the sight of their own bleeding fingers and carried smelling salts around, all the time, to meet just such emergencies as bleeding fingers? (1977: 117)

Sissy emphasizes her childhood in a village "over two hundred and fifty miles away from the coast" with uneducated rural parents to stress that her upbringing was not Westernized. This authorizes her insistence that the idea of meek African womanhood is borrowed from the British colonial gender system. Aidoo relativizes by contrasting Ghanaian and British women, but for her, strength and fortitude, rather than rights or sexual autonomy, are the relevant markers of woman's status. Although Sissy nowhere mentions cutting, it is interesting to note that Aidoo portrays the British women's inability to withstand blood as a marker of their weakness. While Ghanaian women danced after cutting, British women fainted at the sight of bleeding fingers.

Nearly forty years have passed since the publication of Aidoo's book, but the nostalgia for an ostensibly traditional patriarchy in the form of control of woman's sexuality is strong again. Sissy's voice punctures this nostalgia, beckoning us to indulge in her "big mouth" and blasphemous courage. Women from the Upper East Region would agree with Sissy about the importance of strength and fortitude, as I discuss in chapter 5; they say that they can no longer get cut because their bodies are weak. In contrast to those who emphasize the loss of cultural values that safeguarded sexual morality, northeastern women critique structural conditions that sustain scarcity and thus deplete them of blood, health, and energy. What they wish for is not the return of cutting but the ability to sustain their strength and fortitude, as well as more governmental care. Circumcisers who have stopped cutting agree with the women.

COLONIAL MADNESS: WHEN CUTTING COULD HAVE ENDED BUT DID NOT

Azure never wanted to be a circumciser. "I refused to do it and ran to Kumasi. It followed me there with madness, so I came home," he told me. When I met him in 2004, he was sitting beneath a baobab tree outside his compound and surrounded by his family. His daughter-in-law was braiding the hair of another young woman; one of his sons and two of his three wives, who were much younger than Azure, were resting in the shade.

The old circumciser was now content, but his life had been one of tumult and trouble. As a young man, in the Gold Coast era, he went to work in Kumasi. His father and grandfather were circumcisers, and his departure, he says, was a refusal of cutting. His migration was a new twist on a tradition imposed by slavery and the colonial regime of forced labor: three decades before Azure's journey, men had been ferried away in chains to forced labor assignments in the South, and two decades before that, children, women, and men were stolen and sold into slavery in the South and in neighboring countries. For men of Azure's generation migration was a welcome and chosen path, one he preferred to staying at home and following his father and grandfather into circumcision. He spent fifteen years in Kumasi, where he worked in railway maintenance.

But if Azure was ready to take leave of cutting, cutting was not ready to let go of him. In Kumasi Azure went mad and, unable to sustain a life on his own, returned to Bongo. His family, seeking answers to his affliction, took him to the soothsayer (diviner).[10] "When I came home," he recounts, "we went to the soothsayer and the thing said if I don't use the *yabega* tools to work, my madness will not go." "The things"—gods of cutting—had caused the madness, and they would be appeased only if he took up the vocation demanded by his ancestors.[11] Azure had to carry on the work of cutting, so he picked up the tools of his vocation—the knife and the pouch—and began circumcising.

The madness stopped immediately, he says, as soon as "I agreed to do it, before I even started cutting," and it never returned. As proof of his well-being, he points to his wives:

> This is my first wife, my second wife, the third wife is there. Five of my wives left me before I left for Kumasi. That's why my wives are young—they can be my children. If the madness had not stopped, and if I hadn't done the work very well, would I have gotten these three wives? They were given to me.

If life before cutting was a life of loss—of sanity and of friends and family—and a life of agony and bad luck, his return to the North and to cutting meant a life of health, fulfillment, and wealth, conceptualized as wealth in people (Bledsoe 1980; Guyer 1993). He was respected for cutting, and one of his wives was given to him in marriage as a countergift for his services. Because he was married, he was able to eat well: "Does a bachelor get *sagebo* [millet porridge] to eat?," he asks rhetorically. One of the wives, a lively participant in the interview, cheerfully confirms Azure's story: "It's out of happiness that he got all of us. He was alone, but now he has all of us." She, too, is happy.

She wants to tell me more and prods Azure to divulge his full story and to show me his knife and pouch. "You should say all," she says, interjecting: "He also helped women deliver. You should add that when your father cut, your mother was dressing [the wounds of the cut girls]. So when you took over, I was dressing." For Azure and his wife the act of cutting was collaborative—she examined the cut to make sure that it was complete, and he had to remedy incomplete cuts on the spot: "If you have not cut everything, she tells you and you cut again."

Azure said he learned how to cut from the knife itself. Like other circumcisers, as a young boy he had accompanied his father and watched him cut, though only from a distance. It was the *pulungo,* the small knife, that really showed him how to cut. Azure mimics the movements that the knife taught him, but he does not take the knife into his hand when the women bring it out of the house. It is safe to show the knife to me now, he says, because he is no longer cutting, but the knife is still potent and must be treated carefully. Even though it is no longer in use, the knife has a power granted by the gods. I refrain from taking a picture of the knife but make a sketch of its shape in my notes.

Cutting was a dangerous business, and Azure was obligated to thank the gods for keeping him and the cut girls safe: "When you finish cutting for the season, you kill a goat and a dog for them." Other circumcisers poured libations before each circumcision or sacrificed fowl afterward. He describes the sacrifice as a feast: "You kill fowl, goats, and a dog, and brew pito. Call people to come sit with you and eat." He likens the feast to *sarega,* by which he means the Muslim celebration of Eid.

His daughter-in-law breaks in—"Now they're arresting those who cut"—intertwining stories of the end of cutting with the stories of cutting. Azure has made peace with this but jokingly says to me, "I'll cut you today." He laughs amiably, adding that he did not realize that I was white, as he is blind.

"Now I can't go to any place, I stopped it six years ago," Azure said. That was in 1998, after the circumciser in the nearby village of Sirigu was arrested and jailed. But Azure says he knew nothing of the arrest and stopped simply because he was old. He heard about the law only later, when it was announced at the market and at the chief's palace. Azure recalls that there were no explanations of the legislation, only an imperative: "They only announced that we should stop cutting. That is what we heard."

Azure is old and blind, and many of the circumcisers of his generation are dying. This is one reason that cutting is ending but not the only one—circumcisers have always faced mortality, and even in Azure's generation youth had little interest in cutting. Even though he tried to "run away from it," Azure had eventually inherited his father's task. His own son might be next in line to cut, and he is the only distressed person in the group. The son defiantly insists that he knows a lot about cutting, as he used to follow his father on his rounds: "We walked with him, we saw what he did. So if we want to do, we can do." The son's words sound declarative; he wants me to know that he could take up cutting if he wanted. I take his words not as an indication that he will but that he, too, feels its loss. He knows that the gods of cutting and the law are on opposing sides. I ask if they consulted the soothsayer about the decision to end the family line of cutting, forgetting that soothsayers are rarely sought preventatively—one typically turns to them after trouble has already occurred. Azure answers: "No, we stopped and we are waiting. They said we should stop. If you have your relative in your house, will you bring her?" (he means that everyone knows that cutting is illegal and that no one requests cutting anymore). Whether the gods are unhappy about this no longer carries as much import, he says: "If they are not happy, will you agree to do it? What if they arrest you?" For now the fear of arrest is greater than the fear of the gods.

We might wonder why potential arrest would outweigh the wrath of the gods. Police and judges can constrain one's freedom, but gods have power over life itself. They primarily engender life by ensuring reproduction (Allman and Parker 2005) as well as rainy skies and fertile fields, but the gods can also turn punitive if they are not tended to and cared for (Fortes 1965). When abandoned, gods can bring madness and death, terminating the lives of circumcisers, their children, and cut girls and women. Azure and others speak of the gods' demands for care in the form of sacrifices, libations, and observations of taboos to ensure successful cutting, prevent the circumciser's blindness and death, and avert harm from cut girls. At the moment, Azure says, the gods are quiet and are not stirring up trouble.

For Azure the problem is not with gods but with sustenance: he and his family no longer earn any income. "It was out of the work that I got money to perform the marriage ceremonies for these wives. We were also eating well. Now all we can do is farm." Farming, I know, does not guarantee basic sustenance, nor can it supply him with money for his son's marriage ceremony. Azure points to the state of his farm to demonstrate his lack of money: "Look at the weeds. Wouldn't I have given money for them to come and weed?"

An NGO had promised to help, but nothing had come of it. Azure tells me that the day before he had been reflecting on the NGO meeting convened by PRIDE that he had made his son attend. Robert had told me about it earlier: NGO personnel had assembled all circumcisers and wound dressers from the district to teach them why it was important to stop cutting. The NGO hoped to start an "alternative income generation project" in the form of seed money for farming and small businesses. At the meeting, the son says, the NGO verified that everyone in attendance was cutting, dressing wounds, or next in line to take up the practice. However, the seed money never materialized—although NGO meetings and sensitization sessions are quite frequent, actual distribution of material resources is not.

Atanga's Grievance

"Show them how I live," Atanga implored when I visited him, urging me to take pictures of a compound so derelict it had only two rooms left standing. He also stopped cutting at the turn of the millennium. His request to me implied a moral claim: because he had to stop cutting, he could no longer appease the gods and was again afflicted by poverty and misfortune. After he quit, his two wives died, most of his children migrated south, and the gods killed two of his children and one grandchild. Atanga now lived a life of destitution, as measured by local standards; his house had fallen apart, and he was alone. The tattered smock he put on when he saw me approaching was his best. When I asked to take a picture of his compound, he told me to take more and vigorously gestured toward the broken walls, cracked plaster, and roofless rooms decorated by yellow-flowered vines making their way through the cracks. He imagined an audience of Ghanaians and whites who needed to be confronted with his suffering, and he saw me as way to accomplish this, as well as to generate potential cash flow in the form of project money.

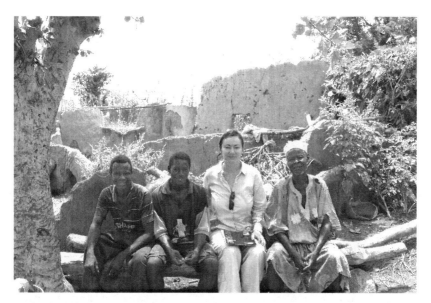

FIGURE 9. Atanga and his nephews.

I had heard about Atanga from his nephew Vincent, a well-liked volunteer for Rural Help Integrated (RHI) who boasted that it was he who had convinced his uncle to stop cutting. The RHI staff frequently mentioned Vincent's success; they were not always confident of the effects of their work, and they welcomed stories that made them feel they had accomplished something. They were eager to put me in touch with him when I informed them I would be moving to Bongo for awhile. Atanga and Vincent told me about their respective lives of service: Atanga was a circumciser and a birth attendant, and Vincent was a health volunteer who helped anyone he could. From the public health perspective, which is structured by what Langwick calls "the colonial separation of belief and knowledge, spirit and substance, and harming and healing" (2011: 58), Vincent and his uncle Atanga are polar opposites—one a campaigner against cutting and the other its practitioner, one who heals and the other who harms. But beneath the surface, their callings are not so different, as Atanga not only cut women but also helped them deliver, while Vincent provides first aid and refers women to the health center. Together they complete the movement of birth medicalization called for by public health administrators, one that opposes indigenous forms of assistance in deliveries and promotes the monitoring of prenatal women by volunteers who are supposed to send them to hospitals to deliver.

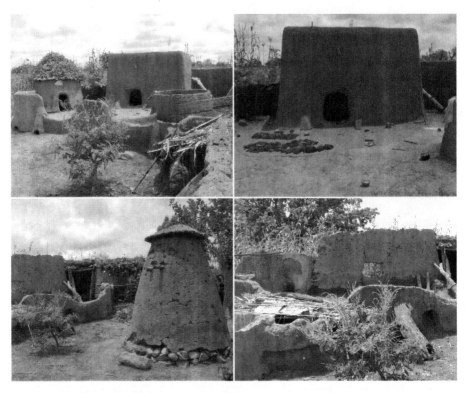

FIGURE 10. "Show them how I live"—Atanga's compound.

Atanga's life mirrored Azure's: Atanga, too, had run away from cutting, tried to build a life for himself in Kumasi, was unsuccessful in his quest, and had to return to Bongo and take up his inherited vocation.

> My father was cutting. He was cutting because someone from his uncle's house was cutting so when he died the thing chose my father. Cutting chooses people. So when my father died, it chose me, but I refused and I ran to Kumasi. But it killed my three children so I decided to do it. Cutting is a god. It chooses people. It was doing good, but not bad.

Atanga spent nine years in Kumasi doing leatherwork, a common handicraft of Frafra men. But then, he says, gods killed his three children and he fell sick. He was violently ill, shaking and convulsing; this, too, was a kind of madness but one that attacked his whole body. His older brothers eventually consulted a soothsayer to learn what was afflicting him and received the verdict that the gods were angry. Atanga would have to return home and take up cutting if he were to be healed. He did, and he was.

Now, decades later, Atanga is indignant about the losses he incurred as a result of the outlawing of cutting, which he experiences as a government-caused injury. He says that he is proud of the work he did as a circumciser and that he was respected and praised because his cutting "was not doing any harm," and the girls he cut healed quickly. He, too, had attended the PRIDE workshop for circumcisers and knows what the government and NGOs say about the dangers of cutting, but they did not convince him, and he questioned the NGO's expertise and authority: "Some of the people who say we should stop the cutting, their mothers and wives are cut. Even some of them have marks on their faces. But now they have read books, and they are telling us to stop cutting, so what can we do? We have to stop." This, too, is a moral claim, for he positions himself as someone who did nothing wrong and who stopped cutting under duress, not because he believed it to be harmful:

> Cutting was good for the girls, it was not destroying them. But now the government says we should stop. That is why we have stopped, but cutting was not harmful. When it comes to giving birth, the girls delivered safely. The cutting does not cause any trouble. It is because we have been asked to stop that we have stopped, but the cutting was not causing any problem. Now we have stopped because we do not want to be arrested. At my age, if I am arrested, it will not be good.

Atanga knew that the government had wanted to stop cutting for a long time. He had first heard about it in the Rawlings era (Jerry Rawlings was Ghana's president from 1981 to 2001), when the local revolutionary organs, the People's Defence Committees (later called Committees for the Defence of the Revolution), had told him that "we cut and harm the girls," to which he responded, "My father never harmed anyone and I never did either." He is also acquainted with the public health concerns about hygiene and the concomitant danger of HIV transmission, so he emphasizes that he used a different knife to cut each woman:

> I used to have about four or five sets of instruments. I would use one to cut a woman and another one to cut a different woman. At the end of the day, I would wash them. But they say we should stop cutting. Someone has been jailed for cutting. His name is Abanga from Sirigu.

For Atanga, like others in Bongo, the law enters narratives of cutting from multiple directions. The arrest and incarceration of the Sirigu circumciser was a crucial impetus for him to quit. The circumciser's death shortly after his release from prison testifies to Atanga's fear that an arrest at his age would "not be good." Everyone is afraid of the law, Atanga tells me: "I was afraid of being arrested. The women are also afraid, but my fear is greater than theirs because they arrested a circumciser, and I don't want to be arrested. That is why I have stopped." By stressing that he was forced, rather than convinced, to end cutting, Atanga wants me to recognize that he was wronged. Something was taken from him without an offer of a countergift or restitution. Without cutting he no longer has any means of appeasing gods who abandoned him again; he has little to eat, much less to sacrifice. On the shrine at the entrance to his room are traces of a cracked egg, not the feathers of fowl or animal skulls. Atanga brings up his loss time and again:

> People used to give me food, but now I can't get that.
>
> My children have run away, leaving me alone. Can't you see what my house looks like? I don't have food anymore, so my children have run to Accra, leaving me alone.
>
> If I were still cutting, I would catch a fowl for you as a guest to send home and make a meal with it, but I cannot even get to eat.
>
> Now that I have stopped the cutting, if I had money I would start the leatherwork again. But where is the money? I could even rear some fowl if I had money.

Atanga, too, told me that PRIDE had promised some form of help but that it did not materialize:

> They said they would call us, but they have not called us. They said that now that we have stopped cutting, they will help us with some money so that we can do some work. But we have not heard from them since then. When they called us [to attend the workshop], they gave us 20,000 cedis [US$2.00] each and that was all. But we can't go and ask them because we didn't ask them to stop us from cutting.

PRIDE was able to secure funding for workshops with circumcisers but not for any subsequent distribution of funds. Atanga does not see himself as authorized to make claims on the NGO, because, like others in Bongo, he sees the government as primarily responsible for social welfare, and because it was the government that had prohibited cutting. Little did he know that NGOs were in fact central to the criminalization of cutting and that the government sees cutting as the province of NGOs. For people outside of

NGO networks, the exact constellations of NGO-government parastatal formations (Geissler 2015) are difficult to trace and make sense of; Azure's son told me that the meeting was convened by "people who had something like a company."

Bereft of the favor of the gods, Atanga has neither protection nor material subsistence. He severed his relationship to the gods once and suffered for it. Whatever colonial capitalism did to produce his madness, it was not interested in curing it or remedying it. Like Azure, he was left to his own devices, and the only recourse he found was in ancestral gods and powerful objects of cutting. By outlawing cutting the government severed his relation to gods a second time, depriving him of their support. But how are we to understand Atanga's demands for restitution? Governmental workers would discount and ridicule it—circumcisers are not owed anything, they stress, as they inflict harm for personal economic gain and need to be stopped. If they were to be confronted by Atanga or Azure, they would hear only the demands for compensation for lost income, that is, for direct reciprocity, rather than the appeal to a form of power that intertwines protection and care. The moral economy and the relationship of subjects to ruling powers that Atanga demands of the government and NGOs are modeled on the power of ancestral gods and their relationship to the living. When Azure and Atanga complain about being abandoned by the state, they are demanding state protection and care, which substitute for the protection and care of the gods. Gods nurture life but can also take it, refuse their care and protection, or turn punitive if they are not tended to and cared for. Azure and Atanga experience state power as punitive and extractive: it takes away, sets limits, punishes but does not nurture or care for them or their social reproduction. The governmental power they wish for would be not only punitive but also, like ancestral power, generative, life sustaining, and caring.

These demands for mutual accountability, and governance that both gives and takes, resonate widely and find expression in the claims of cut women themselves (see chapter 5). Rural women and men from this region are refused governmental care on a much larger scale. While Atanga is exceptionally poor, scarcity is a rule, not an exception. When the state removed Atanga's ancestral protection and means of support, it was repeating a long history of managing northern lives without nurturing them. Atanga had nothing to fall back on when he stopped cutting because he had never been extended governmental care.

Atanga and Azure do not blame migration for their madness, attributing it instead to the wrath of the abandoned gods, but others have done so. In 1963 Meyer Fortes and his wife, Doris Mayer, a psychiatrist, spent three months in Tongo, the village where Fortes had conducted ethnographic fieldwork in the late 1930s. Fortes was stunned by the increase in madness: whereas three decades earlier he had witnessed only "one gross case of madness, as judged by their [local] criteria" (Fortes and Mayer 1966: 19), they now found thirteen cases in Tongo alone. The elders blamed it on gin, but Fortes and Mayer had a different explanation, tying madness to the migration south and break-down of family life. The events that precipitated the psychotic episodes seemed to be unusually traumatic and shaped by stresses of life in the South, a context they interpreted as "circumstances of alienation from the home environment or from the traditional cultural goals and values" (23). Fortes and Mayer did not trace alienation in the South to labor and life under duress in colonial capitalism, such as onerous working conditions and mistreatment of workers, but to alienation from family, home, and traditional values. They wrote:

> It should be understood that for a resident of the Upper Region of Ghana to go to Southern Ghana is still like going to another country; not only is the way of life and of work completely different, but the prevailing language is a foreign one and Northerners are liable to feel at a loss there if circumstances become difficult. (31)

Fortes and Mayer depict the 1930s as time of stability and the 1960s as a period of migration and crisis, a "critical point of transition in [northern Ghanaians'] social history," given that "their traditional social structure and way of life is on the brink of far-reaching transformation" (Fortes and Mayer 1966:17). But data they provide attest to prevalent labor migration in the 1930s, which they chose not to account for. The historians Allman and Parker (2005) have extensively critiqued Fortes's willful distortions of Tallensi life as separate from modernity and free from its ruptures. Certainly the argument about cultural crisis builds on a misleading portrayal of Tallensi life in the 1930s as exceedingly stable, and it ignores colonial violence that had, among other things, displaced entire villages.

Fortes was not alone in his nostalgia for the traditional extended family, ostensibly untouched by migration and colonial encounters. As I discussed earlier, preservation of tradition was the main modality of governance during much of colonial rule of northern Ghana. Contemporary governmental discourses again place more emphasis on loss of tradition than on material conditions of scarcity and dispossession. We should not be surprised that the virginity hypothesis resurrects the colonial desire to preserve tradition as well as Fortes's articulation of the stable extended family as a foundation for social order—and its corollary, the breakdown of the family, as the cause of the dissolution of social order. Anthropological theorizing of culture and social change has shaped popular opinion and governmental culture for nearly eighty years. Yet the notion of a singular threshold of social transformation, of a momentous event that irrevocably shifts the course of social history, is an unsustainable imaginary. Life in the Upper East has been marked by a long history of transformation, violence, dispossession, struggle, and perseverance.

NGO Workers Say

I like your phone.

Go and sit in the front seat with your "husband."

If your grandmother was Muslim, I will be your grandmother.

I need to pay school fees for my daughter. Can you help me?

I want to come and work in America for three to four months.

You're an anthropologist—I know you will write in support of culture. That's what anthropologists do.

She is our anthropologist; she went everywhere with us.

4

Mistaken by Design

BIOPOLITICS IN PRACTICE

Bolgatanga, October 2004. Dr. Adjei's NGO, RHI, is holding a weeklong training session for rural volunteers newly recruited into its community-based reproductive health project.[1] The training session is mostly in English and ranges across medical, public health, development, and gender topics, the discussion of which includes detailed information about biomedical conceptions of the body and reproduction. The volunteers are trained as modernizing subjects who are to encourage family planning and discourage female genital cutting. The second day of the session features a module on the "health consequences of FGM," and I ask Emilia, the RHI worker, how she will teach it, as I am eager to see how Dr. Adjei puts his research on obstetric consequences of cutting to use. Emilia pulls out three wrinkled, yellowed pages of a typewritten document titled "Harmful Traditional Practices" and hands them to me. The pages are worn out from repeated use, having served as the basis of the RHI education for many crops of volunteers. Produced in the 1990s, the document was signed by Madam Munya, a former director of the National Council on Women and Development for the Upper East Region who had for years campaigned against cutting, often in collaboration with GAWW. The document identifies and defines traditions, explains why they are undesirable, briefly discusses widowhood rites and infanticide, and concludes with a lengthy overview of FGM, elaborating, in ethnographic style, the "reasons for the practice of FGM" and the health complications. The discussion of the adverse health consequences of FGM is not purely biomedical but amalgamates popular discourses, development ideologies, and medical conceptions of harm taken from various documents published by the World Health Organization. This means that the document treats FGM as a general category and discusses the consequences of infibulation (for example, women need to be recut at delivery), which is not practiced in the region and is unfamiliar to the workers and the volunteers.

Dr. Adjei often identified his approach as being different from, and superior to, that of GAWW. RHI, he would remark, worked "on the ground" in collaboration with local communities, whereas GAWW never managed to have even an office in northern Ghana. He also fought common public discourses of underground resistance, border crossing for purposes of cutting, and the virginity hypothesis, using his research to refute them—with varying degrees of success. But despite his devotion to challenging prevailing conceptions, he considered Mrs. Munya's old information sheet adequate for the purpose of training volunteers, even though it repeated the very ideas he otherwise struggled against. This also meant that although Dr. Adjei was deeply involved in analyzing data from the WHO obstetrics study and from his own second doctoral project, he did not apply their results in this context. In addition to his lack of interest in correcting the biomedical understandings of harm in the training modules, Dr. Adjei also set aside his deep cultural and historical knowledge about the practices of cutting in the region and of *yabega ŋma* in particular. Rather than drawing upon his own knowledge and his publications, Dr. Adjei used an old document about FGM, a discursive construct with a reality of its own. While most of the workshop was conducted in both English and Gurene, RHI workers explained FGM only in English.

These omissions and occlusions are troubling to anthropologists, and how we think about them is the subject of this chapter. It is one thing to *lack* cultural knowledge, as NGOs are often said to do, but another to refuse to translate popular and official notions about health and harm, as RHI did. How do we make sense of Dr. Adjei's deliberate bracketing of knowledge and refusal of its translation? The fact that the RHI project did not fail to achieve the goals it set for itself, but was understood as successful, challenges long-standing debates in both clinical and critical medical anthropology. This chapter brings these two anthropological approaches into conversation, and it addresses a variant of the anthropological "fallback position" that I discussed in the introduction. Here the fallback position postulates that "without an understanding of indigenous cultures, and without a deep commitment from within those cultures to end the cutting, eradication efforts imposed from the outside are bound to fail" (Abusharaf 1998: 23). This anticipation of the failure of interventions that lack cultural understanding, and do not look the way we, as anthropologists, would like them to look, is a hallmark of the fallback position that articulates a variant of anthropological objections to anticutting campaigns. As my larger goal is to bring a different register of analysis of interventions to bear on anthropological sensibilities, this chapter questions the commonsensical assumptions about the forms of knowledge that are necessary for governing. To that end I bring ethnographic analysis of the place of knowledge in RHI rural outreach programs to bear on debates about knowledge and translation in both applied and critical medical anthropology. In contrast to analyses that emphasize and critique what is *said* in public health interventions, and how it is said, I want to stress that what is *done* and how power is *materialized* matters much more.

For critical anthropologists of medicine and science, the process of translation is especially crucial, because it is said to forge credible knowledge. As Timothy Choy writes, "Translation, thus, through the form of its event, generates the authority and circulations necessary for knowledge to count as expertise. It also enables articulation, or contingent unification across difference" (2005: 11). Ethnographic analyses of public health interventions, most notably of HIV/AIDS prevention programs, illuminate the tremendous amount of work, both linguistic and moral, put into the translation of biomedical concepts and theories (Wardlow 2012; Pigg 2001; Brada 2013). Wardlow asserts that to raise AIDS awareness is to engage in a practice of translation (2012: 407), whereby the public is asked to pay "attention to the scientific and medical terms of explanation" (Pigg 2001: 509). In the context of AIDS interventions, translation means two things: "The unpacking of the English words the letters in AIDS and HIV stand for" and the translation of these English terms into national or regional languages (2001: 509–10), as well as the creation of "the very discursive ground that would make this possible" (Pigg 2005: 45). That is, the larger task is not to translate vocabulary but underlying assumptions about the body, sexuality, and subjectivity. This is said to be particularly important in contemporary postcolonial contexts, where, as Choy writes, "to be credible, expertise must bear universalizing and particularizing marks simultaneously" (2005: 6). I share with these anthropologists a conception of public health education as an effort to bridge interconnected (not fundamentally separate) worlds and to produce something new rather than merely reproduce authoritative original texts and ideas. But I want to show that although public health education always involves performative events, it does not always aim at translation.

As much as HIV/AIDS education involves translation, Ghanaian educational programs about cutting involve a refusal to do so. NGOs are not interested in translating; in fact, we shall see that when lone workers try to engage in this effort, they are sanctioned. How, then, do we understand the refusal to translate? Pigg's notion of public health education as the "social production of commensurability" (2001) is helpful here, and I suggest that NGOs have little interest in rendering FGM fully commensurate with *yabega ŋma* and other regional forms of cutting. RHI training modules assert the primacy of the FGM discourse without bringing FGM closer to the experiences of the volunteers or subjects targeted by the campaign. The question is why.

The typical answer is that NGOs do not know enough. Gosselin writes that those "working to end excision often do not have the benefit" of cultural meanings and social dynamics (2000: 193). Ghanaian scholars also criticize NGO and state interventions by pointing out that their lack of knowledge and inaccurate ideas about traditional practices lead to the projects' subsequent failure. Failure here is assumed, anticipated, and explained by the governmental lack of cultural understanding. At the University of Ghana, Legon, one scholar from the Upper East questioned the authority of the vice president in just these terms: "We have a vice president who is from the North and who speaks against traditional practices, but he is a Muslim. So what does he know about traditional practices?" This scholar leveled the same criticism at NGOs, folding in accusations of opportunism: "And the NGOs, they just chase the money and jump from one topic to another without knowing enough about them. You see, they also condemn FGM without really understanding it." While this scholar contested the construction of the notion of harmful traditions from within the governmental discourse that sees "traditional religion" as barbaric, another disputed the NGOs' mapping of cutting onto Islam: "Some people say, 'These are the reasons for FGM,' but they are all wrong. Clerics give speeches that say, 'Islam says, "Do this to women, and this must be abolished"' when in reality, that's not done at all." This scholar, a Muslim from one of the large groups in the Northern Region that never practiced cutting, saw the misattribution of cutting to Islam as an example of uninformed and ineffective governance. This lack of knowledge, he said, is one of the reasons why NGO projects commonly fail. But, he added, more research was needed to understand why exactly they failed:

> Without people who do research on evaluation and monitoring of how policies get down to the population, how could we know why they failed? The numbers can tell you that they failed, but not why. One reason is because NGOs got on board and preached against FGM in public, but how did they follow it up?

These scholars' grievances highlight the extent to which northern Ghana is misrepresented, and subsequently governed, as the nation's constitutive Other. Yet their assumption that misrepresentation stems from lack of knowledge and leads to failure is, as I note here, shared globally.

Applied medical anthropologists studying public health programs in the global South have long held that the success of interventions depends on a knowledge of vernacular understandings of health and the body. When projects fail, it is assumed that the failure results from the practitioners' lack of knowledge. For example, Robert Hahn and Marcia Inhorn see "the inadequate translation of public health knowledge" as one of the main obstacles to improving public health (2009: 5). Therefore, they argue, public health campaigns need anthropology to supply cultural knowledge and interrogate biomedical assumptions:

> The failure of some public health programs to study and take into account the culture and society of the community toward which the program is being directed has sometimes led to only partial success or even demise of the program. Indeed, for public health programs to be maximally effective, social and cultural differences must be bridged, and communities receiving public health programs must "buy into" program efforts. The participatory research approaches developed in public health are a promising move toward cross-cultural bridge building. . . . But the failure of some public health agencies to reflect on their own cultural assumptions or to base programs on misleading concepts and erroneous theories and information remains a serious challenge to global health in the new millennium. (Hahn and Inhorn 2009: 5)

Hahn and Inhorn testify to the persistence of one of the founding principles of applied medical anthropology, which is the notion that anthropology can and should provide cultural knowledge necessary for improving public health and health care. The assumption linking the failure of interventions to the absence of such knowledge travels beyond medical anthropology. Following James Ferguson's pivotal work (1994), critics of development and NGOs often attribute failure and negative unintended consequences to a mismatch of local realities and intervention designs that ignore them. Thus the analysis of unintended consequences is often tethered to the notions of failure and the negative effects of NGOs' efforts.

In this chapter I contest this tacit consensus, arguing that being misrepresented in NGO interventions does not necessarily stem from being misunderstood (or poorly understood or ignored), that better knowledge does not lead to more accurate representations, and that mistakes built into development designs are sometimes deliberate and can result in projects that are successful on their own terms. Through an ethnography of film screenings designed for outreach purposes in rural areas, I examine how RHI tries to persuade even as it eschews translation. Rather than reading misrepresentations as indicators of a "lack of knowledge," I suggest that they constitute deliberate tactics and refusals of translation. NGOs have their own knowledge protocols, and organizations like RHI continuously generate knowledge—medical knowledge, knowledge of cultural forms, knowledge as evidence of NGOs' effectiveness—and use this knowledge to reformulate or solidify social phenomena as objects and sites of intervention. But they also make tactical decisions about what kind of knowledge will render interventions persuasive and successful. Through an analysis of some of these tactics, I show that rather than figuring NGO practices as failures in the making, we need to recognize that they worked in their own way and were constitutive of the public's acceptance of the NGO's project.

The claims I make here are in no way safe and, in contrast to the fallback position, might offend. But some risk is inevitable, as anthropological predictions of failure have analytical shortcomings and ultimately little bearing on whether NGO projects succeed. Pigg recognized this a long time ago, asking: "Can bad social analysis result in good development programs?" (1997: 275). Without endorsing either the so-called good or bad terminology, I want to account for the fact that RHI was successful, despite eschewing liberal notions of participation, refusing to question dominant assumptions, and propagating a vision of a future that devalued the subjects it addressed.

I take my cue from the anthropology of international collaboration, which shows the productive powers of "difference within common cause," confusion (Tsing 2005: 246, 247), and the indeterminacy generated by the "infinity within the brackets" of agreement (Riles 1998). Riles's critique of the notion that knowledge is "the artifact of transformation of one set of meanings into the next" certainly holds for the construction of FGM as an object of governmental concern whose "patterns are given at the start" (1998: 388). While NGO workers and civil servants talk only to one another in the context of workshops and can simply repeat the dominant knowledge, questions of meaning and representation haunt their interactions with villagers. The NGO addresses these questions, I propose, by making words less important and foregrounding materializing performance (Butler 1993). NGOs like RHI know how to make knowledge matter, but they also know that more than knowledge is needed for the production of authority.

The ethnography that follows shows that RHI operates at multiple registers. To win the rural publics over, the NGO inserts itself into their social and economic worlds, seduces them, and asserts its authority over cutting by visually displaying knowledge of its symbolism as well as an official understanding of cutting as a harm and a crime. Notably, the NGO deploys its knowledge of cutting not by enunciating it but by visually gesturing at it: the film RHI shows represents the symbolism of *yabega ŋma* while simultaneously decontextualizing the practice, distorting it, and reframing its meaning in line with governmental codifications of FGM. Rather than translating words, then, the NGO stages a performative event whose purpose is to remake *yabega ŋma* in the image of FGM. By crafting mistakes the NGO refuses to endorse local understandings of cutting in order to redefine which understandings matter and which knowledge counts as authoritative. The overall strategy is to mobilize different orders of knowledge, affect, and value and to materialize the NGO's power by way of a spectacular appearance and an alignment with state power.

SPECTACULAR KNOWLEDGE: MATERIALIZING
GOVERNMENTAL POWER

Into the Field

On a Friday evening in late April 2004, the RHI team is on its way to a village in the Bawku West District, hoping to arrive before nightfall. Now that its projector has been repaired, the team will be showing educational films about family planning, HIV/AIDS, and female genital cutting every Thursday and Friday, when they do not, as they say, "go to the field" during the day. The film screenings are the centerpiece of RHI projects and the only type of outreach directed at entire village populations.

There are many reasons why a screening, or "show," as RHI workers call it, might be canceled—the fitter [mechanic] is checking the pickup and balancing its tires, the projector is broken and the UN Population Fund has not sent the money to fix it, the driver is taking Dr. Adjei to Accra instead, the roads are impassable because of the heavy rain, a bridge has collapsed, there is lightning. My ethnographic research has its own contingencies—I accompany the RHI workers on these and other field visits but not if I am out of town, sick, or in the Bongo District.

Films are screened at night in deference to the villagers' farming schedules. But driving at night is generally considered dangerous, and many Ghanaians avoid it if they can. Highway robbers, it is believed, are most active at night, and reports about robberies on the Bawku road trickle in daily. For RHI workers nighttime field visits mean long workdays, from 9 in the morning until 9 or 10 in the evening. The field is a distinct space for RHI workers, and travel is a favorite part of their job, though they prefer daytime visits, which rescue them from their routine. They enjoy the movement and action, after days and weeks of lingering about the office, bantering to fight off the suffocating boredom. On visits to the field they have baseline and follow-up surveys to administer, monthly reports to collect from midwives, volunteer supplies to restock, community debates to hold and record. Olivia and Gina, RHI workers, explain the appeal of field visits as follows: "We interact with people, teach them a lot, they feed us, and in the office we just sit."

Field visits are represented as intensely social and intimate; even if interactions with villagers do not materialize, driving to the villages is a social experience in itself. We have to pack generators and the screen and fill up on gas. We stop to buy kebabs in Zuarungu or fried yam at the Zebilla Police Barrier. We pass by the Zebilla market, where the prices are much lower than in town, to buy *dawadawa* beans or onions.

The hills and valleys have turned green from the first rains, and at dusk the landscape is at its most serene. The freezing interior of the pickup, the air-conditioning set on maximum, is less peaceful. Six of us are in the truck, three in the front and three in the back, all crammed in. The RHI staffers argue loudly to pass the time. About Perry's funeral. About funerals in general and how they are a waste of money. About the best brand of mobile phone, a technology that everyone is eager to use but can barely afford. They buy phones but use them sparingly and find ingenious ways to reduce the cost. I get "flashed" by Emilia: when she wants to say hi, she calls me and hangs up before I pick up, saving some credits. The disagreements, however spirited, are forgotten the moment we step out of the pickup.

Each trip brings forth memories of other trips, and today's trip evokes remembrances of Perry, a project officer who died in an accident in January. "This job is dangerous, one of us died in an accident," Gina tells me. Perry's family "didn't act properly," everyone agrees, when it gave him a shameful burial. The family neglected to show his body and interred him at dawn. Emilia surmises that this was because Perry's mother was Muslim. Alima, the only Muslim in the group, becomes upset and insists that cannot be the reason. Muslims, she explains, do not bury the dead before daylight.

They still refer to Perry in the present tense, and apart from the funeral, talk about him as if he were still alive. But Perry is gone, and Martin has been hired to replace him. This is one of Martin's first field trips, but he enthusiastically joins in the banter. Although new to RHI, Martin knows that to partake in an argument is to socialize.

We follow the main road from Bolga to Bawku and then to Togo. The road is paved and in good condition, sometimes bordered by tall trees and forests. Before we reach the White Volta, the boundary between the Bawku West and East districts, we turn left onto a rough road that leads us to the villages. The Burkina Faso border is about ten miles ahead of us.

As the ride becomes bumpy, Emilia mentions a nearby village that doesn't even have a road. To get to the village to supervise one of its volunteers, she and Gina had to get off their *moto* (motorcycle) and ascend a hill. Gina says that in a quarterly report to UNFPA, RHI's primary (and often sole) donor, she once wrote that her group is the "rain beats me, sun dries me team." In the workers' narratives the arduous terrain symbolizes the social distance between the modern NGO and the remote villagers. Emilia and Gina construct this distance not with contempt but with an affability that signals their dedication to their work.

As we approach a market near our destination, the local RHI volunteer, officially called a promoter or a community health distributor, meets us and hops onto the bed of the pickup to show us the way. This is RHI's first film screening here but not its first encounter with the village. The team had traveled here to introduce the program to the chief, solicit his suggestions, and identify "traditional birth attendants." Involvement with chiefs and assemblymen and -women is a cornerstone of RHI campaigns, as the NGO knows what it takes to persuade local authorities to collaborate and to ensure that they are in favor of RHI's campaigns before the film screening. Establishing relationships is the key to gaining acceptance for the NGO, and RHI works closely with both chiefs and elected politicians, offering them respect, gifts, and decision-making power. I was present during RHI's expansion to the Bawku West District and watched how RHI got local authorities to sign on to the NGO's agenda by consulting with them about appointing volunteers—unpaid but highly coveted positions. In addition, rather than simply training volunteers, the NGO first trains the chiefs, politicians, and select "opinion leaders," women and men, from each participating village. They attended a three-day training session on reproductive health, where they listened to lectures, were wined and dined, and received gifts of cloth and cash.

All NGOs in northern Ghana have to be solicitous of chiefs; while chiefs had a limited sphere of influence in postindependence Ghana (Rathbone 2000; Nugent 1995), their symbolic status has grown in the age of democracy. Development projects cast chiefs as representatives of "indigenous knowledge" (Yarrow 2008b), while the constitution charges them with the work of modernizing customs. Dr. Adjei was unusual in how closely he cultivated these relationships; his friendship with the chief of Bolgatanga (the Bolganaba), Martin Abilba III, the most powerful of the Frafra chiefs, lasted more than thirty years. "When I first opened my clinic, I made friends with the chief," Dr. Adjei told me. "He found out I liked jazz and we spent many evenings listening to my albums." This friendship helped secure legitimacy for RHI campaigns, as the Bolganaba was an ardent proponent of anticutting campaigns. In turn, Dr. Adjei employed Gina, the chief's daughter, to work for his NGO. When Gina introduced me to her father, he told me that Dr. Adjei did not have to convince him to advocate against cutting, as he was already in agreement. The Bolganaba said: "Honestly speaking, Adjei virtually became part of the family when he was here. He thought, 'This is a young chief with very modern ideas' that he could tap and utilize for consumption." The chief also appreciated Dr. Adjei's hands-on involvement in providing medical services and public health outreach:

> Though we were working on other doctors, they never showed so much or keen interest in the community like he did. He comes from the South, but he loved to stay in the North and work for the northerner. We can say . . . we can give him credit for that.

As the Bolganaba told it, it was he who "worked on" the doctor, not the other way around.

Village chiefs are less influential than the Bolganaba, unless they are younger, educated, and able to bring in development money. Those collaborating with RHI like having a say about which men and women are chosen as volunteers. The chiefs often suggest their own sons (they would also suggest their daughters, but their married daughters are often in a different village). Given the rate of unemployment and other forms of scarcity, being a volunteer is a coveted position, as it brings various kinds of capital: a bicycle, training, an ongoing connection to the NGO, and per diems, called "motivation," which are minimal but valued. Rural volunteers receive a dollar per day only when they attend trainings or meetings—every quarter, the volunteers were invited

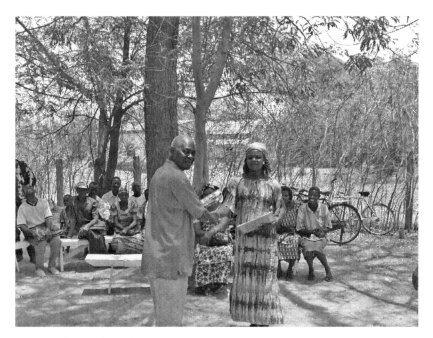

FIGURE 11. Recognizing a volunteer.

to Bolgatanga for a follow-up workshop, where they brought their report cards about services rendered and shared their stories of successful outreach—and received no other remuneration. Furthermore, though volunteering for one NGO can translate into opportunities to volunteer for others, it does not lead to employment.[2] Yet the dearth of jobs and opportunities in the region is such that many chiefs want their sons to be volunteers even if the NGO does not consider them qualified (the requirements include the ability to speak some English, the completion of some schooling, and being married). During RHI's expansion to Bawku West, the workers who had to negotiate with the chiefs were stressed about one who insisted on enrolling his unmarried son.

Those who are chosen as volunteers live in the village, where they are supposed to distribute family planning materials (including condoms), educate the youth and sexually active women and men about HIV/AIDS and family planning, dissuade women from female genital cutting, and provide referrals to clinics and hospitals. For RHI, however, the value of the volunteers lies not only in their distribution of knowledge or care but also in their mere presence in the village. They provide vital connections between the chiefs, the villagers, and the NGO, thus materializing the NGO's advocacy.

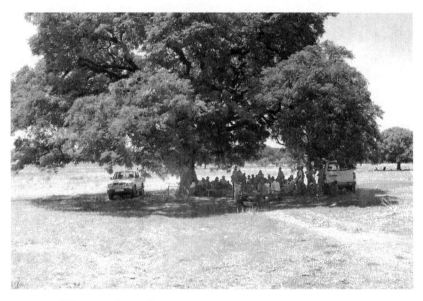

FIGURE 12. RHI community meeting.

The RHI film screening is not the villagers' first encounter with anticutting campaigns. All had heard about the dangers and harms of cutting from "the wireless" (radio) programs broadcast in local languages and English that highlight the health consequences of cutting. These radio campaigns, which range from talk show discussions with nurses to jingles produced by GAWW and other NGOs to audio dramas sponsored by the Navrongo Health Research Center, are imprinted in local memories. Some women have been visited by RHI volunteers in their homes or invited to community gatherings to discuss reasons to end cutting. Rural women also learned of the arrests of circumcisers by radio or word of mouth. While not all arrests were publicized, everyone knew about the arrests of the male circumciser from the Kassena-Nankana District and of a woman from Bawku District. As a result rural women understood that the government was willing to use the force of law to stop cutting.

Anticutting campaigns have not been as extensive in Bawku as in the Bongo, Bolgatanga, and Kassena-Nankana districts, which have been subject to numerous overlapping technologies of persuasion. In the Bongo District nurses in pre- and postnatal clinics regularly target younger women, while everyone is enjoined to discuss cutting at public events. Indeed, advocacy against cutting has become so widespread and deterritorialized that when I asked people where they were told of the harms of cutting, many responded with "at any meeting"—from women's association meetings, gatherings convened by NGOs, political parties, and youth group meetings to after-church meetings. Some of these events are lectures and others are research exercises, during which women are asked their opinions of cutting and its problems.

The Show: The NGO as Entertainment

We arrive in the village at dusk. The RHI workers order the volunteer around, and he does not get much respect—RHI workers do not mask their social position but act in concert with the larger cultural logics of visibly demonstrating and materializing hierarchy. This does not seem to detract from the volunteer's joy and excitement. He takes us to the newly built community center, a round one-room structure where the screening is to take place. The sky is clear and the moon is shining, reflecting off the center's tin roof.

The heat envelopes us as we get out of the frigid pickup, and the workers begin to set up the generator, projector, screen, and speakers. David and Martin haul the heavy equipment, and the women carry the accessories. A number of children gather around right away, but none comes to me or calls me *solemiya, nasara* (a white person, a foreigner). The music and film screening are far more exciting than a white stranger. David puts on a tape with music videos and the children start dancing immediately. Adults gather gradually, reposing on baobab tree branches, wooden benches, and chairs.

In theory the music is the bait. Like many villages in the region, this one does not have electricity, and radios are the primary electronic technology of news and entertainment. In this context RHI's arrival is nothing short of a spectacle. RHI workers first show music and film clips, which they refer to as comedy—things that make you laugh. The films include Nollywood dramas (from the Nigerian film industry) and Japanese action films, and the music clips feature scantily clad West African women dancing to hip-hop. RHI workers say entertainment will be brief, but in practice it usually runs for more than an hour. They consider the real public service to be the shows' entertainment value, and when they talk about the screenings, they characterize the music clips and films as valuable goods. On the one hand, these are an incentive to stay for the public health films, but they also work in conjunction with them to tantalize the rural women and men, compelling them to participate in the consumption of national and international popular culture.

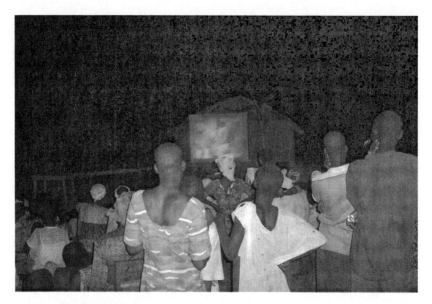

FIGURE 13. RHI's public health drama.

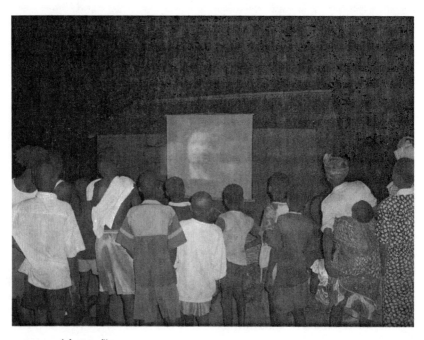

FIGURE 14. A feature film.

The volunteers covet the screenings and implore RHI workers to bring the videos to their village. Given the contingencies of travel and NGO work, the film-screening team does not visit all villages, and volunteers complain when their villages are passed over, pleading with the NGO not to leave them out. RHI workers respond to these complaints by appealing to the moral economy of distributing valuable goods, that is, by detailing the work that lies ahead of them, and noting that they have to show the movie in new communities before revisiting old ones. This involves fine-grained discussions of fairness—everyone deserves a chance at enjoyment, they say, but volunteers must remember that "other people should enjoy as well."

The entertainment videos cut into the time allowed for the subsequent public health films, each of which lasts half an hour. RHI workers therefore rarely show all three, engaging in a kind of triage. If we find ourselves in a village far from main roads and border crossings, RHI workers put away the HIV/AIDS film, since truck drivers are thought to be the main vectors of the disease and the film, which is in English, is the least entertaining. In a village where they know that cutting has ceased (despite official claims to the contrary), they do not show the film on cutting. The family planning film is the only sine qua non, both because the state is worried about the region's birthrate, and because RHI's donor, UNFPA, continues to prioritize family planning despite the official shift to reproductive rights.

The RHI team settles down as the screening begins. Our bodies are confused by the radical change in temperature, and everyone is drowsy. After setting up the equipment, the workers return to the pickup and climb into the bed. They do not mingle with the villagers or talk with them. Social interaction remains confined within social boundaries. Hidden from view, the workers talk quietly to each other for the rest of the evening. Except for Martin.

Martin, who was hired just a month earlier, is concerned about the language gap and is worried that people won't understand the film. RHI is expanding its outreach programs to the Bawku West District, but there is no film in Kusaal, the main language spoken there. The HIV/AIDS film is in English, and the locally filmed dramas on family planning and female genital cutting are in Gurene. Kusaal and Gurene are related and somewhat mutually intelligible, but they are distinct languages within the Mole-Dagbani language family (which belongs to the larger Gur family).

As the film begins, Martin sidles up to the crowd and motions to translate certain parts, so that the audience can follow the story. Martin is enthusiastic about his work. He was hired because of his fluency in Kusaal, and he understands translation as a part of his job. Emilia confronts him immediately, arguing that people will understand the film without the translation. "We can't allow them to ask questions now," she adds. Martin says he is only offering to "translate a bit, not to allow questions" but demurs when he doesn't receive support from the others. Although he is the only Kusaal speaker on the team, he is a newcomer and has not yet earned any professional authority.

Martin was convinced that the words spoken in the film matter and that the dialogue needs to be translated precisely so that it is understandable and persuasive. He is alone in this belief. The other RHI workers treat the plot and visual imagery as communicative and persuasive in their own right. For them the power of the film lies in its visual and suggestive character, not in its transparency. In fact, translation would only detract from the value of the film.

The RHI workers also worried that translation might invite interruptions, which would challenge order and authority. Their objections to translation are in part grounded in a refusal of dialogue, with its implications of horizontal power relations valued in liberal rationality, and attest to the acceptance of hierarchical relations, crowd management, and order. The dialectics of order and disorder govern the conduct of many meetings and workshops; at these events NGOs and donors try to manage crowds by containing them. For instance, when Ghanaian-run donor organizations hold workshops for northern NGOs in Bolgatanga, they rarely allow breaks. They ask, "Can we continue and eat lunch when we finish?" or "Shall we power through?" and proceed without waiting for an answer. To allow the scheduled break, the conveners believe, is to invite an eruption of chaos: "They [participants] would leave and not come again." At the very least, participants would start talking on the phone and return late to the conversation; to prevent the anticipated disorder, the conveners tightly control movement and speech.[3] Given the fragile nature of their authority, RHI workers try to shield themselves from the analytical gaze; allowing people to ask questions would mean subjecting the workers' knowledge to excessive contestation. In short, one reason for refusing to interpret the films is that the RHI workers believe they maintain their authority by controlling the space and the possibility of speech.

Martin is, however, allowed to translate the last film of the evening. When David switches the tape and starts the HIV/AIDS film, which is in English, nobody opposes Martin's announcement that he will translate. This didactic documentary presumes some knowledge of English, which few rural people understand. But Martin has learned his lesson and keeps the translation to a minimum.

The suspicion of dialogue is also apparent in the question-and-answer period. Contrary to RHI's stated plans to hold a liberal dialogue in the form of discussions, actual verbal exchange is brief and predictable. No discussion groups are formed, and the RHI workers do not initiate any debate. Only a few ask questions, and these are elderly men who state their objections to family planning. The elderly men have to object to something, as this is how they perform their authority. Martin responds enthusiastically by mobilizing the modernizing discourse of family planning. Although the relationships constructed in NGO spaces are overtly hierarchical, the exchange is nevertheless playful, and Martin cedes some ground and makes some jokes. There is an art to argument in Ghana, and many people excel at it. Arguing is a form of engaging, and to refrain from arguing is to absent oneself from the social sphere. The RHI workers are instructed to share information and promote open discussion, but they know that innuendo, ambiguity, playfulness, and the mastery of rhetorical contestation are keys to producing persuasive knowledge.

Spectacle as Persuasion

What difference does a visual spectacle make? Why didn't RHI rely on radio jingles, audio dramas, and volunteer activity, like other NGOs and the Navrongo Health Research Center? The volunteers' enthusiasm for bringing screenings to their villages hint at the value placed on this particular form of public health education. I want to suggest that the technological spectacle materialized and legitimized the public health apparatus, as well as governmental power more generally.

The postcolonial state, writes Achille Mbembe, instantiates its power by sharing the symbolism of splendor, indulgence, and theatricality with the governed and by inviting their participation therein (2001). Anthropologists have substantiated this claim. Piot discusses how the Togolese president of nearly forty years, Eyadéma, would, with his cabinet and TV crews in tow, fly his helicopter around northern Togo to attend the annual wrestling matches that constitute male initiation ceremonies (1999). "The reason Eyadéma attends so assiduously to ritual," Piot writes, "is that he understands the power and importance of spectacle—that his power will not be 'real' to his subjects until it is made manifest and visible (in ritual)" (1999: 101). Jean and John Comaroff point to older genealogies of theatrical power in encounters between the Tswana and missionaries; the missionaries bestowed gifts on the chiefs and then staged elaborate feasts in full view of the Tswana (Comaroff and Comaroff 1991). The exchanges began not with words or with translation but "were visual, aural, and tactile, a trade of perceptions" (181). Upon their arrival in a Tswana village, the missionaries displayed their objects—their wagons, tents, and "goods of strange power" (182)—and then feasted, served by black servants, as the Tswana watched them.

Governmental power is materialized in the form of spectacular arrivals, and it is in relation to this production of authority that I interpret the RHI workers' appearance in the village as a performance of technological spectacle. The film screening is more than public health education. The ritualized spectacle communicates to the village that NGOs and the state are authorities with the power to govern the lives of the villagers. After the RHI workers initiate the encounter with gifts to the chiefs, the RHI team materializes governmental power through the staging of their visit, use of multiple technologies, and the visualization of worlds near and far through the films they show. Certainly, the NGO workers are not cabinet members, a pickup truck is not a helicopter, and contemporary Ghana is democratic, neoliberal, and ambivalent about the symbolism of state splendor. The state no longer sponsors grand socialist monuments and authoritarian spectacles as it did in the era immediately after independence. The government at times represents itself as modest, at times as incapable of providing social welfare, and at times as magnificent, and the symbols of NGOs' governmental power are mundane and subdued, enacted in a minor key. But these minor symbols, mobile electric power and visual technology, in the service of producing shared affect, should not be underestimated, as they have the ability to conjure worlds and act upon subjects. The pickup, generator, projector, screen, and the films were seen as an assemblage of artifacts that not only symbolize but instantiate RHI as a powerful and therefore authoritative institution.

Deadly Harm: A Drama in Three Acts

The RHI film about cutting develops national pedagogies of persuasion in the form of cautionary tales about the deadly harm of circumcision. Cowritten by Dr. Adjei and a local playwright, the film was produced in collaboration with a village-based drama group. It is set in a village much like the one I lived in; most characters live in mud huts, wear simple clothes, and speak Gurene. The film presents its case about the dangers of cutting in three acts, each of which follows a different moral narrative.

In the first act a group of villagers arranges for their two daughters to be circumcised. The film shows a family in the midst of a heated discussion, during which one daughter agrees to be cut, and the other refuses. The parents yell at the one who refused and beat her until she relents. On the day of the cutting she sneaks out of the house at dawn and hides in a neighboring compound, where she hopes to be safe. However, the host notifies her parents, who then come to collect her. The next scene is the cutting itself. Five half-naked girls are on the ground, struggling in pain, held down by adult women. The girl who did not want to be circumcised is shown with blood running all over her body; the circumciser's hands are covered in blood as well. The girl does not stop bleeding and dies, devastating her family.

In the second act the film shows an elegantly dressed, Twi-speaking married couple who are visiting the wife's family. Their language reveals that they live in southern Ghana, the more affluent and ostensibly more modern part of the country, where most women are uncut. The wife is weeping, and it becomes clear that her husband has decided to leave her. The husband says that he is divorcing her, because she does not enjoy having sex with him. He claims that she does not enjoy sex because of her circumcision and admonishes her parents for having cut her. The wife's parents fall to their knees and beg him to keep their daughter as a wife, but their pleading is in vain.

In the third act a pregnant woman is trying to deliver a baby. The helper, cast as a traditional birth attendant, announces that the pregnant woman's scars, remnants of her cutting, are making the delivery impossible. The woman and her baby are in danger of dying. The family rushes the woman to a hospital where she safely delivers the baby. Afterward the doctor tells the family that the woman almost died and explains to them that they should not cut women.

A death of a girl, a social death of a woman and her family by way of rejection and divorce, and a near-death of a mother and child. Some of the most grievous social ills—biological death, social death, and shaming—are, according to the film, direct outcomes of cutting. The film reminds viewers about the known dangers of cutting (however rare), and performatively establishes a causal relationship between cutting and death or near-death. But rather than highlighting the bodily harms of cutting in biomedical terms, RHI situates the dangers in local lifeworlds: it is someone's daughter who dies, someone's wife who nearly dies, someone's family that is shamed. Furthermore, the film does not explicitly state the risk or causality, instead inviting the audience to reach its own conclusions. The biomedical narrative about deadly harms is implicit: when the first act portrays a situation in which one of five girls dies after being cut, no voiceover explains that fatal hemorrhage is an immediate complication of FGM or provides a specific calculation of risk, such as "20 percent of girls die from cutting." That the girl who initially rebelled is the one who dies is not coincidental but serves to instruct viewers to respect the girl's agency over her body, for she would have lived had she remained uncut. This act also implicates the neighbors, reminding the audience about the communal aspects of circumcision and the consequences of opposition to it—the girl could have survived had she found support in her village. The film, like Ghana's anticutting legislation, understands the power that wider society wields in regard to the practice.

In the second act marriage serves as a metaphor for the North-South relationship. Every northern family has members who have migrated south, and many of the latter change their habits and tastes. By showing that some women from groups that practiced cutting have married southerners, and by suggesting that others might marry northern men whose own views have changed, the film portrays change as inevitable. It also reminds northern villagers of their role in the nation-state by depicting them as inferior, lagging behind the counterparts in the richer and more cosmopolitan South. The choice of marriage as a staging ground is also a direct response to Ghanaian concerns about the transformation of marriage as a social institution. While young northern men have difficulty scraping together their bridewealth, and women must wait for their boyfriends to do so, the dominant social narrative is concerned with premarital and, to a lesser extent, marital sexual morality (see also Smith 2014). The film intervenes in these debates not by focusing on sexual morality such as chastity and virginity but by promoting new notions of familial gender relations and the place of cutting within them. The father no longer has the authority to arrange a daughter's or a son's matrimonial future. And while cutting once was the prerequisite for a successful marriage, the film argues, cutting now interferes with it, frustrating aspirations for prosperity and social mobility. Cutting is no longer a source of pride but a source of shame and disgrace.

A closer look at the husband's shaming authority hints at the NGO's patriarchal bargain: the film suggests that decision making about cutting should be solely in hands of girls but men should retain all say about sexuality and marriage. To introduce the discourse of sexuality is to enter a treacherous field, which RHI contains by assigning interest in sexual pleasure to the husband. The wife does not enjoy (hetero)sexual acts, but it is the husband who is upset about this. Rendering the husband's control of the wife's sexuality the linchpin of the modern marriage insinuates that marriage should remain a patriarchal institution but one in which the authority has passed from the father to the husband, who may dissolve it at will.

Act 3 is overtly didactic, as it presents a delivery scene that instantiates biomedical expertise and state-backed authority in the person of the doctor, who not only saves the woman and child but also lectures her family about the harmful consequences of cutting. The film reminds viewers of the biomedical power of doctors and hospitals, but viewers are also indoctrinated in physicians' right to lecture them, if girls keep getting cut. The doctor's response to cutting is similar to that of the wealthy husband who considers himself superior and lectures his in-laws, but the doctor's lecture is tempered, and he does not scold them. So, the film implies, the power of medicine is benign and benevolent but demands submission.

Unlike the films shown by GAWW, the affective work of the RHI films is not predicated on disgust or repugnance. Since the villagers themselves are the intended audience, the goal is to make them feel the force of governmental power without being alienated or insulted. The audience laughs when the rebellious girl fails to escape: to hide is to show weakness, and it is antithetical to the fortitude that the girls are supposed to cultivate. The representations of blood loss move the audience to different affective responses: they gasp and cry out loud when the circumciser's bloody hands are shown. The threats of divorce and embarrassment are designed to generate fear, not only of circumcision but also of being disgraced; in response some girls in the audience seem to be subdued.

The biomedical notions of harm favored by the WHO are embedded in the very form of the film, as the three-act structure mimics the categories assigned to the harms of cutting. The scenes focus on the moment of cutting ("immediate complications"), the moment of labor ("delivery complications"), and add a twist to "intermediate complications" in the guise of sexual (dis)pleasure and social death.[4] The first two moments figure prominently in public health campaigns as well as in rural narratives about cutting. One purpose of cutting was to aid reproduction, but women have always known that the act of cutting weakens their bodies and requires long recuperation, as I discuss in chapter 5. If a girl experienced unusual or exceptional difficulties, soothsayers attributed it to the spirits: the difficulties were signs that she was not supposed to be cut in the first place. Circumcisers, too, knew cutting was dangerous but had a different understanding of how to avert complications. They obeyed taboos and performed rituals, ranging from the preparation of the knives to sacrifices of animals. Furthermore, cutting was dangerous not only for girls but also for circumcisers; both needed the gods on their side: "A small boy had to go with me and whistle, as two circumcisers were not supposed to meet on their way," one former circumciser told me; if they met, they would die.

The film's narrative of complications takes the familiar form of cautionary tales, which are usually transmitted orally rather than cinematically. Cautionary tales are forms of persuasion in their own right, as they provide a bounded account of events and their causes. Such stories are one of the main forms of providing reasons and explaining cause and effect in Ghana and elsewhere; these stories purposefully delineate time and social context, placing actions and consequences within a restricted space. Stories, Charles Tilly writes, "rework and simplify social processes so that the processes become available for the telling; X did Y to Z conveys a memorable image of what happened." They establish causality by placing cause-and-effect relationships within a delineated world of individuals "whose dispositions and actions cause everything that happens" (2009: 21). Put slightly differently, stories are a form of knowledge production. As Steven Feld writes,

> Stories create analytic gestures by their need to recall, and thereby ponder, wonder, and search out layers of intersubjective significance in events, acts, and scenes. Stitching stories together is also a sense-making activity, one that signals a clear analytic awareness of the fluidity and the gaps in public and private discourses. (2012: 8)

RHI's cautionary tale establishes many points of contact with the villagers' lifeworlds, but the world of the NGO and rural worlds are not completely congruent. The film contains much that fails to correspond to rural women and men's understanding of cutting, misrepresenting decision making about the practice, girls' agency, and the desirability of cut women. An anthropologist familiar with the actual historical practice of cutting might highlight the following distortions:

It is not the parents who forced girls to get cut, the girls typically organized themselves.

Decisions about cutting were not debated at length and were often spontaneous.

Girls were able to object to cutting or refuse to get cut without being violently punished.

Women rarely die from cutting.

Many men wanted to marry cut women, not uncut ones.

Cut women do experience sexual pleasure.

Men do not object to having sex with cut women.

Cut women do not believe that cutting makes their labor difficult.

A rural birth attendant would not attribute delivery problems to cutting.

A doctor would scold villagers, not reason with them.

I would agree that this list is largely on point, but so would Dr. Adjei and the scriptwriter. Although common anthropological interpretations would contend that such deficiencies and misguided assumptions sap the film of its authority and persuasive power, Dr. Adjei and the scriptwriter would disagree—if they wrote mistakes into the film, it was because they wanted to. Their goal in producing the film was not to hold a mirror up to a historical reality but to performatively bring a new reality into being. Rather than seeing the mischaracterization of some aspects of existing practices as a reflection of the NGO's lack of knowledge or as an indication of failure, we should view them as deliberate strategies.

Why produce such errors of cultural understanding? In doing so, the NGO refuses to mediate between the values that uphold cutting and the NGO's vision of the future. To fully engage with historically contextualized meanings would mean having to endorse them. As Pigg writes, "training programs that present villagers with a theory of the connection between cosmopolitan medicine and local healing knowledge offer to villagers an officially endorsed version of something villagers themselves have been building all along" (1997: 282). By mobilizing erroneous representations of the historical contexts of cutting and the power relations embedded therein, RHI does not need to endorse them in any form. To connect biomedical and developmental understandings of FGM with nuanced cultural descriptions would lend cutting too much credibility.

But there is more to RHI's strategy. The film tries to impress upon the villagers that cutting should end not by recognizing, and thereby endorsing, local conceptions of cutting and their webs of meaning but by reorganizing how cutting is codified for governmental purposes. The NGO was not interested in depicting truths but in transforming values and exercising power. To accomplish the first it painted a picture of rural life, larger Ghanaian society, and biomedicine—not as they are now but as the NGO imagines them and wants to craft them. In that sense the film anticipates transformations that might occur in the wake of governmental redefinitions of cutting. The film teaches the villagers that parents will be seen as responsible for decisions about cutting and will risk being seen as both coercive and violent, thus foreshadowing Ghana's second law against cutting, passed in 2007, which punishes not only circumcisers but also parents (see chapters 6 and 7). It establishes a causal connection between circumcision and death by eliding the influence of ancestral gods and spirits, who were literally not in the picture and who are, many say, indeed being forgotten. Finally, the film depicts contemporary society as a place for interethnic and interregional marriages that nonetheless uphold the primacy of southern modernity.

Together these tactics are meant to demonstrate and assert the NGO's authority over the understandings and values of cutting, social and biological reproduction, and governmental force. To that end they deploy not their knowledge of the historical practices of cutting but their knowledge of locally persuasive rhetorical forms and establishment of authority.

Campaign Memories

The Bongo village in which I conducted my research had two RHI volunteers, but by happenstance this village had been left out of the film-screening campaign. To learn how the RHI film was remembered by its audience, I talked to people I knew from my research in the neighboring market, where RHI had screened the films. Faith had attended the screening, and her memory of the film was centered on the depiction of the act of cutting.

> FAITH: The film they showed, there was a family that was forcing their daughter to go and [get] cut.[5] She ran to the next home, and the people there said she should stay, they would hide her. But they gave her to the parents and said, "How can a girl of your age refuse to get cut!" They cut her and she died.
>
> SAIDA: What did you make of the film?
>
> FAITH: The film had meaning to me.

Faith said the story resonated with her because she, too, had debated whether to get cut, albeit it in quite different circumstances. The story made a lasting impression and had meaning for her, despite the misrepresentations of cutting and the various fabricated details.

Paul, the RHI volunteer in Balungo, drew my attention to the materializing power of the film-screening team: the arrival of RHI confirmed that he and other volunteers had been "speaking the truth." Paul had been a volunteer since 1997 and had carved out a professional niche for himself by volunteering for various other NGOs and government agencies, from the Red Cross to Ghana Health Services. He was one of the people from whom I learned how the films were received in the immediate aftermath of the screening. The RHI arrival caused a sensation, he told me:

> After the film show, it was the talk of the entire community. When people would see me, they said, "What we have been telling them about cutting is true." But on the family planning side, they had some reservations. Some would say, "If you give birth to three children and they die, what then?"

According to Paul, the very fact of the film's screening was persuasive. That RHI arrived in the village in a mobile spectacle, was led by a doctor, and was aligned with chiefs and government officials was in and of itself convincing. The NGO speaks the language of power, and power produces knowledge that counts. More people objected to the film about family planning—public opposition to it is pronounced, especially among older men. In everyday life many young women practice biomedical forms of family planning despite the objections of their male relatives. In contrast, there is little public opposition to anticutting campaigns. By the time RHI started its campaign, cutting had already been devalued and outlawed and was ending. Indeed, rural women and men I knew were afraid of the law, which had an omnipresence. Even though criminalization of cutting and the threat of arrest are purposefully left out of RHI's film and its other educational campaigns, those subject to the law were well aware of it.

Paul told me that he was asked why cutting still occurred in the village depicted in the film, given that it had been outlawed: "People also asked, if in those communities there are no CBDs [community-based distributors], because I and other CBDs in this community tell them if we hear of any case, we will arrest the perpetrators." By saying that people asked "if in those communities there are no CBDs," Paul was talking about himself as much as he was talking about the demise of cutting and the responses to the film, picturing himself as an effective volunteer who was respected for his connection to the NGO. But I, too, had noticed the hyperawareness surrounding the law:

nearly everyone with whom I had spoken about cutting brought up the law early in the conversation. Paul suggested that the volunteers contributed to this awareness and implied that they contributed to the ending of cutting not solely through the power of education but also through threats of arrest and the invocation of state violence. In an important sense, as I demonstrate in chapters 6 and 7, Paul and the villagers were correct—the participation of volunteers and civil servants does make law enforcement possible. So although the RHI film presents their public health campaigns as a benign power, the organization is implicated in law enforcement, not separate from it.

The villagers' surprise at the persistence of cutting is a reminder that NGO interventions are not the only factor in the cessation of cutting but rather are coeval with other social processes. Faith was one of several women who had decided not to get cut several years before the film screening; for her the screening confirmed a decision she had already made. For many others in this village, the RHI project reinforced something they had already been told. As Paul told me,

> People said that what we have been telling them is true. "See how blood is coming out!" As part of the play, there was a point in time, some girls organized themselves and went to get cut. So when they were cutting them, people realized it was painful, so they were wailing. Another session of the film was about a woman who was cut and is now in labor. She was finding it difficult. So people said what we have been telling them is true.

Development projects are often imagined as targeting naive audiences. At the time of my research, for instance, the Navrongo Health Research Center was studying how three different villages responded to three different models of anticutting campaigns. Built into the experimental design was the notion that the villages were isolated from one another and, more important, had not already experienced anticutting campaigns. But the aftermath of the RHI film screening shows that development ideas are part of what Pigg calls a "recursive process," according to which "the representations implicit in every new model recombine with signifiers already in circulation" (1997: 281).

When I asked Paul whether anyone had ever contested what the RHI film depicted about the harms of cutting, he made it clear that my question was misplaced, passionately replying:

> You know that twenty years ago, in this community girls used to get cut. Our mothers are all cut. So when they saw the play, they knew it's true. When one is going to cut, they go with the *bito* [a tree used for food and

medicine] fiber, so that after the cutting, they weave it and put it around the waist. So when they saw those [fibers] in the film, they saw it's true.

For Paul the familiar aspects of the film, such as its cautionary narrative, its visual verisimilitude, and its symbolism, verify the truth of the NGO's claims. The representations of blood and difficult labor justify the FGM discourse—the imperative to eradicate cutting—but representations of the *bito* fibers are proof that the NGO also knows something about the elements of *yabega ŋma*. In other words the film did not need to get everything right in order to be persuasive. And according to the regional style of communicating power, it should not. Persuasive rhetoric does not reveal everything.

In his ethnography of male initiation rituals in north-central Togo, Charles Piot highlights the implicit communicative power of symbols similar to the *bito* fibers. He was told:

> Someone who has *hama*—someone who can do extraordinary things like jump over buildings or, like the president, survive a plane crash—doesn't come out and admit that he has it. *Hama* is not something you talk about. It remains hidden. But at the time of certain dances, and *waaya* is one of these, you can reveal to others whether you have it or not. One way you can do this is through the color of the animal sack you wear around your neck. A red skin [from a fox or a goat] indicates that you have *hama*. (Piot 1999: 93)

Scholars of West Africa have long stressed the different layers of knowledge in the region. Claims on knowledge and truth in West Africa, Mariane Ferme writes, are structured by the "primacy of the concealed in understanding the visible" (2001: 4). In societies organized not only by NGOs and the state but also by the nontransparent and potent powers of gods and material objects, the knowledge that counts often lies in the "underneath of things" (Ferme 2001). Authoritative knowledge does not float on transparent surfaces but resides in the depths (Apter 2005), subject to secrecy and interpretation.[6] Not everyone should have access to such knowledge, as Michelle Johnson found in the Gambia. While she was interviewing an Islamic scholar about passages in the Qur'an that proscribe cutting, she was told that she would not be able to detect them, because it took years of learning before one could do so (2000).

This form of knowledge has pedagogical repercussions, because in this context truths are to be discerned, not stated didactically. As Ferme argues, value is attached to "verbal artistry that couches meaning in puns, riddles, and cautionary tales, and to unusual powers of understanding that enable people to both produce and unmask highly ambiguous meanings" (2001: 4). She continues:

> The skill to see beyond the visible phenomenon and to interpret deeper meanings is, then, a culturally valued and highly contested activity, because on it are predicated all social and political actions and different forms of wealth. It is a skill that bridges a gap between the history and the present, between old and new technologies of communication. (4)

Dr. Adjei and the RHI workers would object to any overt association with esoteric knowledge (Apter 2005), or multiple gods and plural sovereigns (Singh 2012), but he and the RHI workers deploy their understandings of rhetorical styles, assembling the historical forms of knowledge authorized by them and new technologies of communication, such as the film screening.[7] Dr. Adjei and the RHI workers do not need to translate words or produce verisimilitudes because images signal RHI's deeper knowledge of the ritual. The film works rhetorically by inviting villagers to interpret the symbolism, which involves seeing beyond the visible. Hence the film need not be discussed in the form of a liberal dialogue, as officially planned.

RHI knew how to mobilize its knowledge of the symbolism of cutting and that representations of knowledge are only one element in materializing its power. Weaving together the symbolic materiality of elements of cutting (the blood and fibers) and facts of life (difficult labor), these representations loosely link *yabega ηma* as a lived and embodied practice and FGM as a codified object of NGO interventions. While the film misrepresented the contextual aspects of cutting, its depiction of the social object world was suggestive and, for the audience, accurate enough. Villagers recognized the symbolism contained in the film as true and saw it as evidence that the NGO had deeper insights into cutting, thus establishing the organization's claims to knowledge and authority.

Paul would seem to agree that there is something to the argument that persuasive knowledge must both particularize and universalize. As Choy puts it, "Truth must scale down—particularize—at the same time that it scales up—universalize. . . . Universality is suspect . . . at the same time that particularity is insufficiently authoritative" (2005: 9). However, if this claim is to hold in this context, it would need to be extended beyond translation and consider how NGOs draw on a wider range of communicative registers. These include refusals to translate words, deliberate mistakes, and matters of power and performative spectacle. I want to suggest that the NGO's assertions about the harmfulness of cutting were received as true when presented in technological spectacles that materialized and legitimized the public health apparatus, as well as governmental power more generally. But first a note about truth.

Once, while I was walking through the village with Paul, an elderly man from Paul's family joined us and struck up a conversation, repeating what Paul had said about the confirmation of truth. When the doctor arrived and showed the films, the man said, the people knew that what Paul had been saying was true. It was clear that both the screening and Dr. Adjei's presence lent authority to Paul's words, but what exactly was confirmed as true was left unsaid. Was it that cutting was harmful? Or that "the people from Bolga" and "the doctor" said so? Either way, Paul's uncle now knew that people in power understand cutting as harmful and are willing to act on that understanding.

Dialogue and Liberal Fantasies of Care

Anthropologists often focus on the content of public health interventions, since, as Elyachar puts it, we are "used to thinking, perhaps because research is our own native culture, that content is what makes research unique" (2006: 415). However, donors to RHI and other development organizations give form equal importance. They expect that efforts to persuade will take the form of a participatory dialogue. Open and frank discussion (Pigg 2005: 44) and reasoned debate are valorized as model technologies of public health education and social change; coercion and verbal artistry are eschewed. The outreach efforts of both RHI and GAWW are envisioned as embodying and promoting horizontal, liberal dialogue.

In general Dr. Adjei is a proponent of these ideas. I watched him encourage everyone to join in discussions during village visits; he was particularly happy about rural women's participation in group discussions and considered their speech a form of liberation. Unofficially he viewed the NGO as at least partially successful because women were now speaking publicly, whereas in the past, he said, they had been silent. The earlier silence may not reflect women's subordination within the village, as they may have acted upon an understanding that in the hierarchical context of an encounter with an NGO, they do not have a right to speak. But I touch on the issue of speech and dialogue to point to Dr. Adjei's beliefs in liberal ideals; he did not merely profess adherence to them to curry favor with donors. He also knew to present the screenings in terms donors would appreciate, describing the NGO as promoting a "culturally sensitive" approach to the abandonment of cutting that tries to improve "gender equity" by way of "sharing information" and fostering discussion. Consider the following excerpt from an RHI report to UNFPA:

> Under the current 4th GOG/UNFPA programme, Rural Help Integrated has been mandated to strengthen the implementation of an innovative and *culturally sensitive integrated Community Based* Reproductive Health Service delivery in the Bolgatanga, Bongo and Bawku West Districts of the Upper East Region of Ghana. The long-term goal is to have contributed to the improvement of the quality, accessibility, and demand for reproductive health services and improved gender equity in the Upper East Region of Ghana.... Seventeen (17) Video shows were organized in the second quarter of 2004. The films were on family planning, female genital mutilation and HIV/AIDS. After the video shows, the community is grouped into smaller units to *facilitate easy discussions*. During the discussion a lot of *information is shared* on STIs/ HIV/AIDS and other Reproductive Health issues. The patronage in the quarter was very high about 500 community members on the average attended each show *[sic]*. During the Video Shows, the *youth are usually grouped for discussions* on Reproductive Health issues including HIV/AIDS. An average of 500 youth often attend the Video Shows. They are given the opportunity to ask various questions on RH issues and HIV/AIDS and answers are provided. (emphasis added)[8]

Although the report stresses RHI's compliance with liberal norms, in practice RHI workers habitually ignored the mandate to facilitate discussions and promote open dialogue. They saw the screenings as sufficiently educational in themselves and neither formed groups after "the shows" nor left much time for questions or debates. The youth the report mentions were never a specific target audience and never spoke; elderly male villagers were the only people who regularly asked questions. But rather than criticizing the NGO for preventing liberal dialogue, we should recognize that the NGO's materialization of hierarchy is constitutive of its success. The hierarchical structure of interaction and exchange reflects larger social norms that RHI had no interest in disturbing. As Erica Bornstein has shown, efforts to disrupt these larger social hierarchies at times say more about the desires and intentions of those of us with egalitarian aspirations than they do of these efforts' potential for pragmatic success (2012).

The tension between the NGO's liberal ideals and its practices mirrors the deeper structure of anticutting campaigns. While donors write governmental power out of the project designs, Ghanaian NGOs do not hide the fact that there is nothing horizontal about the NGO's relationship to the villagers or the ideas presented in the educational films. To be sure, some campaigns are more coercive than others—hence the opposition by Dr. Adjei and the Navrongo Health Research Center to GAWW's goal of eradicating cutting by way of legal advocacy and law enforcement—but all NGOs must continually navigate between ideal-typic interventions and the forms they take in practice. Anticutting campaigns, in Ghana and elsewhere, are increasingly promoted as primarily benevolent efforts toward social mobilization in the name of "abandoning" cutting. In practice the campaigns rely on overt and subtle materializations of social hierarchy, shaming, and the invocation of sovereign violence in the form of punitive legislation. Although they aim to devalue cutting, not the people who practice it, they end up devaluing and diminishing both. The liberal imagination that many NGOs share with international organizations, such as the UNFPA-UNICEF Joint Programme on Female Genital Mutilation/Cutting: Accelerating Change, is that cutting can be eliminated without the coercive, manipulative mechanisms of shaming, imprisonment, or mobilization of alarm. That RHI belies this fantasy despite its own liberal aspirations is not a testament to a faulty execution of an otherwise laudable form but an invitation to critical reflection about contemporary governmentality that promises to offer care without "casualties" (Ticktin 2011).

RESIGNIFICATION AND NGO-OLOGY

RHI aims to resignify lifeworlds, meanings, and values, not to represent them. The NGO is not alone in this goal: other NGOs focus even less on historical practices, eschewing accurate representations, translation, and dialogue. As we saw in chapter 2, GAWW's method of teaching nurses was not to forge connections between FGM and the various practices of cutting but to teach them about FGM as such. Recall that to illustrate the harms of FGM, Mrs. Mahama mobilized ideologies of modernization, the World Health Organization's *Female Genital Mutilation: A Student's Manual* (2001) and Waris Dirie's book—a ghost-written autobiography aimed at Western audiences about a Somalian woman living in Europe—as well as secondhand stories of suffering and information from newspapers. Rather than asking the nurses to connect FGM to their own experiences of caring for cut women, GAWW asked them to make sense of FGM by aligning it with other "harmful traditional practices." The purpose was not to forge a link between FGM and lived experience but to redefine and reclassify interpretive frameworks.[9]

I want to stress that GAWW's rejection of translation was not caused by its members' lack of knowledge. Although it has not always been the case, the current leadership and workers (except for Hope, the GAWW office worker) are all from northern Ghana, and all are from groups that once practiced cutting. As Musa, the other GAWW employee, put it, "Mrs. Mahama is also from a traditional house."

Interestingly, GAWW, like RHI, also draws on indigenous forms while setting aside indigenous concepts and values. GAWW designed the *ludo* game to inform girls and boys from northern Ghana of the dangers of cutting—part of the recent governmental turn to youth as subjects of intervention—and vernacularized the form of the lesson but not its content. In Ghana *ludo* is played on wooden boards; GAWW deliberately mimicked this form as a platform for the version it designed and distributed in areas where cutting was thought to persist. GAWW's game was printed on expensive laminated plastic sheets and was treated as a special good, to be kept for playing only "under supervision."

The game leaves behind the "harmful traditional practices" model and inserts FGM into a complex of worries about HIV/AIDS, STDs, early sex, and sexual abuse. In their outreach programs GAWW workers sometimes make a case for the connections between FGM and these issues, but they leave them at the level of mere suggestion. The ultimate pedagogical aim of the game is to convey something about the codified concept of FGM as such. One of the question cards that GAWW sends donors as an illustration of its approach contains the following prompts:

> Give the full meaning of the term FGM.
> What is FGM?
> How many types of FGM do we have?
> Is FGM practiced on Boys or Girls?

Note that GAWW does not link FGM to a vernacular, by asking, for instance, "What is FGM called in your language?" Instead youth are to be taught about FGM as a stand-alone concept, a discursive reality in its own right. The game invites young Ghanaians to oppose cutting, and it encourages them to make a leap, jump across the "tracks," and hop aboard the national train.

PRIDE (Programme for Rural Integrated Development), the community-based NGO from the Bongo District, is even less interested in the content of reproductive health education. In addition to teaching villagers about a range

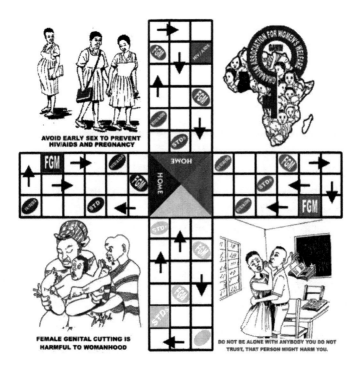

FIGURE 15. GAWW's ludo game (courtesy of GAWW).

of "harmful traditional practices," it focuses on what we might call NGO-ology. Consider the following event. When PRIDE project officers, as their workers are called, arrived at a village primary school to administer a competition for students who had participated in their training, their questions were not about reproductive health but about the meanings of NGO acronyms, general development terminology, and the structure of PRIDE itself. In the first round they quizzed students on basic acronyms, such as NGO, TBA, CBD (readers may know these by now) and others that were used less frequently. Students took turns responding, and the workers and various volunteers nudged them along in good humor. The acronym TBA (traditional birth attendant) means "treatment be faithful," one volunteer joked, referencing HIV/AIDS; the other workers laughed.

Students who advanced past the first round were asked more specific questions, such as "Mention two CBDs in your community." In the final round all the questions were about PRIDE: "Who is the project officer for PRIDE Bongo? How many communities does PRIDE work with in the Bongo District? What year did PRIDE enter your community for family reproductive health?" and so on. A surprising number of students knew answers to some of these questions. On the front table PRIDE workers had spread out notebooks, pencils, and packages of salt. Students who scored the most points received awards that the PRIDE workers distributed with evident joy; they clapped for each student and praised them: "You have all tried." Constance, my research assistant, and I were asked to honor the students by handing out the prizes.

I observed the competition with disbelief and recalled a memory from my own childhood; on top of my ethnographic notebook I jotted down "Titovim Stazama Revolucije," or (Following) Tito's Revolutionary Paths. When I was growing up in Yugoslavia, all students participated in an annual extracurricular competition; we were supposed to learn about Tito's life, his importance, and his participation in Yalta, Crimea, and other historic events and socialist revolutionary organs. The point was not to learn about the deeper principles of socialism or why revolution mattered. I never won this competition and felt ashamed that I did not do better. All this is to say that an ideology that impels participation generates its own meanings, affects, and aspirations.

CONCLUSION

I want to return to Pigg's provocative question: "Can bad social analysis result in good development programs?" (1997: 275). Puncturing the still common anthropological doxa that failure results from a lack of knowledge, Pigg argues that development projects can succeed even if they operate on faulty epistemic assumptions:

> However flawed the development understanding of shamans and their activities might be as cultural description, the comparison they make between shamans and doctors appears to be plausible to all the people involved in the trainings . . . shamans appear willing to cooperate, whether or not they are misunderstood. (1997: 275)

In the same vein, rural women and men have been willing to cooperate with the NGOs and consider their messages, even though the messages at some level misrepresent their values and practices. Misrepresentations of cutting did not detract from the programs' achievements in helping to end it. But I want to push this point further and propose that misrepresentation and poor translation are not always the result of bad social analysis: sometimes they are the products of intentional strategies of communicating which knowledge and values matter and how they matter. We need to uncouple misrepresentation and lack of knowledge just as much as we need to uncouple misrepresentation and failure.

That campaign planners operationalize incorrect assumptions or inaccurate cultural descriptions does not mean that is the only knowledge they have at their disposal. As I have shown, representations of the contexts of cutting were culturally inaccurate by design, and the omissions, misunderstandings, and mistakes were purposeful. While the historical conception of cutting envisions it as a socially productive practice, the film portrays it as socially and physiologically destructive. By refusing to render *yabega ŋma* commensurable with FGM, RHI deliberately devalued historical meanings of cutting, representing it not as what it is but as what it will be in the eyes of authorities and Ghanaian public culture. RHI thus left it up to the rural women and men to negotiate how, with respect to their view of cutting and their place in the Ghanaian social order, they see themselves and how they are to be seen.

The film's "buy-in" was enabled, at least in part, by its mobilization of knowledge about the forms of *yabega ŋma* as well as about locally relevant forms of persuasion and power. The NGO understood some relevant cultural forms and the secret knowledge entailed in them, and the organization knew not to make this knowledge too transparent. Knowledge, as I have shown, sometimes derives its power from innuendo, not from transparency, and the film successfully employed the suggestive power of images, symbols, and cautionary tales.

Although many rural Ghanaians have become convinced of the need to end cutting (not just by the NGO but by many layers of interventions), their understandings of cutting and its harms are not fully congruent with the NGO's. Evaluations of the truth and meaning of the film are both echoed and made more complicated by rural women who affirm that NGOs are right—but not about everything. As I discuss in chapter 5, anticutting campaigns have been successful at achieving their aims but not because NGO discourses are accepted in their entirety. Rather than fully accept NGO advocacy or engage in wholesale resistance to it, rural women evaluate what it leaves unaddressed and refuse the institutionalization of governmental meanings. As NGOs succeeded in contributing to the ending of cutting, the unintended consequence of their projects is not failure but a critique of their platforms.

Women in Bongo Say

If the chief summons you, you have to go, but you can refuse any errand he
  gives you.

Have I spoken well?

Why are you asking these questions?

Thank you for coming to talk to us. It is good to think about these things.

Tell her the truth!

You should stay with us long, long.

Bring Afua a grinding machine.

I will call your mother and I will greet her.

Invite your daughter [my research assistant] to go with you to America.

Blood Loss and Slow Harm
in Times of Scarcity

WE DON'T HAVE ENOUGH BLOOD

Nitu, my housemate in Bolgatanga, came home distressed and puzzled from her job at an NGO called Widows and Orphans Ministry. A widow supported by the NGO was hospitalized and needed a blood transfusion, but the hospital did not have blood available; the doctors, following usual practice, asked for family donations. When the NGO workers went to the village to look for her family, they were rebuked and told: "You give her blood!" Nitu knew that a widow who was supported by the NGO could expect that her extended family—more specifically, the patrilineal and virilocal family she married into—would refuse to care for her, as widows had become some of the most vulnerable women in the region.[1] The family might have reproached the NGO because they suspected that she had AIDS and thus saw her as undeserving of care, or they might have considered the NGO to be the more appropriate care provider, given the inequality between themselves and the seemingly wealthier and healthier NGO workers.[2] One thing was certain: by refusing, the family members acted upon a common understanding that donating blood would compromise their own health.

In contrast to the biomedical narrative that posits the easy replenishment of donated blood, many Ghanaians have come to see blood as precious and scarce. In recent years apprehension about the lack of blood—with respect to both people's bodies, in the form of anemia, and the country's blood banks and hospitals, in the form of meager institutional reserves of donated blood—have congealed into a discourse about *national* blood shortages. Blood shortage is now understood as a collective condition and seen as a public health crisis provoked by the state's biopolitical failures. What is more, in Ghanaian public culture, the semiotics and value of blood speak to more than questions of health and the politics of life: blood is understood as a vital and powerful resource for wealth accumulation (Meyer 2003; Gilbert 2006; Garritano 2012) and is considered a valuable substance that circulates in "occult economies" (Comaroff and Comaroff 1999b).

My own interest in understanding the ties between individual and collective blood shortages, Ghana's biopolitics, and critiques of occult economies is motivated by my research in the rural Bongo District with women who were the subjects of NGO interventions. In 2009 I realized that blood was a key to their narratives about the ending of cutting and the understanding of cutting as harmful. They now understood the ending of cutting through the narratives of blood loss, food shortages, and extraction of vital force that critically evaluate Ghana's present.

This is how Abanga, Mr. Robert's aunt, put it: "You will lose blood through menstruation, you will also lose blood during childbirth, and in addition, when you cut. Yet you won't get enough food to eat. There is no food. But in the olden days you could get enough food to eat." Abanga was the first to speak, as she was the oldest in a group of women sitting on granite boulders under a shady baobab tree, where, during the farming season, they gathered after a morning in the fields to catch the wispy breeze. They kept each other company while working—preparing the bito leaves for the evening meal, threshing and sifting millet, or weaving the hats and baskets that are a source of hard-won, meager income. I often joined them when I was living in their village as the guest of Mr. Robert, a development worker and local politician, and his wife, Afua, a budding seamstress. This time, on a dry June day in 2009, the women had gathered in response to my invitation. I had returned to Ghana to learn more about the shifting meanings of cutting (*yabega ŋma*) in the wake of its demise and the enactment of the new law in 2007. The conversation turned to the waning of cutting, and Abanga emphasized that she was at peace with this change: "Any year that passes by has its own dynamics. It's with time. People no longer put holes in their noses. My own sons don't have tribal marks. It's with time that cutting faded out." Despite her equanimity about the end of cutting, Abanga was, she said, concerned about underlying blood shortages. So were others.

Rather than resisting all NGO interventions or bemoaning the end of cutting, Abanga and other cut women gave meaning to its disappearance by constructing what I will refer to as the "blood narrative." This narrative points to historical conditions that made cutting untenable. "Yes, we did

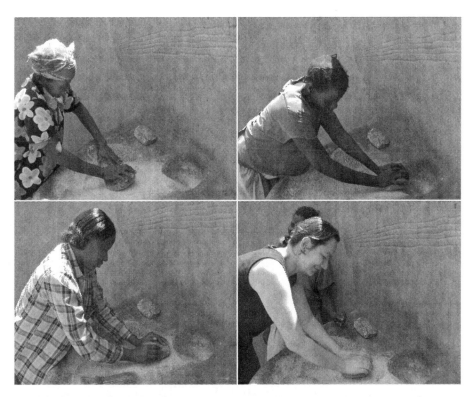

FIGURE 16. "You must learn how we work"—grinding millet.

practice cutting, and, yes, we stopped doing it, but that's not what really matters," women like Abanga say. Their actual concern resides elsewhere, in the underlying condition of their bodies, which have become predisposed to blood shortages because of food scarcity and prolonged structural violence, both of which have become particularly acute in their lifetime. I will suggest that the blood narrative reframes what counts as harm and that it does so not to contest the immediate objectives of anticutting interventions or the premise that cutting needed to end but to critique what NGOs leave unaddressed—governmental abandonment (Povinelli 2011), extraction of women's vitality, and moral economies of obligation and belonging.

The blood narrative is historically situated, not timeless. In Bongo it emerged after cutting ended around the turn of the millennium, and it has since stabilized. In earlier years I had heard concerns about blood shortages from particular women, but a decade after the demise of cutting in their village, a shared narrative emerged: cutting had to end, because women's bodies had become chronically short of blood and blood was no longer expendable. I was struck by the intensification of this notion: *all* women I conducted research with—young and old, cut and uncut—now tied the ending of cutting to efforts to safeguard blood in times of scarcity. They readily included themselves in a shared *we,* a collectivity bereft of blood and opposed to cutting. During the first decade of the twenty-first century, then, the blood narrative spread and consolidated, thus gaining traction alongside, and in response to, national anxieties about blood shortages and the rising popularity of the occult economy as a platform for critiquing extraction, exploitation, and illegitimate accumulation of wealth and resources.

The blood narrative pivots around a particular kind of reasoning about blood as a foundation of health, tying it to food scarcity and larger blood shortages in the country. Abanga's words hint at the narrative's complex logics: cutting is now seen as unworthy of blood loss and as a critical event that generates a lifelong susceptibility to ill health. This narrative addresses the macroeconomic problems that make women in Bongo unable to withstand the effects of cutting by establishing a counterfactual narrative: blood loss at cutting would be tolerable if their bodies were healthy in the first place. While these women understand cutting as causing undue suffering, they see the vulnerability of their bodies as symptomatic of a larger problem. By contrasting the lack of food in the present with its availability in, as they say, "the olden days," the narrative highlights a temporal dimension of concern about blood shortages. Cutting had to stop, they say, given the struggles of the contemporary moment, when women can no longer afford to lose blood.

In this chapter I take concerns about blood, value of blood loss, and cutting as a starting point and examine how women targeted by NGO and state interventions problematize "harm" and make sense of the end of cutting. Rural women in Ghana's Upper East Region have their own critiques of anti-cutting interventions and contemporary governance. By accounting for their perspectives on cutting and its endings, I emphasize those "critical social etiologies" (Comaroff 2007: 211) articulated by ordinary people whose lives are at stake. We shall see that the blood narrative works in concert with, and at a critical distance from, national and global problematizations of cutting and discourses about blood and crisis. I suggest that the blood narrative responds to both the ending of cutting and to the governmental institutionalization of the meaning of cutting as crisis-inducing pathology. NGO and state advocacy have had profound consequences not only for the ending of cutting but also for how the women they target "exercise existence" (Mbembe

2001: 15) and negotiate the values that govern their lives. Women in the Upper East Region know that cutting is publicly demonized and that governmental discourses present it as a symptom of ostensible rural ignorance, outmoded tradition, and resistance to development. To end cutting, Ghanaian NGOs and the state, bolstered by international organizations, have not only criminalized cutting but have also problematized it as a crisis. We have seen how cutting is defined and constructed as both a reproductive pathology—an inherently harmful practice that causes bodily damage, ill health, and death—and a cultural pathology of a people cast as staunchly traditional, patriarchal, and resistant to modernity. State power, writes Achille Mbembe, "attempts to institutionalize its world of meanings as a socio-historical world and to make that world fully real, turning it into a part of people's common sense" (1992: 2). While NGOs and the state seek to isolate cutting in a hermetically sealed world of rural northern Ghanaians who resist change, women in Bongo link the end of cutting to national and pan-African idioms, joining a chorus of voices that critique governance by extraction. Social worlds structured by governmental rationalities think, feel, speak, and act in reference to them without being overdetermined by them (see Biehl 2013).

In consonance with larger Ghanaian understandings, these women see blood not only as a bodily substance but also as social and cultural one, one that amalgamates indigenous and biomedical notions of health and animates a range of social critiques of bodily transactions, scarcity, deprivation, inequality, and the state. When rural women invoke blood loss, they do not define the present as a sudden moment of a biopolitical crisis or immediate threats to survival. They describe an ordinary, systemic crisis that is both chronic and intensified and has made bodily vulnerability and deterioration a constant in their lives. They understand blood loss as what we might think of as *slow harm:* an effect of long-standing practices that produce and materialize bodies as vulnerable, a gradual weakening and dissipation of health during years of reproduction and labor in the context of scarcity.

The notion of slow harm builds on Lauren Berlant's distinction between a crisis and a "slow death." Crisis, Berlant writes, "rhetorically turn[s] an ongoing condition into an intensified situation in which extensive threats to survival are said to dominate the reproduction of life" (2011: 7). In contrast to the shocking, exceptional character of a crisis, slow death results from "crisis ordinariness" (10), that is, from historically situated, ongoing structural forces that imperil life and social reproduction. When the present is cast as a sudden or unusual crisis, select elements of systemic and ordinary problems tend to be seized upon and constructed as exceptional (see also Roitman 2013). In contrast the slow harm of blood loss described by women in Bongo is much more pervasive and deeply entangled in their lives. Like slow death, slow harm results from historically situated structural forces that imperil life and social reproduction in the context of scarcity and governance by extraction. But rural women's bodily attrition points to a *weakening* of health and the dissipation—not the disappearance—of vital force during years of reproduction and labor. There is thus a conceptual distinction between slow harm and slow death: bodily attrition is endemic to life in Bongo, but although it can bring death, death does not define it.

By analyzing the ending of cutting through the prism of groups that have been the main target of NGO campaigns, this chapter turns the lens of the problematization of harm inside out. Exploring how cutting is constructed as harmful from the unusual vantage point of the subjects of NGO interventions, rather than their architects, disrupts knowledge about cutting, rural women, northern Ghana, and political and moral economies of care that often remains unquestioned in the public realm.

Before we proceed, I want to issue a brief reminder that concerns about blood and slow harm are not the sole, or even the primary, reason why cutting ended. Rather, these form a self-standing narrative that emerged in the wake of the waning of the practice. As I have shown, the reasons for the end of cutting, however uneven, include a host of historical factors and responses to NGO interventions. Some circumcisers stopped cutting because of their age, and others ceased taking apprentices because they did not want to pass down a now-illegal practice to their sons and nephews. For girls education and migration have become the preferred modes of coming of age and self-making. The future of marriage, for which cutting was one preparation, has itself become unstable. And even those girls and women who get married embrace NGO messages about family planning and the ending of cutting.

BLEEDING TO DEATH: THE GOVERNMENTAL DISCOURSE ABOUT BLOOD LOSS

Although the claim that cutting leads to excessive blood loss is but one of many health problems presented to rural communities by NGOs and public health workers, it is the one that resonates most strongly even though it means something different to the parties involved. In Ghana and globally anticutting campaigners represent blood loss as an uncontrollable spillage that occurs during or immediately after the act of cutting. Both GAWW and RHI follow the WHO classification of bleeding as an "immediate consequence" of FGM (World Health Organization 2016) and stress its deadly effects. They equate blood loss induced by cutting with hemorrhage: a singular event, an extraordinary life-threatening emergency that entails profuse, instantaneous, and unstoppable bleeding. Indeed, "bleeding to death" is often invoked as a metaphor for the harmfulness of the practice; Mrs. Mahama, GAWW's president, encapsulated her lectures on health by warning that "most of them [cut women] die."

In the visual representations of blood loss in photographs, documentaries, and filmed public health dramas, NGOs mobilize blood as a potent sensory substance in an effort to push the public toward an affective recognition of harm. The RHI film about cutting is a cautionary tale, a locally produced drama that depicts a girl who bleeds to death. GAWW usually shows two documentary films produced elsewhere on the continent that graphically depict the cutting of an infant. Both evoke the desired responses—recall that rural men and women as well as the nurses were moved by the video representations of blood loss, gasping and crying out loud when the films showed circumcisers' bloodied hands.

The communicative potency of the blood idiom is articulated visually and affectively in a variety of other contexts. GAWW posters, brochures, and t-shirts regularly feature blood loss, often depicting a close-up drawing of a bleeding child and her genitals (see figure 17 as well as figure 15). The red ink portrays the oozing blood as an excessive and uncontrollable spillage that occurs during or immediately after the cutting itself. Such representations in photographs, documentaries, and public health dramas evoke affective responses, which explains why the idiom of blood travels well and so impresses multiple audiences.

These representations are not limited to Ghana; anticutting posters from several African countries prominently feature excessive blood loss. In addition, the anatomical model produced in Germany and widely used by all IAC affiliates has a special addition that represents extensive blood loss (see figures 3 and 4 in chapter 2). Unlike the films and pictures, the plastic model did not move the nurses to tears, though it did provoke their curiosity.

Conceptualizations of blood loss as a potentially catastrophic emergency circulate widely in Ghanaian governmental discourses, and nurses, civil servants, and health volunteers portray it as a near-deadly crisis. On Bolga's

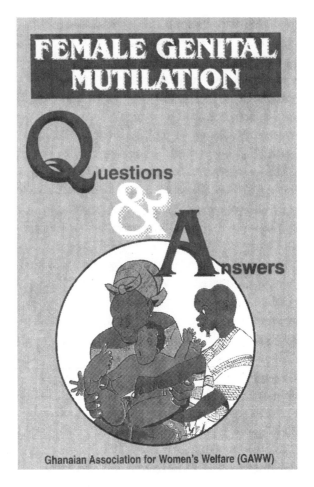

FIGURE 17. GAWW brochure (courtesy of GAWW).

URA radio programs, for instance, nurses often talk about deadly hemorrhage when explaining the health effects of cutting. A nurse giving a radio interview in Hausa stated that the main health effect of cutting was "bleed[ing] to death, because they may not like to send her to the hospital for treatment, for the fear of being surrendered to authorities." According to this nurse, hemorrhage is preventable, though parents often refuse to send their daughters to a hospital. The shadow of law is never far from discussions of cutting, but the nurse's statement places responsibility for hemorrhage on reluctant parents.

The discourse of witnessing deadly hemorrhage has gained spectral dimensions, as it is largely constructed in reference to unspecified rumors.

NGO workers, nurses, and activists regularly mention that a girl had "one time bled to death" after cutting or that girls were brought to the hospital because they were bleeding so profusely that their lives were in danger, and they had to be given transfusions. Ghanaian audiences know not to take these statements literally, just like they know that "most of them die" does not mean that cutting imperils survival for most cut girls.

At the same time hemorrhage is not merely a discourse, as exceptional crises do occur. Albert, a YMCA worker, was one of two people who told me about actual cases of hemorrhage in the Bawku District, where cutting is still practiced. Both he and Fatima, a Red Cross volunteer, said that they intervened when they witnessed a girl who was bleeding profusely. Albert and his team took the cut girl to the Presbyterian hospital in town:

> One time I was in another village—in fact, had we not been there at that time, nobody knows, this little girl could have died. We were there on a YMCA business, we went to meet [a youth group] and talk to them and to educate them about the aims and objectives of YMCA. So in the course of that—the house was just very close, and we could tell there was probably trouble somewhere. Because we got there and we saw people all around. They didn't want to tell us what was going on. They had cut this girl, I don't know what they did, and she was bleeding. She was bleeding, and it got to a time that they realized that, you know, this girl was going to die. So they had to confess to us, and we helped to rush that girl to the hospital. And you could tell they were pleading with us not to identify the parents of the girl to the hospital authorities because they were afraid [the parents] were going to be prosecuted or something, but we encouraged them not to be afraid and just discouraged them from doing it [cutting]. That girl's life was saved because we were there. Nobody knows, maybe she could have died. And who knows how many girls have died out of this whole thing, especially when their knives are not sterilized, and they do not go by the medical procedure to do this, and they have nothing just to stop the bleeding, anytime it happens. Well, we got to the hospital, and they [the hospital staff] were so appreciative. They quickly took her up and really thanked us, because most of the time when this happens, they just try to keep the girls at home and do the best they can, but sometimes their best is just not enough to save themselves. They [the hospital staff] were very appreciative, and they saved the girl's life.

In Albert's account rescuing the cut girl from an emergency by bringing her to the Bawku hospital meant saving her from hemorrhage. Fatima also told me that she had recently saved cut girls from hemorrhaging to death.

She was able to rush by bicycle to a nearby village and locate a doctor who then transported the cut girls to the hospital. They had to be given "two pints of blood," Fatima stressed, conveying the seriousness of their condition and indicating that their survival had been at stake. For Ghanaian NGO workers and civil servants, then, blood loss is a metonym for a near-deadly crisis.

SLOW HARM: RURAL WOMEN'S PERSPECTIVES ON BLOOD LOSS AND THE ENDS OF CUTTING

Cut women in Bongo share concerns about blood loss, but they conceptualize it differently. While they are moved by sensory impressions of hemorrhage, cut women understand blood loss from cutting not as a sudden bodily crisis but as a gradual bodily attrition, a weakening of strength, health, and life force. The blood narrative does not refer to singular events of uncontrolled exceptional blood loss that imperil individual women's lives. Rather, the narrative points to a collective condition: all their bodies have been depleted of blood during years of reproduction and labor amid scarcity. Unlike the crisis of hemorrhage, this slow harm does not kill them but gradually reduces their vitality.

Agnes, the pito brewer, was one of the people from whom I first heard about the relationship between blood shortages and the ending of cutting. When I first met Agnes at a 2004 support rally for the National Democratic Congress (NDC) political party, she was on fire. Invited to speak on behalf of the women, she seized the microphone and, striding into the gathering crowd, railed forcefully against politicians who descend upon the village to ask for votes, only to then forget their promises and obligations. They eat women like rice, she thundered. When I interviewed her later, in the cool darkness of her room, she was self-reflective. She took my questions as an opportunity to reflect about her life and said she enjoyed the way our conversations provoked her to think about things that "we usually don't think about." Cutting had to end, she told me, because of recurrent blood loss: "When you menstruate, you lose blood, and if you cut, you lose blood." My interview transcript shows that I was confused by her statement. "So you lose more blood if you were cut?" I asked. "The blood that comes during the cutting is more than what one loses at the end of each month," she told me. My question about the quantity of lost blood was misplaced, I learned over time—at stake was not the precise amount but its value and the larger understanding of blood as a substance of health.

Blood Calculus and Health Maintenance

Anthropologists working in West Africa have long noted that blood is central to indigenous conceptualizations of health, gender, and reproduction (Bledsoe 2002; Fairhead, Leach, and Small 2006; Masquelier 2011). Some say that blood is analogous to the concept of the immune system: "Whereas the path to good health in contemporary America (and Europe) is often construed as a build-up of immunity," Fairhead, Leach, and Small write, "in West Africa it is a build-up of blood" (2006: 1117). Blood is viewed as the main foundation for health, bodily resilience, and well-being. Masquelier writes that it "structur[es] local experiences of health, illness, and reproduction" in Hausaphone Mawri communities in Niger, where it is said that blood must flow but must also be conserved (2011: 161, 162).[3]

Excessive blood loss predisposes women to ill health and is associated "not simply with depleted strength and reproductive resilience, but also with susceptibility to other dangerous conditions" (Fairhead, Leach, and Small 2006: 1113). In the Upper East, rural and urban women share this understanding and see recurrent blood loss as predisposing them to ill health and making their bodies vulnerable. Josephine, director of a leading gender-focused NGO in Bolga, told me that she often hears this: "'Well, what modern medicine has been telling us is that [cutting] is not good. It is not a good practice. First of all, it makes us bleed a lot, and so we can get sick.' And so on." Blood loss has such powerful connotations that the NGOs' long list of consequences of cutting means little when seen against the backdrop of a lifelong susceptibility to ill health. Other effects of cutting are simply "and so on"—not worth mentioning. This understanding of blood was made explicit when a regional politician suggested that I visit his uncle, a village elder who told me that cutting was outlawed because of blood loss. "They are concerned about losing blood?" I asked. "Yes, but he is talking about entire health consequences," the politician clarified.

Agnes, Abanga, and others evaluate the effects of cutting in reference to an economy of blood that values a calculus of conservation. "You'll lose blood if you're going for cutting," women tell Cecilia, the health volunteer, "but if you're not cut, your blood will still be there, and you'll eat and get more blood and add to it." This blood calculus weighs blood accumulation against blood loss: blood buildup is desired, loss is to be avoided, and much of life is structured by the "struggle for blood" (Fairhead, Leach, and Small 2006: 1112).

This economy of blood embodies an understanding of health as something that accumulates during a long period of time. People continually assess processes that lead to increase or decrease of blood: What, they ask, can I do during the next several years (or even throughout a lifetime) to increase blood and avoid blood loss? Sufficient and protein-rich food, such as eggs, guinea fowl, and groundnuts, is seen as necessary for regaining blood. So is rest. If women lack adequate food and rest, blood cannot be replenished, and chronically depleted bodies are unable to recover. The amount of blood in the body is something to be managed, though in times of scarcity this management remains uncertain and cannot be planned or rationalized, as neither the source of blood nor its expenditure are under individual control.

Tribal marks and cutting are now seen as separate, and particularly objectionable, categories of blood loss. A cut woman who became a widow at a young age many years ago, and who has since suffered from ill health, told me: "They say if we cut, we lose blood, through cutting and tribal marks, in addition to blood lost during childbirth. As a result cutting is not good." Assibi, a woman who is in the last generation of those cut in Bongo, told me that she agreed with the NGOs and the government that cutting and tribal marks were no longer tenable:

> They said that the cutting destroys us. If you do tribal markings, you lose
> blood; when you cut, you lose blood—and all these constitute sickness.
> So government has said we should put a stop to it. And now that we have
> stopped cutting, whether you are fat or thin that is your structure.

Because blood loss raises the stakes of the blood calculus, rural women measure the value of cutting against the backdrop of continually recurring blood loss and the overall shortage of blood that marks their lives.

"Normally Short of Blood": Gender, Scarcity, and Ordinary Crises of Anemia

In the Upper East Region, women are seen as particularly vulnerable to blood loss as a result of their reproductive experiences—the monthly shedding of blood during menstruation, the multiple pregnancies during which their bodies nourish babies and have to produce blood for two, and the deliveries during which they bleed. These recurrent and lasting blood losses are seen as depleting strength, health, and reproductive capacity. As Bledsoe writes for the Gambia,

Having sufficient blood is critical for maintaining strength. Yet blood is also needed to make a baby, and the process of giving birth is considered to be a major cause of blood loss for a woman, particularly when intensified by hard work and inadequate diet. . . . Such problems are intensified because blood, unlike strength, is replaceable only with great difficulty. (Bledsoe, Banja, and Hill 1998: 37)

Gambian women also see reproductive capacity and health as eroding as a result of the "wear and tear on the body, particularly in the wake of obstetric traumas" that diminish women's bodily resources, including muscles, strength, and blood (Bledsoe, Banja, and Hill 1998: 16: see also Bledsoe 2002).

That women are thought to be more susceptible to blood loss is manifested in the noticeably gendered character of blood donations in the Upper East Region, where donors are almost exclusively men.[4] The preexisting gendered disposition to blood loss has intensified because of concerns about the inability to replenish blood and strength as a result of diminished sustenance. As Agnes put it, she was unable to rebuild her blood and strength from multiple pregnancies because she lacked food:

When I was young, I was very strong. But, you know, when one gives birth to two [to] three children, she can't be so strong. I've given birth seven times; two are no more. So I'm not as strong as I used to be; now I am weak. Here our problem is food, how to get food. After giving birth the way I did, I should be able to eat what I want, to grow strong. But it's hard to get food; we can't feed well. This is our main problem, how to get food and eat. When we farm, we don't get good yields.

Bodies that are chronically depleted of blood now cannot replenish it. Although Agnes had a steady income, food was scarce for her, too, and she saw this as contributing to blood shortages. I came to understand that the recurrent blood loss places women at a particular peril of weakening their health in the context of scarcity. This is how a woman who returned from working in southern Ghana put it:

Our problem is that our husbands don't have white man's jobs to do, so we only engage in farming, and when we are through with farming, we weave hats. If you are not able to weave hats, it becomes difficult for you. We are always poor and when we are sick, you can't buy medicine for yourself because you don't have money.

To explain their bodily condition, women cite scarcity, deprivation, and the long-term effects of both on health, situating these issues historically.

They note that the struggle for food has become more acute in their lifetime because of erratic rains, infertile land, decreased crop yields, and the lack of wage-paying jobs in the region. Their most bitter complaint is that their harvests do not yield enough grain and legumes to last them the whole year and that they have no money to purchase food. Women I got to know share the narrative of decreased crop yields but also regulate its forms. When one farmer who was the head of her household told me that in the past she would get eight bags of groundnuts from planting one bag of seeds, her daughters laughed and asked her rhetorically, "How much did you get?" They agreed that the land used to yield more, but they thought their mother had exaggerated. Meanwhile food has become prohibitively expensive as a result of a staggering level of inflation—between 2005 and 2011 food price inflation in Ghana "eroded real household purchasing power by 47%" (Osei-Asare and Eghan 2013: 27). As I discussed earlier, the decline in livelihoods does not have a single cause but results from a compendium of forces, including climate change, austerity-based structural adjustment programs, and the rise of inequality that followed.

Food also has its own semiotics and is used to construct metaphors for happiness, well-being, and social harmony. *Dia maa* (food only) or, more simply, *dia* (food) are common positive responses to the question "How are you?" "Food only" stands for "everything is well, we are only looking for food"; this response indicates a state of contentment and well-being. This expression is also used to describe social harmony. For instance, one woman in a polygamous marriage described her friendship and good relations with her "rival" (a cowife) by saying that they looked for food together. Similarly, *mam poore pee me* (literally, "my stomach is washed") is the primary way of saying, "I am happy." Recall also that Azure, the former circumciser, had told me that taking up cutting had meant that he got to eat *sagebo* [millet porridge], thus indicating that he was happily married. For rural women scarcity-induced anemia is the new normal. As Napoka, a trader and farmer from Bongo, put it: "Even as we are there, when some small sickness attacks you, you are normally short of blood. If we do that [cutting] in addition, what are we doing to ourselves?" Women who attend pre- and postnatal clinics are told that they are "short of blood" and that their blood is not "good enough." The pervasiveness of anemia has been made visible through blood tests and public health outreach. Nearly half the women and 90 percent of the children in the region are anemic, and 36 percent of children are stunted (too short for their age) (ICF Macro 2010b). Urban Ghanaians often use blood tonics, produced by urban enterprises specializing in "traditional medicine," as a remedy for anemia; these have been shown to stimulate the production of red blood cells, increasing the amount of hemoglobin. Few rural women can afford them, and they prefer food as a means of building up their blood and rest as a source of strength.

UNICEF intensified its child survival interventions in the Upper East in 2004, offering all pregnant women attending prenatal clinics vitamin A, iron, folic acid, deworming medication, and preventative antimalarials (UNICEF 2004). Pregnant women are supposed to receive these medications for free, but access has been inconsistent and restricted to the duration of pregnancy—anemia does not generate lasting access to resources by way of "therapeutic citizenship" (Nguyen 2010: 7), and vitamins, mineral supplements, and blood tonics are costly. Women who are not pregnant live under the shadow of knowledge that they have anemia but no access to nourishing food or treatment.

Child survival interventions have begun to reduce infant and maternal mortality and legitimized biomedicine as a source of authority about pregnancy and child survival, but the dispensation of treatment has also heightened preexisting concerns, making women acutely aware of their "blood shortages." Against this backdrop cutting has turned into an instance of unaffordable blood loss. As Akolpoka, a young woman who falls sick every pregnancy and has lost three of her four children, puts it:

> In the olden days cutting was a good thing but today I think—remember what I told you, that each time I am pregnant I have to be given drips. If you are cut, you lose blood, this is in addition to the monthly menstruation. This is why I think that cutting is not good.

Akolpoka was so anemic that doctors deemed regular supplements insufficient, and she had to be given intravenous fluid replacements. At a time when women have to be "given drips," and the gendered, already vulnerable body has been pushed to the threshold of survival and viable reproduction, cutting is deemed untenable.

Reproduction and the Shifting Value of Cutting

Blood loss is assessed in accordance with its value. The loss associated with reproduction and fertility—a source of wealth in its own right (Awedoba and Denham 2014)—is tolerated, whereas blood lost at cutting and scarification is now seen as wasted. This question has been at the crux of NGO interventions. For blood loss to be conceptualized as wasteful, cutting itself had to be stripped of value by being severed from fertility. Cutting used to be understood as beneficial to social and bodily reproduction in the sense that it produced an appropriately disciplined child. Children of cut mothers were thought to have proper social skills, while the term *clitoris child* (*zankaberε bia*) was applied to stubborn, disobedient children of uncut mothers. Whereas in the Sudan, infibulation ensured what Janice Boddy refers to as "moral motherhood" (2007: 111), here it ensured "moral childhood" by transferring the mother's bodily discipline to her children (see also L. Thomas 2003: 33). In addition, some women told me that cutting was seen as enhancing women's bodily reproductive capacities: it "prepared the womb" and "reduced the clitoris," an obstacle to childbirth.

These positive associations have been severed, and cutting is no longer viewed as beneficial. The shift in values was explained to me as resulting from new knowledge. "In the olden days, people didn't know that the clitoris doesn't prevent childbirth," Abanga told me, and another woman added, "Things have changed for the better. Back then, in our time, we didn't know, but now we know that it has no use. Whether you cut or not, you will be able to give birth." Since cutting is decoupled from reproduction, the associated blood loss is no longer justified. Asibi, an elderly widow whom I got to know well as she was my hosts' neighbor, had a particularly difficult experience with cutting and came to see her blood loss as wasted: "I went through bitter times and was in bed for a whole month. I wasted a lot of blood. It made me feel weak." These understandings are outcomes of migration encounters with uncut women, anticutting campaigns, biomedical reproductive health outreach, and the forgetting, as some put it, of the reproductive power of ancestral spirits.

Note the wording that Asibi and others use: although they see blood lost at cutting as wasted, they do not say that cutting is harmful or deadly. They do not say that cutting obstructs childbirth but that it "doesn't prevent" it and has "no use." These turns of phrase reveal a devaluation of cutting, coupled with a subtle refusal to accept public health and NGO framings of cutting as a bodily and cultural pathology. Rather than seeing cutting as *destroying* women's reproductive capacities, cut women describe it as *not improving* them. In contrast to the biomedical conceptualization of cutting as *deadly*, they deem it *not useful*. The blood narrative does not demonize the practice and the knowledge and values embedded in it but instead points to historically situated bodily vulnerability: cutting has become a liability in particular conditions of slow harm. Asibi and others think of blood loss as a gradual weakening of health and bodily strength during years of reproduction and labor in the context of scarcity. Unlike the crisis of hemorrhage, slow harm does not kill them but gradually pushes their bodies to the threshold of viable life. Cutting, they say, needed to end because the effects of gradual blood loss harmed them all. Their point is not that cutting should have been preserved but that bodies should be healthy enough to be able to withstand it, recuperate from it, and emerge stronger from the experience.

Short of Blood, Short of Food: Times Have Changed

The temporality of blood loss and bodily attrition is a crucial feature of the blood narrative. "Now, blood is scarce," I was told repeatedly. Faith, a young woman recently returned from southern Ghana, told me that her husband convinced her not to get cut because "in this era, it's not good if people cut." Cutting was not always bad for their bodies, the women say. It is only

> now
> these days
> in this era

that cutting is no longer useful.

As I have noted, the past is marked as the time when women did not know that cutting "has no use." But what is the present? The current era is a time of struggle for food that is associated with a shortage of both blood and food. In the group conversation I mentioned earlier, Abanga and others detailed the historical differences in blood, health, and bodily constitution. Azuma said:

> The world has changed. In the olden days, if you were grown up to that age, blood will be too much in your body so if you don't cut, the blood would not reduce to be all right for you. Times have changed, and now we don't get good food to eat, so if you cut and bleed, if you are not lucky, you may not survive and you might die. That is why we have now forgotten about the cutting.

The women I spoke with were constructing their account of change and a critique of the present for each other as much as for me, and Azuma's depiction was applauded. "Azuma has said it all, is there something else?," one person asked while another affirmed what she had said:

> What I have to say is that what Azuma has said is true. When we did cut, there was no problem. It used to be fine for us, to the extent that if you lost weight [after cutting], you would grow fat [later on]. Because when you cut, they pamper you and give you good food to eat so that you can regain the blood you lost. But now things are not like they used to be. We don't have enough blood. So if somebody cuts, even if they give her good food, she won't be healthy, she will be malnourished. That is why they have stopped cutting.

This reasoning situates the issue of cutting in relation to rural women's main concerns about the present: the intensified lack of blood and food. In the past, it is said, women were able to recuperate after cutting because they had enough blood built up, and temporary weakness could be remedied through proper nourishment. But *now/these days/in this era,* their bodies are constitutionally weak; privation has rendered them vulnerable and anemic, and their "bodies do not get peace."

These are all said to be new problems. In the past, the women say, they were able to recuperate after cutting because they had enough blood built up. People always knew that cutting would weaken the body—hence the long recuperation period during which girls rebuilt their strength and ate nutritious food to regain their blood. "If you eat good food [after cutting], you will heal fast," is how one woman put it, and "when you start going out, you will change and be very fine, but if you don't eat good food, when you go out, you will be lean because of the blood you lost." Girls were supposed to be given gifts of groundnuts, eggs, and meats and were freed from performing labor until they recuperated, which was up to three or four weeks. Relatives, as well as potential suitors, used these gifts to demonstrate their investment in the girls' well-being. Because food was sufficient, if not abundant, recuperation was possible, and the loss of blood and bodily strength was neither permanent nor irrevocable. Blood lost at cutting caused a merely temporary weakness and could be regained through proper nourishment. Today the effects of food scarcity are such that not even proper nourishment meant to replenish blood lost at cutting can counteract the effects of slow harm. Now, even if a girl receives good food, I was told, she will not be able to regain her health. This understanding has reshaped the way women evaluate blood loss and has made cutting unappealing.

Rather than simply asserting that chronic blood loss has weakened their bodies, many women ask *why* this is so, analyzing worsening economic and environmental conditions that structure how they live and labor, and contrasting the present to a more favorable past. In doing so, they map social problems not onto culture, as NGOs and the government commonly do, but onto scarcity, which they then attribute to poor land yields, unemployment, and extractive governance. They figure the past as a mirror of the difficult present, and the difference between "olden days" and "this era" serves as a critical response to pathologizing discourses.

We should not mistake this narrative for a mere adoption of NGO advocacy.[5] Although both rural women and NGOs agree that cutting does not belong to the present, they stand on opposite sides of a discursive divide: they share the same vocabulary, but their words "mean something different" (Tsing 2005: xi). NGOs situate the present in linear time, at the threshold of a national modernity that cannot accommodate what they regard as outmoded practices. For rural women subjects of NGO interventions, the present is a time of struggle and scarcity; cutting does not belong here because it is no longer feasible or affordable. Their time is, in Mbembe words, "time as lived" (Mbembe 2001: 8).

These accounts of worsening material conditions and the attrition of their own bodies are worth taking seriously. I do so not only because of their intrinsic value but also because they constitute a viable account of history. Put more provocatively: that this particular aspect of the past is idealized does not mean it was not better. Because scholars have not proved rural women's understandings of the historical dynamics of scarcity right or wrong, at the very least we must not dismiss them. This is particularly important in the larger context of food production in sub-Saharan Africa, which is less now than it was in 1960; since 2007 food prices have been at record highs, provoking protests across the continent, and drought has persisted since the 1970s.[6]

Africanists are familiar with narratives of decline and tend to understand them not as reflections of historical trends, but, in deconstructionist terms, as mobilizations of narratives of the past for purposes of constructing new meanings, moralities, and claims to authority and power (Lund 2013). I take a different approach, emphasizing the character of the blood narrative as *both* a mobilization of history for contemporary purposes *and* a possible testament to historical change, and I do so for both political and analytical reasons.

In the Ghanaian context development narratives of cultural pathologies as causes of economic decline and imperiled livelihoods have the imprimatur of the media, the state, and donor organizations, and these narratives are reinforced by repeated utterances that count as knowledge, whereas rural women's narratives are labeled as superstition and ignorance. Rather than limit my analysis to renarrativizing the historical claims of those already marked as suspect and untrustworthy, I feel the political imperative to address what feminist philosophers refer to as "hermeneutical injustice" (Fricker 2007:1). This requires staying alert to how power relations structure our own epistemic practices and economies of credibility. Hermeneutical injustice occurs when there is no readily available discourse or a conceptual apparatus that would render intelligible the experiences of subjects who are contesting their disenfranchisement. The blood narrative disrupts this injustice by advancing a nonpathologizing critical understanding of gendered bodily attrition and decline in livelihoods.

THE NATIONAL SHORTAGE OF BLOOD:
HEALTH, TECHNOLOGY, AND THE BODY POLITIC

For women in Bongo blood loss is more than an indigenous idiom of health. Both historical and public health understandings have shaped how these women think about cutting and the gendered character of blood depletion. I suggest that their notion of blood loss amalgamates and absorbs both indigenous and biomedical understandings, as well as popular notions of blood circulating in Ghanaian public culture. Theirs is a mobile and elastic meaning-making framework that must be situated within a wider set of scientific and popular discourses and practices about blood. The notion of blood as a foundation of health and the concern about the general shortage of blood are the result of cross-pollination between indigenous and biomedical understandings of health, new medical technologies, and the rising value of blood.

This also means that rural women do not simply accommodate NGO messages about blood loss within preexisting understandings, indigenous or biomedical. The proximity of the blood narrative to NGO discourses is not a local adaptation or translation of hemorrhage but a richly embedded, culturally resonant framework in its own right that is nested within national conceptualizations of blood and its shortage. The blood narrative has stabilized after two decades of interventions, and I noticed both its spread and consolidation between 2004 and 2009, when Ghanaian discourses about blood and its shortage intensified and the overall value of blood increased.

National blood shortage is seen as a public health crisis and a crisis of biopolitical governance. Technologies that materialize concerns about lack of blood and make its paucity visible include the spread of anemia tests and the increasing number of research studies that rely on drawing blood. The news media regularly publicize Ministry of Health statements about vital statistics, such as the rates of anemia, malnutrition, and maternal and child mortality. The popularization of this biopolitical knowledge has generated a sense of peril so resonant in public culture that Miss Ghana 2003 chose anemia as her public service theme, embarking on an "awareness and prevention campaign" titled "Your Blood Is Your Life." For this nascent celebrity, along with many in the public health establishment, anemia and other "blood shortages" could be combated with behavior change and "sensitization." In this view the problem is that people lack knowledge about which food is nutritious, while traditional taboos prohibit women and children from eating it.

The increased attention to anemia in the bodies of citizens has been accompanied by media reports about an inadequate "national supply of blood": "Koforidua Hospital Runs Short of Blood," "Patients in Danger as Korle-Bu Blood Bank Dries Up," and "National Blood Bank Empty" are examples.[7] The need for transfusions is mounting because of the effects of HIV/AIDS, car accidents, and increasing numbers of women who deliver in hospitals. Ghanaian scientists and the government are trying to devise ways of ensuring a more adequate supply. Radio stations and newspapers report that hospitals cannot provide blood transfusions to all patients, sometimes noting that mothers and infants are dying because their anemic, malnourished, and malaria-ridden bodies are depleted of blood and bereft of care. New exercises in civic engagement and private-public partnerships try to ameliorate the consequences of national blood shortages. Radio stations, including those popular in Bongo, organize blood drives for the Ghana blood bank, sometimes teaming up with herbal clinics that provide blood tonics to all donors.[8]

Hospitals often require patients to replace the blood they receive with donations from relatives, thus making family visits a site of tension. Patients are also concerned that they will be asked to pay for transfusions, although the government denies this, stating that hospitals do not charge for blood itself but for storage and processing fees and special safety tests. In the face of depleted blood banks, in the Korle-Bu Teaching Hospital, the country's largest, supplying some of the blood is outsourced to what the media have dubbed "blood transfusion contractors"—private individuals who sell their blood directly to patients and their families.[9] Scarcity and commodification of blood have augmented its value, and blood is no longer seen as affordable. Hence, neither is blood loss.

Public debates about the national shortage of blood serve as social diagnostics of the present and are used to critique the state. Ghana's ascendance to middle-income status has visibly stalled since 2011, but even before that, blood shortages brought into stark relief the state's neglect of the social body and citizens' welfare during Ghana's economic and political boom. Some government critics also see the state's failure to secure enough blood as an index of its inability to govern. A conversation with Susan, an Accra-based feminist lawyer who works for the government's Commission on Human Rights and Administrative Justice (CHRAJ), clarified the potency of the blood discourse. She posited that blood management is the most fundamental duty of the body politic and criticized the government's refusal to adopt a gender policy (a national framework to improve the status of women) and design a blood policy. The government, she said, has had a draft gender policy since 1999: "We've been making nice about getting it adopted because it affects, you see, it affects especially blood policy." Without the gender and blood policies, she explained, "it means there isn't proper monitoring of blood donations, blood, giving of blood, all those things. And of course women are most vulnerable, you know, because they lose more, and then [there is] the issue of HIV/AIDS, you know." The relationship of gender, blood loss, and blood donation might seem to be surprising terrain for a critique of the state, but for Ghanaian feminists like Susan, the problems here were both serious and self-evident. Moreover, at a time of profound activist dissatisfaction with the newly created Ministry of Women and Children's Affairs, the critique of the minister's ineffectiveness was most poignantly expressed in biopolitical terms. The government's failure to regulate blood donations, protect women from unnecessary blood loss, and provide blood transfusions figured as a larger indictment of the state. If the government was unable to regulate the gendered aspects of blood donations and was negligent about the body politic, it was not fulfilling its basic functions. Susan shared rural women's view that the vulnerability caused by blood loss was gendered and particularly acute in the present moment, but she saw this as stemming from her concerns about HIV/AIDS, rather than issues of scarcity, labor, and the inability to replenish blood.

The Ghanaian state attempted to address some of these concerns by passing the National Blood Policy in 2006, which established the Ghana National

Blood Service and mandated coverage of blood products in the National Health Insurance Scheme.[10] The insurance was also supposed to facilitate access to health care; it was introduced by the Kufuor government in an effort to provide affordable, but not free, universal health care. Posters for the insurance touted blood and blood products as covered benefits and featured them prominently, immediately after prescription medicine. This did not alleviate social anxieties, nor did it help those who cannot afford the premiums—for destitute Ghanaians and the ordinary poor, both health and health care are out of reach, and the insurance itself is facing insolvency.[11] The seemingly paltry contribution required, equivalent to eight to ten U.S. dollars annually, is a fortune even for those who have some cash income. For example, weavers in Bongo who are able to sell their baskets earn about one or two dollars in profit per basket, which takes them a week to produce. Gaining access to health care is even more prohibitively costly for farmers. Atampoka, an unmarried thirty-year-old woman caring for two children but with no social support, complained explicitly about being unable to pay for insurance:

> When they started registering [for the National Health Insurance Scheme], that year I had money and I was able to register for myself and my child. A year after, I fell sick, and since then I have not gotten money to go back and renew it. So for some time now, I have not gone to the hospital because I have not been able to go and change my photo. So I have to be with my sickness.

Anthropologists of humanitarianism and global health have argued that we are today witnessing a form of a minimalist biopolitics that aims not at improving lives but saving them (Redfield 2013). Ghanaian concerns about the unavailability of blood point to something more sinister: even the very saving of lives is imperiled. Noting that the national insurance system is facing insolvency, government critics emphasize the state's biopolitical and regulatory failures, such as the absence of life-saving treatment and institutions that would secure it. Women who have stopped cutting take these critiques of the body politic and inequality in the social order a step further: they mention scarcity and blood shortages in one breath and are less concerned about biopolitical measures or legal frameworks than about bodily attrition and imperiled health. They point to the state, which saps their vitality, and do so by way of metaphorical references to occult economies.

Like many Ghanaians, women in Bongo critique contemporary governance by extraction in the language of vampirism and blood sucking, illustrating how the political semiotics of blood inform their critiques. Blood has material and symbolic importance for national and global politics, economic and ethical regimes, and social organization. To understand the cultural underpinnings of Ghanaian concerns about blood, we need to consider the wider semiotics of blood and its value in Ghanaian and pan-African public cultures. Stories about the theft of blood, ritual murders, and colonizers as vampires have long been tied to questions of political economy and were used to critique the violence of colonial extraction and exploitation (White 2000; Comaroff and Comaroff 1999b; Moore and Sanders 2003). In East and Central Africa, White writes, "no one knew exactly what Europeans did with African blood, but people were convinced they took it" (2000: 5). In colonial Ghana, stories of ritual murders and blood as potent ritual medicine served as the terrain of inter-Ghanaian power struggles (Gocking 2000: 198).[12]

This discourse has returned and is resurfacing in proliferating invocations of an occult economy that equates "people and their body parts with commodities, their life-force with ill-gotten wealth and their fertility with immoral consumption" (Moore and Sanders 2003: 15). The rich scholarship on discourses of occult economies explains them as "moral frameworks" (Moore and Sanders 2003: 15) that critique the "disparities of power and wealth" (Ferguson 2006: 74). Invocations of the occult help make sense of the violence of late capitalism and the production of inexplicable wealth by distilling "complex material and social processes into comprehensible human motives" (Comaroff and Comaroff 1999b: 286).

In Ghanaian public culture, films, theater performances, and newspapers have popularized stories about ritual murders and the occult economy (Meyer 2003; Gilbert 2006; Garritano 2012; Gocking 2000: 200).[13] Notions about the spiritual and symbolic power of blood and vital force have recently intensified, and blood has come to mediate competing desires and struggles for wealth, health, power, and moral virtue. The occult economy is at the heart of widely circulating representations of blood as a substance with great spiritual power. Nigerian and Ghanaian films and theater performances (known as concerts) have popularized fantasies of ritual murder: moral tales about the stealing of blood and body parts that juxtapose wealth against virtue and life itself. Blood, according to these representations, can procure wealth but at high cost, endangering both life and moral integrity.

As I discussed in chapter 4, RHI served as a harbinger and mediator of this moral critique, bringing popular culture into rural lives by screening films and video clips. Campaigns against cutting are not restricted to public health messages about hemorrhage or the negotiation of "moral positions" about reproductive health (Pigg and Adams 2005: 26) but supplement public health pedagogies with popular culture. This, too, is a type of moral pedagogy, but its concerns are the crisis of *social* reproduction, inequality, and extraction of vital force, and its medium is the occult semiotics of blood and body parts.

NGOs' Moral Pedagogies

On a dusty evening during the dry season I observed how RHI workers shared the semiotics of the occult with their workshop audiences in Zebilla, the capital of the Bawku West District. RHI had been judged successful in the Bolgatanga and Bongo districts, where family planning had increased and cutting had largely ended by the turn of the millennium, and the NGO received funding to expand its reach. Located halfway between Bolga and Bawku and bordering Burkina Faso to the North, the Bawku West District is one of the most neglected in Ghana. The workshop was designed for a new crop of volunteers, rural chiefs, local politicians, and influential women whom the NGO dubbed "opinion leaders." For several days the attendees were housed in a nice hotel, treated to rich meat-laden meals, and given gifts of cloth and cash. The educational program was also considered a gift, as opportunities to learn are rare.

At dusk, after a long day of lectures and discussions about reproductive health, the workshop participants gather under the thatched gazebos in the courtyard of a small hotel catering to NGOs and tourists. RHI workers are busy setting up a projector to screen films about family planning, female genital cutting, and HIV/AIDS, but they first want to treat their audience to some entertainment and have chosen a popular film "just for a little while, to get their attention." The Nollywood film, *Billionaires Club*, is about Zed, a man who submits his infant son to ritual murder in exchange for wealth— a moral tale about the conversion of blood and life into wealth by witchcraft. The plot is familiar. Zed wants to join a club of rich men with big cars, big houses, black suits, young and glamorous wives, and fashionable American accents. One evening, on the pretense of taking his sick infant to the hospital, Zed hands him over to club members. The scene is graphic: Zed is anointed by the ritual master as the camera zooms in on a large mortar and pestle wielded by a scar-faced woman who is pounding Zed's son bloody. Zed also allows the club members to murder his wife and is rewarded with cash and human capital—influential friends and a young cosmopolitan wife. Soon, however, Zed is tormented by his wife's ghost and his dead son's cries; when his own body turns against him and he develops sores all over, death becomes the only avenue to peace. The moral lesson is clear: the boundless desire for wealth accumulation that urban Ghanaians often term *greed* is costly. Extracting wealth and power from blood and bodily matter places a higher value on individual enrichment than on sustaining familial and social relationships, and those who do so pay dearly.

The audience readily joins in the animated moral commentary that accompanies film watching: "Ah, you foolish man!" "Greed, it is all greed!" "Tsk, tsk, tsk, you wicked woman, don't go for him!" Like many Nigerian and Ghanaian films of its genre, *Billionaires Club* compellingly cautions against illicitly pursuing fast money (Meyer 2003; Garritano 2012) and expresses the sentiment that "the single-minded pursuit of money [is] patently amoral" (Smith 2008: 138). Blood is represented as a potent and valuable substance that mediates the perils of increasing wealth at the expense of one's physical and moral integrity as well as the well-being of the family. The occult exchange is invariably condemned, and perpetrators typically die by the end.

By the time *Billionaires Club* concluded, it had gotten late, and RHI workers decided not to show the NGO's films. At the time I felt the object of my inquiry slipping away. In theory rural screenings of public health films were the cornerstone of NGO encounters with their subjects, but I had yet to observe them after half a year at GAWW and RHI. This soon changed, when RHI repaired its projector and resumed its rural outreach, and I realized that RHI's entertainment appetizer often overshadowed the scheduled programming. I began to think of the films and music clips as pebbles thrown in the way of ethnography that thwarted my ethnographic desire and generated the pleasure of excess and surprise that are the stuff of fieldwork.[14] Years later I understood that tantalizing audiences is a part of the NGO's appeal, as well as that the screenings of popular films that critically evaluate the extraction of vital force in contemporary Ghana were consequential to women who were the subjects of NGO campaigns. The moral narrative of

Nollywood films was part of the assemblage about blood and crisis that informed rural women's narratives about the ending of cutting.

Insofar as they construct cautionary narratives about inequality, representations of the occult in films such as the *Billionaires Club* display political undertones. As Daniel Smith argues, they are "partly expressions of anger and discontent about the consequences of corruption" (2008: 140). They have also been celebrated as powerful critiques of neoliberal capitalism as they "act out [the] transformation of human life into surplus value" and point to "the human costs of prosperity, which is never achieved without the exploitation of another" (Garritano 2012: 61). It can also be said that, at least in fantasy, they provide resolutions to the violence of extraction that are elusive in everyday life.

I see such films as more ambivalent, as explained later in this chapter, but my main goal here is not to critique them but to analyze the work they do in shaping popular oppositional discourses. Nigerian and Ghanaian films fetishize the aesthetics of capital, embodying the fantasies of enrichment and social mobility (Meyer 2003). They also soothe social anxieties by exalting a narrow, and frequently conservative, conception of morality and the good life. Often aligned with intolerant forms of Christianity, they portray non-Christian spiritual practices, or "traditional religion," as sole sources of morally compromised wealth and locate the good life within the bounds of Christianity alone.[15] Finally, they share the neoliberal trait of hypermoralization in that they explain social ills in reference to individual moral behavior (Brown 2003). Audiences respond accordingly and join in scrutinizing the protagonists, especially when they are women. When I watched these films with friends and colleagues, commentaries on their morally reprehensible behavior were prominent: "That woman, I'm afraid she will get in between the couple." "And she thinks she is a marital woman." "Yes, just because the man did her a favor, she invites him to go to her house in the night. And look at her now, she is insulting him!" Thus, rather than implicating regional and global economic forces, these films pivot around gendered and individualizing moral lessons.

Wendy Brown (2003) pushes further the argument made by James Ferguson that neoliberalism disavows its own moral basis in the name of technical principles of scientific capitalism (2006: 80). While Ferguson's focus is African critical responses that understand, for example, the increase in food prices, as morally illegitimate, Brown's is on fleshing out the tacit moral logics of neoliberal rationality. She writes:

It figures individuals as rational, calculating creatures whose moral autonomy is measured by their capacity for "self-care"—the ability to provide for their own needs and service their own ambitions. In making the individual fully responsible for her/himself, neo-liberalism equates moral responsibility with rational action; it relieves the discrepancy between economic and moral behavior by configuring morality entirely as a matter of rational deliberation about costs, benefits, and consequences. In so doing, it also carries responsibility for the self to new heights: the rationally calculating individual bears full responsibility for the consequences of his or her action no matter how severe the constraints on this action, e.g., lack of skills, education, and childcare in a period of high unemployment and limited welfare benefits. Correspondingly, a "mismanaged life" becomes a new mode of depoliticizing social and economic powers and at the same time reduces political citizenship to an unprecedented degree of passivity and political complacency. The model neo-liberal citizen is one who strategizes for her/ himself among various social, political and economic options, not one who strives with others to alter or organize these options. A fully realized neo-liberal citizenry would be the opposite of public-minded, indeed it would barely exist as a public. The body politic ceases to be a body but is, rather, a group of individual entrepreneurs and consumers. (2003)

Popular critiques of illegitimate accumulation such as those presented in the *Billionaires Club* reveal the violence inherent in producing the "model neo-liberal citizen" who strategizes how to accumulate wealth and destroys, rather than fosters, social relations. But while such films also place primary blame on individual women or men, rural women critique the entire political system that positions them as prey.

The Social Life of Occult Economies

Discourses of the occult serve as critical "diagnostics" (Moore and Sanders 2003: 4) for terms of exchange and modes of governance across wider social domains—from media representations of corruption to public understandings of medical and ethnographic research. "You don't need an ethics approval for your project, you are not drawing anyone's blood," a Ghana Health Service official in Accra once told me.[16] Indeed, researchers have noted Ghanaian reluctance to participate in medical studies involving blood drawing and parents' fear that babies' blood is "collected for sale abroad for transfusion into the aged" (Newton et al. 2009: 498).[17] These refusals reveal critical awareness of potential exploitation in national and transnational research transactions and the inequality between giving and taking (Hayden

2007). A recent study that required drawing blood from infants illustrates this well:

> Many of the children are anemic, so some parents believe the blood samples for the study (1 mL) contribute to the babies' anemia or make them more suscepti-ble to illness. One father reasoned the blood samples caused his baby to fall sick three times afterward. Another mother suggested her baby wouldn't be as strong as an adult because of the blood samples.... Some parents of children who required transfusions for their anemia expected the study to pay for the cost of the blood when they were unable to find a replacement and reasoned the blood samples led to the need for transfusion.... This is a particularly difficult issue to address when participants don't understand that the small amount of blood required for the study would not necessitate transfusion.... Most inter-esting was the belief that the study was selling the blood or using it in rituals.[18]

The parents' statements address health concerns similar to those articulated by women in Bongo, as well as apprehension about the illegitimate com-modification of blood for ritual purposes. From the scientists' perspective, such worries are the result of a lack of proper understanding, that is, of an irrational overestimation of the value of blood. As Latour (1987) reminds us, accusations of irrationality hinge on naturalizing the scientific worldview and disavowing the scientists' own lack of understanding—in this case, of social evaluations of research transactions as potentially exploitative.

Representing as it does a combination of health concerns and apprehen-sion about the theft of vital force, blood is a visceral substance for expressing public dissent about extractive economies and exploitative terms of exchange. The global forces implicated in these processes are not always made explicit but at times take shape in references to differences between African vitality and Western lifelessness (White 2000; Aidoo 1977). Many people are aware that their country's demographic pyramid is upended in the global North, with many more elderly people than young people. Young Ghanaians there are eagerly hired as nurses and aides in retirement homes. So close is the association of the West, death, and suspect economies that in Twi second-hand clothes sold in markets are referred to as *obruni wawu*— "a white per-son has died." Economies of extraction and exploitation govern Ghana's place in the global world, but regional and national processes are more apparent to rural northern Ghanaians for many reasons, such as that they primarily migrate within the country, not internationally.

The idioms of blood and its illegitimate extraction have joined other bod-ily metaphors, such as "politics of the belly" (Bayart 1993), for critiquing the state. Ghanaian media and popular songs rely on idioms of both eating and bleeding to critique corruption in public and private sectors (Shipley 2012). While she was working for a Ghanaian newspaper, the anthropologist Jennifer Hasty found how prevalent such idioms were and how easily she adopted them herself: "Government offices and businesses riven with corruption are said to be 'hemorrhaging' while those responsible may be portrayed as vampires" (2005b: 278). In Bongo these accusations are leveled locally at politicians who are seen as sucking blood and "chopping" (eating) state resources that rightfully belong to the public. If during colonialism Africans saw the colonizers as vampires, today they portray local politicians in those terms—they are seen as "chopping" not just money but, as Agnes put it, people themselves.

At the NDC rally I mentioned earlier, Agnes had inveighed against politicians who eat women like *mui* (rice). She later explained her sentiments:

> They play us and eat, but when they win, after the voting, they forget of us. After the voting, they forget of us. When it's time for another election, they come to organize us and we vote. When they win, they forget of us again. I also said that as we are about to fast, if they're not able to tell us what they'll do for women if they win, we women should not vote. We are suffering to take care of our children, this schooling and so on. So I said if they win, while they're enjoying themselves, they should think back, we're human beings.

By mobilizing prevalent bodily metaphors about predatory consumption and extractive governance, Agnes highlighted the inverse relationship of the fattening of the country's leaders through "bingeing on state resources" (Hasty 2005b: 275) and the thinning bodies of its impoverished citizens. She recast and dramatized this critique of the state in gendered terms, by stating that the politicians were eating, that is, misappropriating and abusing, not only state resources but women and their vitality. Agnes is among the many people who see themselves as exploited by the "carnivorous" state (Mbembe 2001: 201), which cheats them of the benefits of citizenship. Many shared the view that state abandonment ceased only when politicians showed up to ask for their votes. One of Afua's peers said that the politicians never delivered the help they promised: "When they were campaigning, they told us to snap pictures and they will help us, but we have waited in vain."

Agnes repurposed the counting of people and votes—symbols of democracy and rote technologies of biopolitical power—to new ends, appropriating the state's own metrics to emphasize the profound inequality of governmental transactions. Although the state claimed the rural women counted, for Agnes the politicians' routinized forgetting meant that women had minimal political value. Politicians failed to treat them as fully human. So, she implied, Bongo women had to be healthy enough to cast a vote every four years and respond to the census once every ten but were disregarded in the interim. They were neither *zoe* nor *bios* (Agamben 1998) but had to maintain their existence as bare citizens on the threshold of biological and political life.[19]

Rural women would be right to criticize regional NGOs in such terms as well. The NGOs' extraction economies are subject to both popular criticisms in Ghanaian cities as well as scholarly theorizing (Mohan 2002) but are less visible to rural subjects. Although Agnes and others point to the NGOs' broken promises, they see politicians as the main parties responsible for the abandonment. As a result of decentralization and locally intensified political campaigning, Agnes and her neighbors have come to see politicians as representatives of state institutions that are able act on their behalf but choose not to and instead get rich and fat at their expense. This critique is itself an assemblage of historical and indigenous discourses, as well as, strikingly, the state's own opposition to illegitimate accumulation that privileges wealth over social relations. It was, after all, the former president Jerry Rawlings who instituted a campaign against exploitative capitalists whose bodily size was indicative of their exploitative practices (Nugent 1995).

CONCLUSION: WHERE IT HURTS

My main goal in this chapter has been to explore how cut women problematize the ending of cutting and thereby redefine its public meanings. To conclude I want to ask two questions: What makes the blood narrative desirable for cut women, and what work does it do for them? Also, what work can anthropology do with the blood narrative or what kinds of pebbles does an ethnography of slow harm throw in the way of theory? With Biehl (2013) I agree that ethnography's force takes shape not as a contribution to theory but as being "in the way of theory." Ethnography refuses to neatly order the world and issue final judgments, and my analysis testifies to the unfinished and ever-evolving character of the social worlds we study. In that spirit I want to conclude by highlighting how this ethnography of the blood narrative interrupts putatively stable understandings of power and resistance as well as analytical categories of a world in crisis.

Feminist scholars have argued that the body is in a fluid, continual process of materialization through practice and regulation (Butler 1993; Taylor 2005). In Janelle Taylor's words, the body is an "-ing" (2005: 745)—less a noun than a verb. She writes: "Not simply the inert objects on which mind and culture perform their meaning making, bodies take shape and take place through practices of all sorts: feeding, legislating, training, cutting, explaining, beating, loving, diagnosing, buying, selling, dressing, and healing, among others" (745). Women who ended cutting agree and draw attention to processes of blood depletion that materialize their bodies. While their bodies have taken shape through the practices of cutting, feeding (or the lack thereof), legislating, and diagnosing, they raise a concern about absent materializing practices. Increasing scarcity is weakening their bodies. Anticutting interventions have intervened in one aspect of materializing their bodies— cutting—but have not made them less vulnerable; likewise, reproductive health programs helped them survive childbirth but abandoned their bodies after pregnancy.

I want to suggest that the blood narrative renegotiates cut women's place in the Ghanaian polity by shifting the content, scale, and tenor of concerns about cutting. In contrast to public discourses that set cutting apart from the polity proper and relegate it to the unruly and ungovernable North, the blood narrative locates the ending of cutting within the national body politic, along with shared concerns about blood shortages, governance by extraction, and a national crisis of obligation and belonging. The blood narrative also enables cut women to delegitimize cutting on their own terms and to make sense of its ending. It could be said that it allows them to preserve dignity and save face in response to governmental and public shaming and to NGOs' claims that the women and their ancestors had no knowledge of bodies and reproduction and that cutting is a bodily and social pathology.[20] All this stands in stark contrast with their lived experiences of cutting as a former point of pride. But this narrative does more: it responds to prevailing discourses about the cultural inferiority of groups that are seen as resisting incorporation into national modernity and are faulted for their suffering. Cut women explain the ending of cutting within widely shared conceptions of health as well as within the national discourses about blood as an index of social concerns about inequality, crisis, and state failure. The ending of cutting is thus resituated within shared concerns about the perils of bodily and economic transactions in times of struggle. By mapping harms onto not culture but scarcity and abandonment by the state, the subjects of anticutting campaigns refuse the institutionalization of governmental meanings and reconcile perspectives otherwise seen as incompatible.

Anthropologists have long examined how social relations and political economy contribute to health and illness (Scheper-Hughes 1993).[21] By accounting for rural women's perspectives on cutting and its endings during a time of systemic crisis, this chapter highlights the immanent critique articulated by the "ordinary" people whose lives are at stake, showing that analysis of political etiologies of bodily attrition and imperiled social reproduction does not belong to scholars or social justice activists alone (see also Hamdy 2008; Nordstrom 2009).[22] The blood narrative offers a new answer to the question of where and when it hurts.[23] The wounds that plague women in Bongo are not the effects of hemorrhage or the cultural pathologies of tradition but the gradual yet newly acute loss of blood in the form of slow harm.

Nor are scholars the only ones who question the governmental institutionalization of meanings or the popularity of representing the present as a time of sudden crisis. Rural women agree with other Ghanaians that blood is precious and scarce, but their blood narrative offers a critical take on public understandings of local and national crises. Prevailing concerns about blood shortages ultimately criticize *bio*politics, pointing to the state's failures to secure supplies of blood and the resulting inability to save lives in moments of crisis. In contrast rural women want more than having their lives saved, so they criticize the political class that feeds on them and the structure of contemporary governance. Slow harm points to the historical production of scarcity and questions the morality of a carnivorous governmental politics that extracts their labor and votes and then abandons them or eats them alive.

Their critique of the present refigures the understanding of Ghana as a nation in a moral crisis and draws attention to the gendered dimensions of commentaries on what counts as a desirable future. Dominant social commentaries focus on loss of public morality and loss of culture, pointing to changes in organization of sexuality, kinship, and migration of girls, and generate a nostalgic discourse that romanticizes cutting and patriarchy. As I discussed in chapter 3, the virginity hypothesis is constructed as a national concern because public and governmental discourses amplify masculinist and conservative voices. As a result the "loss of culture" and traditional values

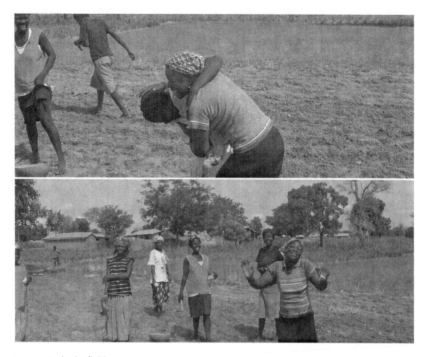

FIGURE 18. In the field.

appears to be the dominant anxiety in the Ghanaian postcolonial and neo-liberal context. Although the blood narrative partakes of the common discursive strategy of assessing the present by contrasting it with a more favorable past, this narrative departs from prevailing concerns about biopolitical and moral crisis. Rural women articulate political causes of social and bodily ills, and, rather than judging the sexual morality of women, they question the morality of governmental politics.[24] They thus disrupt nostalgia for what Povinelli calls "the prior" culture, meaning governmental ideas about unadulterated traditional ways of life, and also challenge the notion that their lives inhabit "the tense of the other," which is ostensibly delayed and not of the present (2011b: 14). Women who have stopped cutting instead foreground issues of obligation and belonging. They are critical of their abandonment by NGOs and the state in times of worsening economic and environmental conditions that structure how they live and labor. They do not aspire to turn back the clock or wish for everything to remain the same. Some "things have changed for the better," they say, such as the delay of marriage until after puberty and the availability of education for girls, which, however inadequate, used to be entirely out of reach. These women do not want the return of cutting, but they do want the ability to regain their blood, strength, and fortitude, which would require NGOs and the state to offer governmental care, not concern or sensitization.

Finally, the blood narrative accounts for the complexity of embodied life in the interval between the politics of life and "necropolitics" (Mbembe 2001). In contemporary Ghana liberal governance "does not exercise itself through the spectacular display of drawn and quartered bodies" (Povinelli 2011a: 134). The state can no longer be described as literally necropolitical—as my Accra host once told me, "The Rawlings regime committed human rights abuses, but the current regime kills on paper." Yet popular films dramatically depict gruesome killings, and critics of the state draw attention to otherwise invisible violence. Agnes's protest against politicians who eat rural women like rice highlights how neoliberal democracy "kills on paper" by extracting their vitality even as it invests in their survival. Women in northeastern Ghana are subject to intertwined forces that both save and diminish lives. They attribute deadly force to the state that "eats them" and saps them of blood, and they never fail to mention the deaths of their unborn children, but they do not construe the present in the affect-laden language of the time of death. Not "slow death" (Berlant 2011), not living "when the time to die has passed" (Mbembe 2001: 201), nor, as those close to them say, bleeding to death, death by occult forces, or death by forces that restore morality. Their complaints about bodily attrition are serious, but their vitality is also palpable.

Cut women's formulations of bodily attrition as an intensified but ordinary crisis are politically consequential, providing the grounds for collective assertion and self-cultivation. We might read their reformulations of bodily and economic vulnerability as a steady and quiet politics (Farquhar 2009). But, to borrow again from Povinelli (2011b), they may also constitute a counterpublic in potentiality, one that lacks institutional traction and might or might not bring about political change but one that endures, persists, remains in motion, and, by insisting on reformulating the world, may well surprise us all.

Government Officials Ask

Who is funding you?
What kind of a report will you produce for them?
What will you do for our women?

The Feminist Fetish

LEGAL ADVOCACY

TOWARD "ZERO TOLERANCE"

In July 2002, I accepted a last-minute invitation to attend a GAWW workshop on reforming Ghana's legislation banning cutting. Although cutting was ending in Ghana and had been criminalized in 1994, GAWW and its allies found the law insufficient and were finalizing their efforts to reform it. This workshop, held in the elegant Bayview Hotel in one of Accra's upper-class enclaves, was meant to introduce the proposed amendment to GAWW collaborators and "stakeholders" and gather their input. Invited were GAWW board members, feminist lawyers from the working group that drafted the proposed legislation, and other NGO, donor, and government representatives.

I was glad to see some familiar faces. Across the room Mr. Yahaya from Muslim Family Counseling Services smiled and gently nodded. I was seated next to Bethany, the administrator in charge of the U.S. Embassy's Human Rights and Democracy Project, which was the main funder of GAWW's campaign. She was pleased to see that the room was full of "important people," which to her meant that GAWW had not wasted its grant. She had lived in Ghana for nearly three decades and had adopted local metrics: if people showed up in numbers, particularly people who mattered, the project was a success.

Ghanaian NGO events are always ceremonial and ritualistic, laden with accolade-laced introductions, opening speeches, prayers, and participatory exercises, but the kinds of rituals that take place are stratified by class and region. Unlike workshops in the Upper East Region, which are sites of tightly controlled disciplinary encounters—no one is allowed to leave the room lest they take a long break or fail to return—those in Accra are dignified and interspersed with lavish service. Here we listened to opening prayers—Christian and Muslim, both said in English—and to the donor Bethany's brief remarks. During the midmorning break, we were invited to have coffee and pastries on the hotel terrace. Afterward, the legal experts arrived and distributed the draft memorandum that outlined the proposed changes to the law along with the rationales for them.

GAWW's first director, Gloria Aryee, and the current director, Mrs. Mahama, were the first to present the case for reform. The 1994 law, passed with GAWW's help, was failing, Mrs. Mahama said: it was supposed to deter girls and families from cutting, but research by Emma Banga and colleagues had shown that the law had no significant impact. Evidence for the failure was that FGM continued to be performed in Ghana, Mrs. Mahama said, and that newspapers reported that three in five babies in the Upper West Region were circumcised. "How can the vulnerable like the three babies report to be protected?" she asked and concluded, "The act of FGM is an inhuman treatment which denies the basic rights of women."

Mrs. Aryee, who was no longer active in public issues because of her age, gave an impassioned speech about the urgency of reform. She waved a report on the ostensibly rising rates of cutting in the Sudan, raising her voice to emphasize that time was of essence because of the imminent danger that cutting would increase in Ghana. "This has set us back! This has set us back!" she repeated several times, implying that because cutting was spreading, albeit on the other end of the continent, the legal reforms sought by GAWW were desperately needed.

Whence this desire for reform? The original law was not actually failing: some circumcisers were arrested and imprisoned, some stopped practicing cutting because they feared arrest, and some stopped encouraging their sons to take up cutting; meanwhile ordinary people knew about the law and its enforcement, and many women and girls were afraid that they would be arrested even before passage of the reform that would make them culpable. Not everyone stopped cutting, and not everyone stopped it because of the law, but the law played a large role in redefining public understandings of desirability of cutting.

For GAWW these historical transformations mattered little. The purpose of GAWW's advocacy was to improve and perfect the law by making it more punitive and more expansive. In concrete terms GAWW proposed bringing more people within the law's purview, an increase in punishment, and a shift in terminology from "female circumcision" to "female genital mutilation." The sentences for circumcisers were to be lengthened from three years to a minimum of five years, and culpability was to be extended to anyone "concerned with" the act of cutting, including parents and relatives. This advocacy ultimately led to passage in 2007 of the Criminal Code (Amendment) Act, 2007 (Act 741). In keeping with GAWW's reform proposals, the revised law extended the culpability beyond circumcisers, but it also increased punishments more than what GAWW had recommended, with sentences ranging from a minimum of five years to a maximum of ten.

The main ethnographic puzzle I address in this chapter is how and why advocates understood this harsher punishment as a productive force, not a repressive one. Musa, a GAWW employee, was one of many advocates who told me that the law was not intended to be punitive but rather to "*broaden . . .* the minds of people to know that this practice actually is not acceptable." As will become clear, although advocates successfully argued for more punishment as a central aspect of the law, they never wanted people to be imprisoned. I will suggest that the notion that law's power is exercised by broadening minds and compelling people, rather than constraining them, exceeds the advocates' intentions and speaks to larger feminist aesthetics of reform as well as Ghanaian cultural understandings of law as primarily educational and communicative. The Ghanaian public sees the force of law primarily as productive despite competing ideas about its social and political efficacy.

My second object of analysis is the exploration of why, given the waning of cutting in the country, the GAWW tactic to construct the law as failed had enough traction to get the amendment passed. Mrs. Mahama's remarks about human rights violations and failure of the original law were emblematic of the larger strategies that GAWW used to argue for the necessity of reform. Existing anthropological studies have stressed the *actual* failure of development projects to meet their stated goals and analyzed such failure as instrumental in the ongoing production of the need for development, as well as the expansion of state power and its depoliticization (Ferguson 1994; see also Miyazaki and Riles 2005).[1] That NGO and development projects will fail in their stated intentions has become a common ethnographic trope. Something entirely different is at stake in GAWW's pronouncements of failure: failure was a performative construct. The question I address is why the notion of failure resonated so readily in this context and why Ghanaian social scientists were among those who interpreted their data in ways that supported it. I will suggest this was a result of an assemblage of several discourses—the ostensible attachment to tradition and people's unruliness in northern Ghana, the indictment of the state as weak, and the dialectics of postcolonial order and disorder.

My main theoretical interest is analyzing the intimate relationship between violence and law. This and chapter 7 work in tandem and should be read against one another. They focus on lawmaking and law enforcement, respectively, illuminating how advocates' initial enthusiasm for a law turns into a rejection of it, that is, how the "fetishism of law" (Comaroff and Comaroff 2006a: 22) leads to a "disidentification" with it (Muñoz 1999). Together these chapters bring ethnography to bear on the interstices of two theoretical orientations: the globalization of feminist "left legalism" (Brown and Halley 2002b) and the fetishization of law in postcolonial Africa. I will suggest that context matters and that subjects matter, meaning that people's reckoning with the force of law produces unexpected outcomes. In this chapter my analysis of the social life of law focuses on Ghanaian feminist advocates' deep faith in law's potential in light of cultural understandings of law as productive. I attend to the instability inherent in the fetishization of law and the advocates' own reckoning with both the power of law and the tensions within humanism and feminist liberalism, namely, those between protection and punishment, freedom and violence.[2] In chapter 7, I show that the collusion of feminism and sovereign violence is contested even when it seemingly wins the day and that NGO workers and civil servants themselves turn "against the state" order (Clastres 1989).

My theoretical aim is to expand the analytico-affective grounds of feminist critiques of governance feminism and legal advocacy. To that end I want to return to something that feminist theory once knew but has since forgotten and read one of Judith Butler's earlier claims against recent feminist concerns about the feminist attraction to law. Analyzing the formation of sexed subjects in *Bodies That Matter*, Butler pushes Foucault's analysis of the juridical in a different direction, writing that Foucault does not sufficiently "address the ways in which 'repression' operates as a modality of productive power" (1993: 22). Law, Butler stresses, produces that which it represses, and juridical power is not separate from regulatory power—a point Foucault made but gave too little attention.[3] In the contemporary moment when state law becomes a central object of feminist interest and critique, we hear little of law's productive power. Feminist theory now emphasizes that the recognition and protection offered by state law come at the cost of regulation, exclusion, and punishment. That is true, as my own analysis will attest, but I also show that law's repressive mechanisms of power are productive.

By illuminating the productivity and instability of the repressive character of law, I suggest that the postcolonial fetishization of law is never simply what it declares itself to be—a desire for "punitive rationality" (Foucault 1984: 337) that authorizes increased criminalization and punishment. The logics and effects of feminists' attraction to legal remedies need to be studied in their performative aspects and seen from multiple angles. If we took the Ghanaian supporters of law reform at their word, we would have to conclude that they wanted to imprison as many circumcisers, parents, and cut women as possible in order to end cutting. But although they justified their efforts in reference to the repressive power of law and a "zero tolerance to FGM" approach, their goal was a more productive law, one that shaped, rather than constrained, the desires of legal subjects.

"INFUSED WITH THE SPIRIT OF THE LAW": THEORIZING LEFT LEGALISM IN THE POSTCOLONY

Popular depictions of African states figure them as existing largely outside the law. Descriptions both internal and external to the continent represent Africa as violent, lawless, and corrupt, which strengthens the grip of overdetermined discourses regarding its criminality and disorder. As Jean Comaroff and John Comaroff write, "lawlessness and criminal violence have become integral to depictions of postcolonial societies, adding a brutal edge to older stereotypes of underdevelopment, abjection, and sectarian strife" (2006a: 6). Lawlessness, we might say, is another discourse that places Africa under the signs of "lack" (Mbembe 2001) and "absence" (Clastres 1989), consolidating the image of the continent as bereft of order and civilization.

In contrast to these representations, the empirical manifestations of the social lives of law paint a picture in which the African states and public cultures are "infused with the spirit of the law" (Comaroff and Comaroff 2006a: 19). Rather than an absence of law in African states, we see complex legal regimes and a saturation of everyday life with juridical imaginations and aspirations. Law is central to postcolonial governance and social worlds. Far from construing law simply as a foreign imposition in the form of liberal governance, postcolonies "seem to make a fetish of the rule of law, of its language and its practices, its ways and means" (Comaroff and Comaroff 2006c: vii). The fetishism of the law, Comaroff and Comaroff write, "has to do with the very constitution of the postcolonial polity" (2006a: 32).

Empirically, one major manifestation of the fetishization of law is evident in the faith placed in new constitutions. Since the end of the Cold War, more than one hundred constitutions have been written or rewritten, mostly in the postcolonies; in Africa alone thirty-six states are now governed by newly revised constitutions (Comaroff and Comaroff 2006a: 22–24). Just as important as the number of revised constitutions are the near-magical qualities attributed to them, the "almost salvific belief in their capacity to conjure up equitable, just, ethically founded, pacific polities" (22). Constitutional democratic order, including liberal ideas about the rule of law and human rights, are imagined as ushering in a break with the violent past and the disappointments of postindependence governance. Jean Comaroff and John Comaroff situate the fetishism of law as a response to, and a foil for, historical wrongs such as the violence of postcolonial military regimes, the conclusion of the Cold War, and the end of apartheid, and the rise of neoliberalism and the concomitant waning of state sovereignty and its guarantee of social order. Analyzing the fetishization of law therefore requires us to attend to the dialectics of order and disorder, as well as to the associated material economies and geopolitical trends.

Scholars have shown that the fetishization of law follows many different paths into the capillaries of the cultures of postcolonial governance and everyday life: the emergence of law-oriented NGOs, the judicialization of political processes (Couso, Huneeus, and Sieder 2010), proliferating sites of arbitrage and adjudication such as truth and reconciliation commissions and community tribunals (such as the Rwandan Gacaca courts), and the International Criminal Court (ICC).[4] This proliferation also means that the cultures of legal fetishization know no national boundaries and traverse geopolitical terrains: we now see national and pancontinental forms of legal advocacy, such as the movement against domestic violence (Hodžić 2010, 2011), as well as the increasing relevance of international law for Africans. As Kamari Clarke puts it, "The global reach of international law is now becoming relevant to the micromanagement of daily life. In postcolonial African states, everyday actions and their meanings are being opened up by the expansion of national jurisdiction into international jurisdiction" (2011: 13–14), often with punitive effects. Meanwhile both domestic and international NGOs have brought law to bear on everyday life; as the Comaroffs put it, there are now "lawyers for human rights, both within and without frontiers; legal resource centers and aid clinics; voluntary associations dedicated to litigating against historical injury, for social and jural recognition, for human dignity, and for material entitlements of one kind or another" (2006a: 25).

Although the centrality of NGOs to the fetishization of law has been recognized, less is known about the dynamics of their participation in the dialectics of order and disorder. As Moran writes:

Left unexamined in most instances is the role of global non-governmental organizations in orchestrating and structuring much of the obsession with legal language and institutions that is ascribed to the postcolonial condition. Do the recourse to courts and appeals to universal human rights arise from within the contradictions of postcolonial nationalism, or do powerful actors claiming legitimacy beyond the individual state impose them from without? (2011: 194)

NGOs that foster conditions for recourse to courts are not only global, as Moran rightly suggests, but also domestic, and it is the latter that have the most profound social consequences. This chapter offers a detailed ethnographic analysis of the dynamics of the workings of domestic Ghanaian NGOs and in doing so also develops an alternative analytics of their unintended and productive effects.

Anthropologists writing about the judicialization of politics and legal fetishism have cast doubt on its ability to deliver on its promises (see contributions in Comaroff and Comaroff 2006b; Couso, Huneeus, and Sieder 2010; and Benda-Beckmann, Benda-Beckmann, and Griffiths 2009). Sally Merry makes a provocative point about the limits of this critique. She agrees that law has "replaced revolutionary violence" with a "politics of reform increasingly reliant on working within the existing structure" and that "this approach is likely to fail." But, she adds, revolutions have also failed, and neither reform nor revolution has "managed to diminish practices of unequal accumulation of wealth and power" (2008: 684). I take this intervention to mean that we have much to learn if we sidestep the reform-versus-revolution paradigm and that anthropologists can do more than document or predict failure. Failure, as I discussed earlier, is already spoken for by the actors we analyze.

With this in mind, my alternative analytics consists of exploring those unintended consequences of criminalization that are productive, turning the NGOs' own construction of failure into an ethnographic object and examining the materiality of everyday life where law meets its subjects. Ethnographers, we shall see, are not the only ones who question the law's capacities or who wrestle with its fetishization. By paying attention to how those who make and enforce Ghanaian laws deem them failures, successes, in need of reform, or, eventually, in need of curtailment, I highlight how Ghanaians address the limits of law's fetishization.

Ghanaian advocacy for the criminalization of cutting is a particularly poignant site for examining and historicizing feminist fetishization of law, because its very premises complicate the neat distinctions between reform and revolution or between politics and the political. Implicit in this is that *politics* is understood as policies and practices that create and maintain order and reinforce the status quo, whereas "the political" is "the disruption of an established order" (Ticktin 2011: 19). As Ticktin clarifies, "Radical change is the result of *political* action, not politics" (19). While in this rendering the political has radical potential that politics quashes, my research shows that the study of any given political project ultimately has to contend with the desires and effects that are simultaneously radical and normative. As Povinelli puts it in reference to Jacques Rancière, every dissensus threatens to become a consensus. She understands the possibility of the political as quite fragile and as consisting of the moment in which dissensus has emerged but has not yet produced a new consensus (2016). Rather than separating politics from the political, I suggest that we think of them as deeply entangled, not because they supersede each other in time, as Povinelli suggests, but because they are both present.[5] Challenging one order often means upholding or erecting another. There is no single established order, but orders in the plural, and we are yet to see a political force that can or strives to subvert them all. What we see historically is much closer to Merry's depiction of the historical limits of revolutions (to which I would add the pitfalls of existing socialisms, whether they did or did not go by this name).

Feminist activism that takes place at the interstices of NGO-driven governance feminism brings these dynamics into sharp relief and reveals the intertwined character of politics and the political. There is more to the desire for law than the maintenance of order. Ghanaian advocacy appears in both guises: as politics, in that it seeks to maintain a national order—saying no to cutting and harmful traditions, yes to an orderly, civilized state—and as the political, in that feminists challenge a gendered social order that makes women subject to cutting, the political order that constructs them as second-class citizens, and the state that refuses to work on behalf of any Ghanaians. Feminist scholars do not agree on the hierarchy of these goals, and I sympathize with those who see the activist challenge to the social order as insufficiently political, especially, as is the case here, when NGOs and others misapprehend "where it hurts" (chapter 5) or when they reduce the site of feminist struggle to culture while reinforcing class and regional inequalities and reanimating the civilizing mission inherent in the governmental politics of development of northern Ghana. Despite these objections I find it difficult to completely invalidate the political character of activist challenges to the state and the social order that work from within and that develop immanent critique. The analytical imperative, as I see it, is to think carefully about the intersections of politics and the political and to chart which politics is most dangerous and to whom in any given historical context. For leading feminist theorists the current answer is the feminist desire for law.

From a Distance: Feminist Critique of Desire for Law

In recent years feminist theorists have critiqued the widely dispersed advocacy that places uncritical faith in the transformational and liberating power of law, whether in reference to prohibitions on gender and sexual violence such as domestic violence and wartime rape, the legalization of gay marriage, or criminalization of human trafficking. Most notably Janet Halley, Wendy Brown, and their collaborators have taken issue with the pitfalls of "left legalism" (Brown and Halley 2002b) and "governance feminism" (Halley et al. 2006), highlighting the limits of their aspirations and their pitfalls and unintended consequences. The critical challenge for feminist jurisprudence, Srimati Basu writes, is that "institutionalizing feminist reform ... may fall short of enacting gender justice" (2012: 470). What is worse, feminist legal advocacy converges with regulatory and punitive forces, as well as with neoliberalism and imperialism. This scholarship powerfully demonstrates that there is much fodder for concern. The critiques of feminist advocacy against human trafficking and sex trafficking have shown that rather than protecting or empowering victims of trafficking, the criminalization of trafficking has produced "carceral feminism" (Bernstein 2014), replete with anti-immigrant policies, reduced labor rights, curbed possibilities of legal migration, and securitization as a dominant policy framework (Halley et al. 2006; Warren 2012).

I share the analytical interests of these scholars: I examine the interstices of feminist liberal advocacy and punitive criminalization, the unintended consequences of the fetishization of law in governance feminism, and the dominance of U.S. feminism. But I do not share these scholars' premises, affects, or their conclusions. One of my sources of discomfort with feminist critics of left legalism is that they understand it as a predominantly U.S.-centric phenomenon that is globalized outward, as if from a center.[6] Meant as critical responses to the dominance of U.S. feminism on the global stage, their analyses have posited U.S. feminism as an originary source of feminist legal liberalism and have tried to show how it has distributed itself around the world, combining women's rights frameworks with neoliberal technologies of securitization, policing, privatization, and individual empowerment.[7] They are right to note the massive influence of American feminist legal activists, but they overemphasize it and credit it with too much power, thus inadvertently replicating the very geopolitical inequality they want to challenge (see Hodžić 2009). Their conception of left legalism as diffused from the core to the periphery limits their methodological and analytical perspectives, rendering invisible the work of feminist legal activists in the global South. As a result they erase the agency of the very women whose political subjectivity forms their object of concern and whom they do not want to see reduced to victimhood.

By analyzing legal advocacy "from the South," this ethnography shows the interdependence of Ghanaian legal logics and international policies such as the legislation proposed in the U.S. House of Representatives in 2015 for a zero tolerance for FGM act. I aim to show why punitive rationality is ultimately opposed in Ghana but not in the global North. Second, by considering law as productive, my ethnography opens a space for analyzing how and why Ghanaian NGO workers and civil servants craft themselves as subjects and citizens. Productive does not equal positive: I show how advocates' fetishization of law generates desires for greater punishment and enacts state violence on those whom it aims to protect, in their terms, from cultural violence. Analyzing the productivity of legal advocacy means noting that its logics and unintended effects both *entail and exceed* the negative ones. As I discuss in this chapter and the next, NGOs' engagements with law enforcement eventually led to a meaningful reckoning with the force of law and the forms of recognition and subjectification it offers. My goal is not to vindicate the feminist fetishization of law, much less to celebrate it, but to show how Ghanaians wrestle with Janus-faced liberal governance that invests life with both surveillance and violence, as well as with hope for stability, justice, modernity, and effective governance. I will show that the complexity and instability of legal fetishism provokes critical reflections, leads to surprising acts of disidentification with the normative colonial order of things, and generates new forms of ethical imaginaries and social relations. My main contention is that by paying attention to how Ghanaian NGO workers and civil servants reconcile their protean, internally fraught, waxing and waning faith in the power of law, we can learn much about the forms of critique that propel locally meaningful action and social transformation.

In the introduction to this book I suggested that feminist theorists studying governance feminism have taken up ethnography as a method but have not embraced the ethnographic commitment to proximity and thinking *with* or the postcolonial feminist commitment to writing "nearby" (Chen 1992). Feminist critics of legal advocacy write about it from a moral and affective distance; they consider the turn to law and its unintended consequences to be bad objects. Critique, then, stabilizes these negative effects and leaves little room for understanding whatever is not determined by punitive rationality. In contrast thinking with and writing nearby entail methodological orientations as well as affective dispositions. I see this form of feminist anthropological ethnography as striving against putative a priori knowledge of the outcomes of social processes. Unlike theories committed to normative analyses, feminist ethnography need not render "final judgments" (Fortun 2001: 350). By "bracketing" my critique, as Ara Wilson puts it (2010: 87), I do not dispense with critique altogether but stage an analysis from *within* a recognition of the complexity, contingency, and indeterminacy that arise from people's reckoning with the force of law. Rather than writing from a constructed distance, I explore what emerges in close-up encounters, those of NGO workers and subjects, as well as mine.

Before proceeding I want to situate this focus with respect to the remainder of the book. My ethnographic attention to law stems from its importance as an object of intense interest and problematization for Ghanaian advocates, as well as from the resonance of the law among women who were made to fear it. But Ghanaian lawmaking and law enforcement also speak to deep-seated questions about theorizations of power. Alongside a more complex Foucauldian trajectory (Butler 1993; Hunt and Wickham 1994), I analyze how law and desires for legal regulation operate in the economy of productive power. My ethnographic analysis shows that Ghanaians understand law as both/and: both of the state and the capillary, repressive and enabling, normalizing and self-constituting.

FETISHISM OF LAW IN GHANA'S PUBLIC CULTURE

Ghana is one of the countries in which law has become central to public imaginations about justice and equality as well as to national politics of the day. At first, enthusiasm for law spread across the polity in the wake of the Cold War when Ghana shifted from socialist and military authoritarian rule to constitutional and neoliberal democracy. In 1992, after adoption of its constitution, Ghana's fourth since independence, spirits of reform were high, and law held out a promise of a more stable future and a break with wanton rule and social privation. Approved nearly a decade after Ghana's economic collapse and subsequent adoption of austerity measures and structural adjustment policies imposed by the World Bank and the International Monetary Fund, the constitution was more than just another in a series of government documents. It was a legal, political, and cultural phenomenon that fostered the fetishization of law and, as I will demonstrate, made possible the legislation against cutting.

Ghana has experienced a slew of legal reforms propelled by the country's engagement with global technologies of rule: the concomitant rise of neoliberalism and good governance has necessitated laws seen as facilitating privatization and enabling foreign investment. But the passion for women's rights was also integral to the constitution-making process and the subsequent fetishization of law. NGOs focused on women's rights are among the major institutional forces that have turned to law as an instrument of social change and of governance of everyday life, creating new laws and legal institutions that have saturated everyday life with legal imaginaries. The agencies based in Accra and run by lawyers believe in a nearly salvific, transformational force of law, and they work on infusing public cultures with aspirational visions of social justice and social change by legal means. The rise of feminist lawyers as leaders in the larger women's movement has invigorated advocacy, most notably for the Domestic Violence Act, and fashioned law into a prime terrain of political struggle—not only about gender and sexuality but also about sovereignty and political subjectivity (Hodžić 2009). To say that this and other laws are fetishized does not point to the absence of critique but to the extent of public preoccupation with law. The national mood ranged from endorsement to mockery, opposition, and rage, but contestations about this and other legal transformations became central to the political life of the country, expressing and generating anxieties about wider-ranging social transformations.

Ghanaians have also learned to live with the polyvalent character of law, evident in the formation of new institutions mandated by the constitution such as the Commission on Human Rights and Administrative Justice and the National Reconciliation Commission. Their configuration is peculiar in that it wears the symbols of law but does not enjoy its full force. Although neither institution has the authority to dispense justice or ensure redress, Ghanaians act as if they do. Many women turn to the human rights commission to seek economic justice and spousal maintenance, hoping that law can help them where family and the state have failed. Indeed, the commission serves as a preferred alternative to courts for many women who seek a formal, legal mechanism that would compel their husbands to pay maintenance and upkeep. Although the primary purpose of the commission is investigative and it has few enforcement powers, its appeal stems precisely from this "soft power." Women I knew well in Bolgatanga, along with those who came to Elizabeth's or Nitu's NGO for assistance with their problems, were reluctant to "take their husbands to court," as they said, lest they be ostracized by their community. They would turn to the human rights commission, Legal Aid, and NGOs as nonpunitive institutions and would file reports with the police unit that keeps track of domestic violence.[8] What they want from law is the power to compel, not to punish; as I will show, this desire is central to Ghanaian understandings of legal force.

THE HISTORY OF ADVOCACY FOR LEGAL REFORM

GAWW's advocacy for law reform is a prism for understanding the shifts in Ghana's fetishization of law during the transition from the quasi-military regime to democratic, neoliberal rule. In 1994, when cutting was first outlawed, the notion of rule of law held out a promise of stability, but law was also viewed as a technology whose force needed to be curtailed and supplemented with so-called education. A decade later the faith in Ghana's rule of law had dissipated but not the faith in perfecting the legal system, which would then make up for the weakness of the state. The legal imaginaries in the campaigns to criminalize cutting reveal a trend toward a heightened dialectics of order and disorder: over time, greater power for social and governmental change is attributed to law despite the simultaneous lack of trust in the efficacy of *any* law. "The law doesn't work, we want new and stricter laws," the logic goes. "And we want not only new laws but also more punishment." These dialectics are inscribed in Ghana's history of postindependence coups that toppled democratic regimes in the name of social justice, as each regime change was an attempt to restore order by overthrowing a government seen as corrupt. What is new is the turn to law: the more the state was seen as incapable of governing, the greater became the desire for legal reform and punitive law.

The passage of the 1994 law against cutting was accompanied by somber statements qualifying its power and emphasizing that it was not a magic bullet. GAWW never expected criminalization alone to end cutting. As GAWW officials wrote in their reports to the Inter-African Committee on Harmful Traditional Practices Affecting the Health of Women and Children (IAC), they planned relentless "massive educational campaigns" to "prevent the practice of F.G.M. [from] going under-ground."[9] By mentioning "underground" continuation of cutting as a potential outcome of the legislation, GAWW construed law not as an antidote to disorder but as its potential cause. Education was a remedy that was supposed to ensure that the law would find a welcoming environment rather than compelling people to hide from its force.

By depicting the law as an imperfect mechanism that requires "educational programmes" as its accompaniment, GAWW may well have wanted to secure funding and support for its future campaigns, ensuring the NGO's own survival. For GAWW it was of paramount importance that criminalization of cutting not be understood as an endpoint of its campaign. However, self-interest cannot account for the desire to inaugurate an education program after passage of the law, because the understanding of law as a necessary but insufficient tool for ending cutting had wide traction. Whenever the law was mentioned, it was stressed that it alone would not end cutting and that further interventions were necessary. As Mr. Yahaya from Muslim Family Counseling Services told me: "But the law, as it stands right now, will not achieve much, without a vigorous campaign, you know, against the practice. People will still have to be educated."

The government agreed with this sentiment. The attorney general's office was especially reluctant about criminalizing a traditional custom. In a memorandum that GAWW touted in Ghanaian newspapers after passage of the bill, the attorney general and the minister of justice, Obed Asamoah, wrote:

> It has been emphasized by the Law Reform Commission and elsewhere that the abolition of female circumcision by force of law though it may deter some practitioners may not eradicate it due to the deep traditional belief in the custom. In order to achieve any realistic impact on the problem other means in addition to legislation will have to be found. It has to be acknowledged that it is *only* through education that the tradition, superstitions, and general lifestyle of the people can be changed, but nonetheless it is incumbent on the government to proscribe the practice by legislation. (emphasis added)

Law, yes, but only when accompanied by "other means," that is, education. Education was necessary for law not to fail and not to turn against itself. These were often performative statements: the power of law not only was but *should* be limited.

Making Failure

I cannot trace the exact moment when GAWW decided that the law was not only insufficient but failing, yet I noted that the very passage of the 1994 law marked a departure in GAWW's self-representation. Earlier GAWW had emphasized its successes, but after the law was enacted, the NGO's leaders began to highlight their challenges and obstacles, discussing the intractability of cutting. NGOs usually represent themselves as successful, but GAWW began doing the opposite, disavowing success and stressing the limits of interventions. I suggested earlier that what became intractable was not cutting but the joint discourses about its intractability and the law's failure. Here I focus not on contesting GAWW's claims but on analyzing the logics of its advocacy, which require construction of the law as a failure. While their donors might have liked GAWW to tell them stories about its successes, the NGO wanted to convey that its work had just begun.

As soon as the statute took effect, GAWW began to portray it as inadequate and started discussing reform. Its leaders gathered institutional allies among police and civil servants throughout the country and then applied for funding to collaborate with feminist lawyers on the NGO's advocacy platform. In 2000 GAWW received the aforementioned grant from the U.S. Embassy's Human Rights and Democracy Fund for revising the legislation to increase sentences and culpability.

The stated purpose of the reform was to make the law functional and successful—because it was said not to work in practice, its text had to be emended. GAWW constructed the existing law as deficient and raised questions about the number of arrests and the rates of cutting, telling the U.S. Embassy: "The question here is how effective this law has been since it was passed seven (7) years ago. How many people have been arrested? Has the cutting of young girls and babies ceased?"[10] These questions were rhetorical and not to be answered in reference to actual arrest data or diminishing rates of cutting. GAWW knew that some circumcisers had been arrested and sentenced, that the watchdog committees had succeeded in preventing cutting in some instances, and that cutting was waning in areas where scientists were measuring change. GAWW leaders knew about the sharp decreases in cutting from the Navrongo Health Research Center and from Dr. Adjei's research, but they put this knowledge aside to argue for reforming the law. They claimed that cutting was intractable, that circumcisers continued their practice unabated, and that resistance to the law was widespread.

These statements eventually became a common sense, as repetitions lend truth to utterances. "People do not report," and "do not tell," I often heard from civil servants, "because of ignorance" and "because they don't know." The ostensible failure of the law to compel people to report cutting to authorities became a mainstay of arguments for reform. As Mrs. Mahama told me:

> But what, actually, eh, inspired us about the law is that, you know, since the law was enacted in 1994, not many people ... it's very difficult to get people ... arrest people on FGM, because nobody will report in the first place, you see? Nobody will report. And so we feel that maybe the law was too narrow. If, actually, the parents or the close relatives realized that if they are caught doing it, they will also be sanctioned, you see.

For Mrs. Mahama and others the alleged lack of reporting—as we shall see, people eagerly reported instances of cutting—would be remedied by changing the law. The existing law was "too narrow" in that it punished circumcisers but not families who requested their services; as Mrs. Mahama put it, "Right now, it's only the exciser who faces the music." A law that made more people culpable would make more people feel addressed by law and ready to report cutting to the authorities. The solution was to "broaden the scope" of the law by extending culpability to parents and all those involved in cutting.

Susan, a GAWW affiliate and one of Ghana's leading feminist lawyers, explained this logic as "roping in more people" to ensure that they "would report these things":

> Because then, you see, you have the circumciser who you can get under the regular criminal code as the main, um, let's say the criminal, the person, yeah. But then you have the parent who took the child, and then you have all those people around who danced and made noise so that nobody will hear.

All those who made noise at the ritual of cutting should now face a different music—the music of the law.

Ordinary Disorder: Rule of Law in Postcolonial Ghana

One reason why GAWW was successful in depicting the law as failed was the recent public consensus that few Ghanaian laws are functional. A public health nurse and administrator from Bolgatanga put it succinctly: "In Ghana, our laws—they're made but nobody seems to be very strict about them." The view of the state as uninterested in being strict became acute in the wake of disappointments in democratic governance. Since neither the legal system nor the state had lived up to the promises made after the transition to democracy, faith in the power of law was subsiding. Ghanaians counted on the state not to act on its laws or policies and were surprised when it did, yet many responded not by turning away from law but by wanting to improve it.

Feminist lawyers saw the letter of the law as something they *could* perfect, given that they could not perfect the state. Theirs, too, was a dialectic of order and disorder. Jane, one of the lawyers who drafted the reform, told me that the problem was the Ghanaian "system":

> I had also noticed the gaps in the legislation and thought that so many people fell outside of it that it wouldn't have been effective, being that kind of system that we have in Ghana. So we wanted to use that bit of legislation for social change, but it didn't go far enough.

I asked Jane to tell me more about the system she was referring to. She connected the desire to perfect the letter of the law to the context of a flawed judiciary and police; the system she described was one in which "you don't have sensitized judges and law enforcement officers." The way to make the law work was to "tighten the framework so that it actually is able to bring in all those who are concerned with the practice." No gaps should be left to the interpretation of reluctant police and judges. In other words, the perfect law should be a counterpoint to the malfunctioning state. She elaborated: "A piece of legislation is only as good as the paper on which it's written, if nothing else happens, you know. And we live in a country that is very, you know, very good at passing legislation if you like, but with a very weak enforcement system." Advocates wanted to make an ideal law to counteract the state's incapacity. I understand this incapacity not as a symptom of a so-called weak state but as a compound effect of material incapacitation, a preference for nonpunitive legal rationality, and a masculinist reluctance to prosecute that is masked as a performance of incapacity.

Susan shared Jane's understanding and saw the new law against cutting as enabling activists to "network and get as many people interested as possible" in order to set up alternative structures. As will become clear in chapter 7, this would mean sensitizing the police and the judges, expanding the domestic dispute unit, and training new kinds of citizen enforcers. The feminist response to the dialectics of order and disorder was that the state's "very weak enforcement system" would be counteracted by compelling laws and civil servants who are mobilized to action. They saw the law not simply as an agent of the state but as an institution that remedies its weakness by drawing society into law enforcement.

GAWW coupled references to the weak state to the notion of unruly and ungovernable northern Ghanaians, promoting the idea that northern populations resist the law, state governance, and development. Since northern Ghanaians ostensibly circumvented the law by going underground and crossing state borders, GAWW proposed that the northerners needed to be governed by a particularly stringent set of laws. Circumcisers were seen as the paradigmatic unruly subjects, mobile and ready to escape the rule of law, especially when protected by villagers who helped them cross the border. This is how Mrs. Mahama characterized this context:

> You see, so they protected them, particularly those they go to bring from other areas to come and do it. So by the time you even get to know that, "Oh, there is something, this thing [cutting] has gone on here," where is the this thing [circumciser]? She is gone. You can't get her.

Edna, the GAWW worker, added, "They don't stay at one place; they keep on moving." With the revised law, she said, "You, the parents would be held responsible" even "if the circumciser is not there." Edna reasoned that the reformed law would at least hold *somebody* responsible.

This imaginary of mobile circumcisers, I will show, belies the extent of their extraordinary compliance and submission to authorities. Circumcisers sought by the police were found at their houses, willingly reported to medical authorities, allowed NGOs to take pictures and videos and to record interviews, took the police to the cut girls' houses, and appeared in court even after they had been released on bail. In other words those pursued by the police did everything *but* evade the law. Nonetheless, given the public consensus about the shortcomings of the weak state, ineffective law enforcement, and northern violence and unruliness, GAWW's narratives about failure found a fertile ground and became public opinion. This effect was achieved with the help of social science.

I first heard about the study of the ineffectiveness of law the summer I arrived in Ghana. My hosts in Accra, as well as Elizabeth, the NGO director I met on a plane, had many words of praise for Mrs. Banga, a former member of the GAWW board who was a professor of nursing at the University of Ghana and head of the Ghana Registered Nurses Association. Elizabeth introduced us; Mrs. Banga was her aunt, she told me—as I learned later, by virtue of being married to a man from a neighboring village. I was eager to learn from Mrs. Banga about GAWW's history, but she really wanted to talk to me about a research project she had completed for an international agency. Titled "A Study on the Effects of Legislative Abolition of Female Genital Mutilation," the research had commenced in 1997, only three years after the law was enacted. "We found that most people don't know about the law," Mrs. Banga told me when we met. "So how can the law work, if people don't know about it?"

Hers was the study that Mrs. Mahama referred to at the Accra workshop as evidence of the failure of the law. Mrs. Banga did not have a copy on her computer but called her three coauthors to try to locate it. The fate of reports commissioned by international agencies and NGOs is such that they often disappear. Some are never completed, some are never shared, and others vanish over time. The authors themselves rarely have them, and they hold on to them tightly when they do. "You must write about this loss of knowledge," Dr. Patrick Twumasi, a medical sociologist, told me after his unsuccessful search for a copy of a study he had conducted for GAWW. But what for him was an indictment of Ghanaian bureaucratic cultures and their malfunctioning was for me a telling illustration of the place of knowledge in governance. Knowledge, we see time and again, is not used to guide the course of interventions but helps construct their scale and legitimacy. Commissioned studies matter most if they confirm popular beliefs and common sense. Those that can be interpreted as affirming existing discourses have a long afterlife, even if they leave few material traces, such as Mrs. Banga's, whose fragments were located on disks and flash drives.

None of the authors who searched for this particular report was able to locate a complete final version, but over time I received different drafts from two of the authors. These reports reveal that the discourse of the failure of the law sits next to data that show its grip. Contrary to its own findings, the study bolsters the discourse of the law's failure and underground resistance to NGO campaigns. The report shows that 87 percent of respondents stated that "FGM should be banned by law in this country" (Banga et al. 1999: 51), and 72 percent stated that "the law has stopped FGM in this community" (54), but the authors concluded on an alarming note that the law had failed. "The revelations from the study are disturbing," the report states, as "most respondents have never heard of the law and therefore were unaware of it" (Banga et al. 2001: 62). The proposed solution was to use nurses as vectors of public education about the statute, but Mrs. Banga did not receive funding for such a public education project. Instead, GAWW relied on the report to support a more punitive law.

Researchers from the Upper East Region, including the Navrongo Health Research Center and Dr. Adjei, were opposed to the criminalization of cutting and the stricter legislation sponsored by GAWW. Dr. Adjei objected to the general fetishization of law and thought that "community engagement" was a more suitable strategy for ending cutting. In one of our conversations he told me: "I'm not saying [the law] is bad, but all that I'm saying is if you are able to do the proper thing with the little money you have, the practice will stop, because in Ghana it's not serious." Navrongo researchers were even more perturbed; they saw the law as an unwanted variable that tainted their data by introducing fear as a factor in people's responses to their research questions. I also heard from the Ghanaian and American staff at the U.S. Agency for International Development, the U.S. Embassy, and the UN Population Fund that they knew about and at least partially agreed with these objections.

Dr. Adjei, a consummate modernist, hoped that he could use his research findings to demonstrate the faulty premises of GAWW's advocacy for reform. Just as he had tried to reason with groups that practiced cutting by staging experiments that showed that a pumpkin bears fruit even if an uncut woman jumps over it, he wanted to convince GAWW and others that the existing law had not failed and that cutting was indeed ending. The opportunity came when he was invited to give a presentation, "FGM and Its Health Implications on Women," at GAWW workshops on reforming the law. This was part of GAWW's series of "consultative workshops" titled "Review the Law on Female Genital Mutilation and Advocate for Law Reform." Convened after the amendment and memorandum were drafted, the workshops were held in Accra and in Bolgatanga from October 2001 to July 2002; Accra was chosen because it is the capital and seat of the national government and Bolgatanga because it is the center of anticutting campaigns in the North. The purpose of the workshops was to authorize the proposed reform by convincing the invited government officials, UN workers, and NGOs that the existing legislation had failed. I arrived in Ghana at the end of this process and observed the last of the workshops; I reconstructed GAWW's earlier advocacy from conversations, interviews, and GAWW documents.

Dr. Adjei was invited to the workshops to present the results of his research. But instead of discussing the health implications of cutting alone, he wanted to convey that a stricter law was unnecessary. Given the norms of public decorum, he could not oppose GAWW directly, so he discussed his findings about "FGM prevalence" that testified to its ending. In the Bolgatanga District prevalence had dropped to 6.3 percent among "in-school" girls and to 27 percent among "out-of-school" girls. Workshop participants learned that efforts to end cutting were succeeding in districts where sustained interventions had taken place for two decades and that cutting was least practiced among girls who had received formal education.

As a talented speaker who presents complex findings in an accessible way, Dr. Adjei made an impression on the audience but was unable to counter the prevailing discourse of the law's failure and the intractability of FGM. One reason is that reformers did not consider failure a literal statement of legal malfunction. Rather, GAWW and other advocates saw the law as not living up to its potential.

When I interviewed Jane, I learned that she had great faith in Dr. Adjei's approach but saw no contradiction between the statements about failure and the waning of cutting in areas where his NGO worked. Jane singled out RHI as a successful NGO because it not only educates but also "engages the community" reminding everyone of the force of law:

> I'm very happy about the work that Doctor Adjei does, in Bolga, for example. You know, he, he has chosen a participatory method that engages the community. So while he's engaging with them, you know, mending the wombs and all of those things, he's getting chiefs to now say, "You can't do this in my jurisdiction." He's getting community elders to say, "We signed on to this thing; we're not going to get it done." And at the same time they are able to tell their people, "If you do it, the law will get you." You see? So it's a combination of, of approaches. It's a combination of methods and approaches and it works. It works! It works!

To Jane, her admission that interventions had been successful and her endorsement of Dr. Adjei's efforts ("It works!") were irrelevant to the debate about the proposed legislative revisions. He had taken the question of the law's failure too literally, just like he had taken the question of the pumpkin's reproductive capacity too literally, not acknowledging its aesthetic resemblance to a woman's womb. For the reformers failure meant a deviation from ideal legislation: the future law needed to be not just better but perfect.

FEMINIST AESTHETICS AND THE DESIRE
FOR PUNISHMENT

A perfect law has a specific form, and I want to suggest that the advocates were moved by passionate formal concerns. Following Marilyn Strathern, I understand the "persuasiveness of form" and "the elicitation of a sense of appropriateness" as aesthetics (1991: 10). Extending this concept, Annelise Riles argues that transnational legal collaborations hinge on the sharing of aesthetic, rather than substantive, concerns (2001). Her work shows that the shared aesthetics of form and design enabled agreement about international norms and platforms for action on women's rights. I want to show that the aesthetization of legal form is also at the heart of feminist fetishization of law. For the advocates the instrumental functions of the law were intertwined with the formal qualities of the letter of the law. This aesthetics made possible punitive imaginaries of law by smoothing over concerns about the excesses of punitive rationality.

Feminist lawyers and GAWW considered existing legislation a failure because they saw it as having an inherently flawed *form*. It was "too narrow," they said, had "too many gaps," and did not resemble other laws. They wanted the reformed legislation to be neatly aligned with other Ghanaian laws and international treaties they were passionate about. This alignment would perfect what the law looked like, what it resembled, how it sounded. The law against cutting should *look* like other "model" laws, they said, such as Ghana's law against *trokosi* ("customary servitude") and Burkina Faso's legislation against FGM.[11] The proposed law should refer specifically to *female genital mutilation,* not *circumcision,* so that it would echo the term used by GAWW and other campaigners. By using the term *female circumcision,* the existing law was outmoded and in need of updating.

African NGOs and activists regard Burkina Faso as a model country for campaigns against cutting because of the strong political backing for the national IAC chapter. Chantal Compaoré, wife of the long-serving (1987–2014) head of state Blaise Compaoré, was the honorary chair of the Burkinabe IAC chapter and was later named an IAC goodwill ambassador. As a result the Burkinabe campaigns against cutting have been visible across the continent and beyond. In addition, Susan had lived in Burkina Faso for several years and found the Burkinabe law against cutting to be appealing because it was "more comprehensive":

> We realized the [Ghanaian] law was there, but it wasn't comprehensive, as comprehensive as it was in Burkina Faso. . . . In Burkina, you all get roped in and then with the Burkina law, if you were in a community and you knew this was going to happen, and you did not report it, you were, you are an accessory as a matter of course. . . . They have a higher incidence [of cutting in Burkina Faso] and their law, as I said, is more comprehensive and it's working.

Susan was right that Burkinabe laws are regularly enforced against circumcisers and parents, fining or jailing them. By 2005 eighty-eight cases had been brought to court and more than four hundred people were said have been punished.[12] Susan attributed this not to political will but to the letter of the Burkinabe law.

Jane made similar claims about the Ghanaian trokosi legislation. Passed in 1998, the trokosi law extends culpability to a wide range of people, namely, to whomever "participates in or is concerned with a ritual." As Jane told me:

> Now, if you read that piece of, that part of, the criminal code amendment, it's, it's wide in its code, you know. It covers not only direct practitioners or perpetrators but those who even encourage the practice, those who take people for ritual enslavement, those who receive people for ritual enslavement—you know, it's a whole run of rights.

For her and others the law against cutting needed revision because it *could* take a more comprehensive legal form and *could* address a greater number of subjects. Thus the trokosi statute became a formal template for reforming the law against cutting.

A basic but important point bears explicit mention here: the advocates' push to model the FGM legislation after the trokosi law were not motivated by how the trokosi law was enforced by the state. Trokosi practitioners did not face criminal charges, nor, to my knowledge, is the law enforced even today. When Jane and others claimed that the trokosi law was more enforceable, they meant that by holding parents and guardians responsible, the law encompassed a greater number of subjects. This shows that the valorization of the trokosi legislation had to do with its formal characteristics, mainly its scope and its breadth—it left no gaps. The proposed amendment closely followed the trokosi statute, replicating its language word for word to enumerate those who could be held directly and indirectly responsible: "Whoever participates in or is concerned with a ritual or customary activity . . . commits an offence and is liable on summary conviction to imprisonment."

Annelise Riles's analysis of the construction of NGO as well as UN documents about women's rights shows that activists deem those documents most successful that most resemble existing forms and extend them in a new direction (2001). Extending her analysis to Ghana, I suggest that GAWW and other reform advocates wanted to replicate the form of model laws. This reasoning and the desire for formal resemblance is common in a legal logic that seeks commensurability. Thus Ghanaian advocates sought to align the proposed amendment not only with laws they regarded as proximate, such as the trokosi law and the Burkinabe law against cutting, but also international laws and treaties.

In Step with the World, Ahead of the Curve on Zero Tolerance

Advocates wanted the law to align with Ghana's Constitution and with a wealth of laws, policies, and conventions from the larger world of global governance, such as African human rights instruments and international treaties. These alignments should be understood as performative strategies: GAWW and legal advocates mobilized the desire for Ghana to be "in step with the world" but their goal was to do more than that: they wanted to shift the campaign against cutting toward zero tolerance. This entailed two strategies: affirming and legislatively authorizing the terminology *female genital mutilation* and demanding greater punishment for a wider range of people held liable for its practice.

To justify reform to the appropriate authorities (the attorney general and the parliament), the memorandum outlining the proposed changes details the opposition to FGM in Ghana-ratified treaties such as the Convention on the Elimination of All Forms of Discrimination against Women (CEDAW) and the Convention on the Rights of the Child, international policies contained in various UN and WHO resolutions, and in national policies on reproductive health, population, and the empowerment of women. By enumerating these, the memorandum reminds the lawmakers that they need to keep Ghana in step with the world. This argument is particularly important in the case of cutting since FGM commonly mediates

Africa's global image, from which Ghana strives to disassociate itself. Aligning itself with the world meant casting FGM outside the nation.

The desire to change the name of the offense from *female circumcision* to *female genital mutilation* took center stage in the advocates' argument for reform. The terminology was one of the "gaps in the existing law" that needed a legal remedy. At the level of substance the difference in nomenclature appears minute—although the existing law did not use the capitalized phrase *Female Genital Mutilation,* it did use the verb *mutilate.* But for the advocates the law "lacked" the discursive bundle entailed in the notion of female genital mutilation, or FGM. FGM indexes a complex discursive assemblage of knowledge, affect, and interventions. In Ghana's public culture it connotes a "harmful traditional practice" that is a source of national shame.

It is not surprising that language becomes so important in debates about cutting, given the discursive wars fought about nomenclature. But that the terminology would be considered important enough to justify statutory revisions reveals something about the desire to perfect the form of the law, as well as about the status of cutting in Ghanaian society. GAWW had grown emboldened and able to count on public opposition to FGM, so the organization could now afford to take a tough stance. The language change was a symbolic maneuver meant to signal the unapologetic tenor of the paradigm "zero tolerance for FGM."

In turn, the memorandum about reforming the cutting law stated that Ghana could not afford *not* to take such a stance, as it had to be aligned with the global consensus:

> The present law refers to the offence as "Female Circumcision". However, the World Health Organisation and other bodies acknowledge that excision and infibulation constitute actual mutilation of normal organs. . . . It is therefore being proposed that the name of the offence should be changed from "Female Circumcision" to "Female Genital Mutilation" (FGM) to reflect its actual nature.

Participants at the Accra workshop agreed with the proposed change to "Female Genital Mutilation (FGM)." The term is used regularly by those who speak English, even though I have sensed discomfort in many because they hesitated before saying it or prefaced it with the common phrase "the this thing." Mrs. Mahama knew that everyone in the room considered the acronym acceptable, and she capitalized on this view by telling a story that ridiculed the liberal sentiments of those who objected: "Recently, we were at a workshop where it was referred to as *cutting!* It's like appeasing those who could be offended!" "Yes, yes, yes," the participants rejoined. "Even in the UN people say that," someone chimed in, and the participants shook their heads in disapproval. Why would they want to appease cut women? And why would they follow the lead of "politically correct" feminists and as Morissanda Kouyate, the IAC's director of operations, later put it, "somber anthropologists"? Mrs. Mahama continued, "Surgery can be cutting, but this is not therapeutic and [the language of the law] should reflect its nature. So it should be FGM until the world decides otherwise."

Codifying FGM in law was a complex task, one that on paper aligned Ghana with the world while in practice wrested the authority over anticutting discourses from those in the global North. Although the memorandum drew on WHO documents and Mrs. Mahama made references to international authority ("until the world decides otherwise"), the desire for a terminological shift to *FGM* should not be understood simply as GAWW's attempt to align Ghana with international discourses but as asserting the advocates' own place with respect to them. Mrs. Mahama knew that many international organizations had already shifted from *female genital mutilation* to *female genital mutilation/cutting,* or *FGM/C. FGM/C* is now the term of preference at UN organizations (with the exception of the World Health Organization) but not for GAWW or the IAC. Mrs. Mahama sought to change the terminology to *mutilation* not because of but *despite* the emerging shifts in global governance of cutting. Together with the larger IAC network, GAWW was Africanizing the global discourse.[13]

The advocates' logic of aligning FGM with trokosi was equally complex. They presented the reform of the law as integrationist in the sense that cutting was to be synchronized with trokosi and the larger world of feminist governance. But while the reformed law on cutting followed the form of the trokosi law in the name of aesthetic alignment, commensurability, and a perfected legislation, its substance was different. Cutting was deemed a crime so grave that it called for greater punishment, and the sentences for the two practices have never been similar. Trokosi is punished by three years of imprisonment, whereas cutting was already punished by three to five years; the reform called for increasing the sentences for circumcisers to a minimum of five. Like female genital cutting, trokosi is stratified by class and ethnicity. It is not practiced among the wealthy or the powerful but on the relative margins of the state and is often called backward, harmful, and traditional. But trokosi has not come to define the Ewe in the way that cutting defines the North, figuring it as a site of violence, barbarism, and disorder, and trokosi was not subject to harsh punishment.

In Accra I observed how the desire for greater punishment was fueled. Supporters argued for longer sentences, which would "reflect the nature of the offense," as the lead lawyer put it. She meant that the length of prison sentences needed to be commensurate with the harms of FGM. Anyone who "sends to, or receives at any place any person for the purposes of excising, infibulating, or mutilating" would serve sentences of "not less than five (5) years," and those who "coerce another person" or participate in the ritual of cutting would receive a sentence of "not less than three (3) years."

Notably, these proposals culminated in calls for punishing cut women themselves. At the Accra workshop I attended, the director of the national office of the National Council on Women and Development (NCWD) introduced the issue of cut women's culpability: "My issue is with the victims themselves. There have been instances where grown women decide to do it themselves. What do we do with them?" The call for punishing them resonated with several workshop participants—those who consent should not be exempt from prosecution, some said. "Suicide is also a crime," one person pointed out, adding, "It's an offense, even if you do it yourself." Others, however, wondered whether cut women ever have the ability to make decisions for themselves: "Sometimes men will suggest it to women, so the question is, Who really decides freely?" After a brief debate the group agreed that the "victim would have to be punished, because otherwise it would encourage the society to practice it."[14]

Harsh sentences for harsh people living in a harsh environment.

Not everyone agreed with demands to imprison cut women or with calls for greater punishment, but the loudest voices carried the day. I would learn later that some of the people present were firmly opposed to the reform, but that July day they were silent.

The Silencing of Regional Publics

Feminist scholars who have analyzed the making of the legislation against cutting in the global North, including Australia, Canada, and in the United States, have highlighted the contradiction in the ostensible inclusion of African women that ultimately results in their being silenced (Macklin 2006; Rogers 2007; Gunning 2002). The problem, these scholars stress, is not that African immigrants were left out of the legislative advocacy but that their priorities were sidelined even when they had lobbied for the legislation. Consultations in Ghana were similar in that they consisted of staged public debates that produced only the appearance of consensus. GAWW traveled to Bolgatanga to solicit the views of those whom it considered representative of local views, such as regional NGOs and civil servants, but exercised complete control of the interpretation of these debates. As a result officials closest to those who practiced cutting were impelled to speak but were ignored.[15]

GAWW had to contend with government officials and civil servants who had little appetite for the project of perfecting the law by increasing punishment. Those northern Ghanaians consulted about the reform were ambivalent at best. However, they did not have the option to state their objections publicly, as explicit utterances of opposition are not a welcome form of speech in public contexts, where agreement and rhetorical finesse are the dialogical norms. Understanding the complex reception of GAWW's advocacy therefore requires listening not only to what was said but also to what was not. Opposition was not expressed in terms of overt objections but in the form of silence and proposed alternatives.

For GAWW the failure of the law was not to be questioned. At each workshop GAWW devoted only one presentation to the question of the law's efficacy and depicted it as having failed. The participants' task was to elaborate on the reasons for the failure. They were not to recall when and how the law actually did work—whether by preventing cutting or by the arrest of circumcisers—but were to specify and illustrate the failure.

But rather than asking for more punishment, civil servants and NGO workers from the Upper East Region wanted to make the existing legislation work through more "education" and "mobilization." As the regional director for the Ghana National Commission on Children told me, "It's rather better to appeal to the conscience of the people." She and others proposed a wide range of educational strategies to enhance knowledge of existing legislation (from "translation of the law" to "propaganda" and "cartoons") as well as "motivational" strategies to aid in its enforcement (from forming watchdog committees to rewarding those who report instances of cutting to authorities). By doing so, civil servants and NGO workers placed the law where they thought it belonged—in a compendium of strategies that compel subjects to comply with the injunction to stop cutting. The GAWW report states: "All participants identified education as the best way forward in the enforcement of the law of FGM and the eradication of the practice. Participants were silent on the merits of the law itself with regards to whether the penal provision was punitive enough."[16] To be clear, the education they proposed consisted of outreach campaigns, not schooling, but they also called for financial aid in form of microcredits that would allow girls to stay in school rather than be "given out" in marriage. These proposed alternatives and silences were the sole traces of dissent.

In Parliament: "Whether to Deal Humanely or Otherwise with Practitioners of FGM"

Once the debate moved into the heated space of the Ghanaian parliament, the desire for a stricter law and punitive rationality won the day. The tug of war between politicians who wanted to modify the proposed legislation and increase punishment even further and those who wanted to rein it in culminated in sensationalized debates in which fetishization of law turned into fetishization of punishment.

The proposed legislation wended its way through bureaucratic channels between 2002, when the bill was submitted to the attorney general, and 2007, when it was debated and passed by Parliament. In contrast to the much-debated Domestic Violence Act, neither the government nor the media voiced any objections. What ensued when the proposed anticutting bill reached Parliament surprised everyone. The attorney general's office had reduced the lengths of sentences proposed in the draft submitted by GAWW, but the tide moved in the opposite direction in Parliament, where the calls for more punishment multiplied and got louder.

The impassioned debates did not center on whether to pass the bill or the practical problems involved in widening the range of culpable people to the point that whole villages could be held liable. Rather than discussing whether the proposed reforms were needed, MPs discussed *how much* to increase the proposed sentences and, as they stated, "whether to deal humanely or otherwise with practitioners of FGM."[17] High-ranking MPs, mostly from southern Ghana, thought cutting so intolerable to Ghanaian society that they proposed sentences ranging from ten to twenty-five years. A few legislators, primarily from northern Ghana, opposed such a large increase. The ensuing disagreements were well captured by the media, with the government-backed Accra newspaper, the *Statesman,* reporting the following:

The Speaker of Parliament, yesterday stood down a proposed amendment to a section of the Criminal Code (Amendment) Bill that was seeking to increase the sentence of persons engaged in Female Genital Mutilation to a minimum of ten years and not less than 25 years instead of the four years that was initially proposed in the committee's report. The Chairman of the Committee on Constitutional, Legal and Parliamentary Affairs, Kofi Osei Ameyaw had sought to amend the bill, which is at the consideration stage, to make the punishment more severe as a deterrent. He, with the support of Alfred Agbesi (NDC, Ashaiman) and some female MPs wanted an amendment to provide punishment commensurate with the pain—physical, emotional, etc. suffered by the victims of FGM. But in a sharp reaction, Haruna Iddrisu, (NDC, Tamale South), Abubakari Sumani (NDC, Tamale North), Doe Adjaho, Deputy Minority Leader and Abraham Ossei Aidooh, Deputy Majority Leader, strongly opposed the amendment, saying that instead of the 10 years and not less than 25 years the chairman of the committee and others were proposing, it should rather be five years and not less than 10 years. They argued that since it was a cultural practice of particular ethnic groups in the three Northern Regions of the country, it would rather be beneficial to use educational campaigns to combat and eventually eradicate its practice, rather than the imposition of harsh punishments. Harsh punishments will rather encourage perpetrators to move into the hinterlands to engage in the practice, they added. Ruling, Speaker Ebenezar Sakyi Hughes stood the proposed amendment down and referred it back to the Committee and urged them to come up with a solution acceptable to all sides.[18]

The calls for more punishment took on a life of their own, and the proposal to exponentially lengthen sentences structured the parameters of the debate. The upshot was that prison sentences proposed by the MPs and initially understood as harsh were now figured as the more humane alternative, with the vote in Parliament showing that the majority supported a "humane sentence of five years minimum sentence and 10 years maximum sentence."[19] The larger public welcomed the new legislation, agreeing that cutting had no place in modern Ghana.[20] Newspapers celebrated the law's passage, sending "kudos to parliament on the female genital mutilation amendment."[21] In the Upper East Region the public was silent.

Liberal Love: Law as Benign

Feminist lawyers and GAWW could not have anticipated the political enthusiasm for punishment and were unable to account for it. Rather then reckoning with the behemoth they created, they used the discourse of liberalism to minimize the law's repressive force and refused to represent it as anything but benign. By *minimize* I mean their refusals to contend with the political implications of the discrepancy between the sentences for trokosi and cutting, as well as the punitive repercussions of the new law. They took recourse in a range of liberal notions, including women's rights, protection of the vulnerable, survivors, community ownership, empowerment, and dialogue.

Jane described the revised legislation as an ethical measure that would save vulnerable Ghanaian girls:

> Now that legislation says: "Look, we're not only looking at the one who does the act, but we're looking at the whole society, more holistically, more system-wide kind of approach." Because we know what it is like for a survivor to be faced with the whole system—for one little girl to be faced with a system like that.

For Jane the ultimate beneficiary of the proposed law was the hypothetical little girl who was a victim of her society and who needed law to protect her from the the cultural and social structures that shaped her life. By extending the force of the legal system and making more people subject to punishment, the proposed reform imagined an alternative system as ready to come to the aid of the cut girl.

But who was the subject of the reform efforts? As we saw at the Accra workshop, the cut woman written into the law was an adult woman or a girl old enough to consent to cutting who needed to be made subject to punishment. In contrast Jane represented this subject as a little girl, an innocent and vulnerable person who needed to be protected from her parents. Thus the law and its representation bifurcated the image of a cut person: the law could now punish an adult woman who wants to get cut but was legitimized by reference to a little girl devoid of agency. While the adult woman perpetuates the system Jane referred to, the young girl is subjected to it.

Like Jane, Susan minimized the repressive effects of the proposed legislation by saying that it would have beneficial effects, such as empowerment of girls—"the same empowerment that Burkina Faso has"—and community ownership whereby "everybody is involved, and everybody could get caught so there's a bigger reaction, and then you have so many women out there who are talking about it and actually dealing with it." Having the "people themselves involved to own the issues" would also ensure the law would not be perceived as imposed: "Sometimes we are seen as, 'Oh, those women from Accra who don't know what our culture is are interfering again,' you know."

Susan's comments reveal her anxiety about her place in the campaigns against cutting, as well as her unlikely solution. Making more people culpable, she hoped, would displace the burden of opposing cutting from "those women from Accra" to northern women themselves. The seeming contradiction between a law that would make more people subject to punishment and Susan's vision of community ownership and dialogue bears scrutiny. Susan claimed that the proposed legislation would make people "talk," and get "involved"; for her the value of dialogue and engagement exceeds the fact that both would take place under duress and threat of sanction. Left unaddressed is that people in the Upper East region "have to live within the limits of the law," as an NCWD official told me, and that these limits are not of their own choosing.

For Susan the benefits of producing liberal subjects engaged with the state outweighed such concerns:

> But the idea is to get community responsibility eventually for handling these issues, you know. Because if you know that about five, six, seven people could all get into court and be dealt with seriously, the issue dealt with seriously, it's likely that one of them will make an effort. At least they will discuss, they'll discuss it: "What do we do now?"

The reformed law would produce new kinds of social relations governed by liberal dialogue, Susan hoped, as the force of law would induce a crisis so grave that people would have to discuss what to do. As I will show in chapter 7, law enforcement did bring about a crisis that led to change, but it was not the change that Susan imagined.

While Susan framed community ownership as resulting from people's ability to handle the consequences of the law, rather than their having a say over it, GAWW represented northern Ghanaians not only as the beneficiaries of the law but as its authors and the agents behind the advocacy. Although women and men from northern Ghana had little say in the reform, Mrs. Mahama and Edna cast it not as GAWW's brainchild but as a result of demands from northern Ghanaians themselves. The following interview excerpt shows how they displaced desire for reform to people "in the field." As was increasingly becoming the case, Edna worried that Mrs. Mahama was aging and becoming less articulate, so Edna supplemented

Mrs. Mahama's words; Mrs. Mahama in turn corrected Edna, whom she found imprecise. The result is a tapestry of words and statements that reinforce one another:

MRS. MAHAMA: And it was at the insistence of the this thing that we had with . . . thought that that law had to be reviewed. Because anytime—

EDNA: It was in the field.

MRS. MAHAMA: It was in the field, particularly the chiefs.

EDNA: The people complaining.

MRS. MAHAMA: The people complained that "Why?"

EDNA: The scope was too narrow.

MRS. MAHAMA: That "Why?" Because, I mean, after all, it is the people who take the children out to be done [to get cut]. So why should they be left free and the circumcisers alone would be targeted? You see?

EDNA: After all they are sitting down.

MRS. MAHAMA: After all they are sitting down.

EDNA: You brought your child.

MRS. MAHAMA: They bring the child for them to do it and it is their work. So if they bring the child and then they do it, why is it that they [the circumcisers]—Aha!—should be the only people to be this thing? That is how it came about that we said, okay, then let us—

As we shall see in chapter 7, Mrs. Mahama and Edna are referring here to one objection to the 1994 law that was indeed common in the Upper East Region. Many people found the 1994 law ill conceived and unjust because it held only the circumcisers responsible. However, people in the Upper East did not call for more frequent punishments or longer sentences but questioned the legitimacy of the legal process. GAWW repurposed this regional critique for its own ends.

The strategic twisting of locally meaningful objections make the legitimizations sound hypocritical, and to an extent they are. For instance, although Jane and others legitimized the law in reference to cut girls, the advocates not only did not ask the cut girls and women what kinds of interventions they wanted but made them afraid of the law and made them subject to prison sentences. The answer the cut women and girls invariably gave when I asked what the law against cutting said was "If you go for cutting, they will arrest you." Indeed, their encounters with the police seemed much like arrests: girls taken into custody as witnesses were examined by doctors; interrogated by the police, civil servants, and NGO workers; and shamed. The five young girls brought to the Bolgatanga hospital after the arrest of the circumciser from the Kassena-Nankana District in the late 1990s were put on display as they sat on a wooden bench and nurses and NGO workers stood above them and videotaped them. Despite the elision of law's actual force, the advocates' basic belief—that the power of law is benign and works through discipline rather than repressive punishment—is not an outcome of hypocrisy but an apt description of how Ghanaians want the law to work.

ON BEING TORN: THE INTERVAL BETWEEN EDUCATION AND PUNISHMENT

What do Ghanaians want from law and how do they understand its workings? The answer is important, because the logics of advocacy and Parliament's decisions are less consequential for the social life of law than popular aspirations. Nobody wants the law "to remain on paper," as one legal activist put it, but how law should work is less obvious. At first glance it would seem that Ghanaians see the force of law as repressive; the ideal-typic notion of law is enforcement by "sanctioning, imprisoning, and punishing." As a Ghana Health Service nurse and administrator from Bolgatanga told me, she had faith in the law because "once they've started sanctioning people, imprisoning, and, uh, I mean, punishing people for it, I believe that within five, the next five years, it will be stopped, yeah." Or listen to Mr. Yahaya explain the history of his NGO's engagements with the law:

> But not so many people know about the law. We actually had to, you know, talk to people about the law. Any time we organized a, you know, a forum, that was part of the education, to know that the law exists, and, you know, people who were caught practicing it would be, you know, maybe prosecuted, and, you know, imprisoned, you know.

The health administrator and Mr. Yahaya both offered an ideal-typic understanding of the law, or "law as if," whereby law is understood as enforced if it leads to arrests, trials, and punishments. But if we listen to their statements carefully, we hear not only the official discourse about the law "as if," or the langue of prosecution and imprisonment, but also the underlying hesitance and ambivalence. The administrator's suggestion that law would sanction people by "imprisoning, and, uh, I mean, punishing" them was interrupted by a moment of hesitance. The easily overlooked "uh, I mean" is a telling sign of a distance from and uncertainty about the ideal-typic understanding of the law. Likewise, when Mr. Yahaya talked about the circumcisers who would be "maybe prosecuted, and, you know, imprisoned, you know," he seemed to doubt his own words. His *maybe* and *you know* hint at a logic of law that is not encompassed by official understandings but references Ghanaian parole of law enforcement.

I am here borrowing Jean and John Comaroff's adaptation of the Saussurean concepts of langue and parole (2006a: 24). Theirs is a loose adaption that understands *langue* as the stated, official system of rule of law and *parole* as its social life. I understand *langue* as the officially stated notion of law, law "as if," and *parole* as actual hopes vested in law and as cultural understandings that permeate legal advocacy and largely go without saying. I take both to be systemic and collective; they are at times in concert and at times in tension with each other. Ghanaian advocates invest law with productive power; even when they profess what appears to be adherence to langue, what Hunt and Wickham refer to as a "positivist formula of jurisprudence" whereby "law = rules + sanctions" (1994: 41), the advocates are aiming at something else. In the section that follows, I describe in further detail the cultural logics of the compelling and disciplinary force of law, the parole that goes unstated.

When Ghanaians imagine the workings of "law enforcement," they do not necessarily envision the police or arrests, trials, and sentences. What, then, does enforcement mean? They agree on one thing: to work, the law has to be actively used and has to serve as a deterrent. Deterrence takes precedence over justice, retribution, or punishment of those who transgress the law. According to this logic, when the law is transgressed, it has already failed. Ghanaians from many walks of life strongly prefer the law to serve as an instructive, rather than a punitive, mechanism. The same can be said for punishment, which, anthropologists have long noted, is not the primary mechanism of discipline in the Upper East Region. Fortes and Mayer single out what they call the benevolent character of discipline here, writing: "Corporal punishment is rare. Obedience to parents is built into the domestic routine and the value system rather than enforced by coercion" (1966: 9). Punishment was administered when merited, Fortes writes, but was extremely rare; families trained their children not by corporeal punishment but by "constant supervision" (1970: 209).

The belief that law should not depend on punishment was shared by feminist lawyers. Although Jane is one of the feminist activists described to me as "radical," and her leadership in Ghanaian legal advocacy is a prime example of what feminist scholars refer to not only as governance feminism but as carceral feminism, Jane did not see law as punitive. Its purpose, she said, is to provide "the balancing part" to educational campaigns by forcefully communicating new norms of behavior:

> I believe in the carrot-and-stick approach. It's like getting a rabbit to do something. So you wave the carrot before it, which the rabbit likes, but because it's so much induced with the carrot, eating the carrot, it forgets that there's a job to do. So you have the stick to, you know, prod. So it's like doing the education, persuading, you know, advocating, lobbying, and all of those things must go on. At the same time there must be the law that says: "Look, we're doing all these things, but if you don't stop, the law is going to come, come and get you." And that should be a balancing part that we need.

Jane's notion of the law as the proverbial stick is worth examining in detail. The stick does not hurt or punish—in Jane's account nobody was beaten by it. Rather, the stick prods people and announces that "the law is going to come and get you." If Jane imagined the law as working by sanctioning, imprisoning, and punishing people, the stick would mean the arrest, trial, and sentence. But in her rendering, the stick is a speech act. The law works by nudging people and compelling them ("prodding") by way of enunciating its own power, specifically, the ability to exercise the state's prerogative of sovereign violence. What sets law apart from other speech acts, such as films or health campaigns, is that the law has an inherent force. It compels subjects and regulates normative behavior by its indexing of sovereign power—the threat that law can and will get you.

Jane and others referred to law as a framework and a structure: "It is important for us to have frameworks so that those frameworks can be used by advocates, educators, teachers, and so on and for people to understand why those frameworks are necessary, if you educate people." The seemingly circular logic of her statement points to the Ghanaian logics of parole of law enforcement: advocates use the law to educate Ghanaians about the necessity of the law. Again, the primary force of law, in this understanding, is communicative and instructive. In conversations with other NGO workers, civil servants, and legal activists, I gleaned similarly fine-grained notions of law as an educational and compelling force.

In practice, they said, law is enforced by being announced in public discussions. An official from the Ghana National Commission on Children (GNCC) in Bolga told me that enforcement means talking about the law.

> GNCC OFFICIAL: We talked about the legislation, because we are supposed to see to it that it is enforced.
>
> SAIDA: MMM. How can you do that?
>
> GNCC OFFICIAL: Uh, the only way we can do it is to create awareness. Let people know that there's a law, and if you do this, this will be the repercussion, or this will be the punishment. So advocating and creating awareness, and educating people on the law, for them to know.

Why, then, was the law reform necessary?, I asked women's rights advocates. They told me that because law enforcement needs to flow from the letter of the law, the law needed to be perfected. For Jane the new law was simply a better technology of persuasion whose force is communicative, not punitive. To my question about how she envisioned the enforcement of the second law against cutting, she responded:

> Any organization that is interested in human rights, is interested in women, is interested in children, should take it and use it. For us here it will become part of the training we do on woman's legal rights, you know. So when we have to speak on women rights issues, we will mention that as an example. Um, if we have to go up North to do some work, we'll take it with us.

Remarkable here is not so much what Jane said about enforcement but what she did not say. She did not invoke arrests, prosecutions, trials, or prison sentences. What she and others wanted was for law to work its magic, educating without causing harm. As discussed earlier, advocates see the perfect law as an antidote to an incapacitated and masculinist state, but when advocacy led to heightened punitive rationality, they excused it in reference to liberal and humanist ideals.

They also knew that law does cause harm. I learned about Ghana's prison conditions from Susan, who gave me a copy of an annual report from the human rights commission, CHRAJ, during one of my visits to her office. CHRAJ had conducted an investigation into Ghana's prisons and found them abysmal. Not only were many people "on remand"—imprisoned without ever having been tried or sentenced—but the sleeping, eating, and hygiene conditions as well as disciplinary violence were described as severe human rights violations. In recent years prisons conditions have become a site of activism, media attention, and critique of the state.[22] Like elsewhere in the world, prisons in Ghana are overcrowded (in 2012 they were at 170 percent of capacity), and their provision of shelter and nourishment is far from adequate. The incarcerated circumcisers had to perform hard labor for food.

When I next saw Susan, I asked about her thoughts on the increased prison sentences for cutting in light of the prison conditions. The purpose of the revised legislation was not to punish people, she insisted:

> It's not so much getting people in prison because it's already a criminal offense anyway. Expanding the territory will mean roping in more people, but the idea is not getting all those people in prison, otherwise you'll have maybe a whole community in there. . . . It's absolutely necessary to prevent it [cutting] from happening. I mean there's, there isn't much point catching people after—well, there is a point, because it will serve as a deterrent to others, and hopefully prevent, you know, um, more damage being done to other girls. But the whole point is to stop it before it happens, and the amendments should work that way. So the amendments should help in the prevention. So the idea is that the enforcement will flow from the amendment to the law itself.

For Susan and other advocates, the perfected law will enforce itself. This is a widely shared Ghanaian parole of the law: good legislation enforces itself by making subjects feel addressed by the law. Advocates saw the new law as a better deterrent, because it interpellated a wider range of people. What they misunderstood is the relative insignificance of the letter of the law for those targeted by it. Girls and young women who might have considered cutting, as well as their parents, already felt themselves addressed by the 1994 law.

Susan's slippage between two different logics of the law reveals another blind spot, perhaps a more willful one. She had caught herself midsentence, saying, "There isn't much point catching people after—well, there is a point, because it will serve as a deterrent to others." Despite the desire for better interpellation as a means of prevention, detaining people after the act of cutting and punishing them would give law more credibility as a deterrent. That deterrence depends on catching and punishing people, and not merely hailing them as legal subjects, is the official understanding of the force of law, the law "as if," the langue of law. Susan's midsentence slippage is precisely the interval of uncertainty and ambiguity that structures law enforcement in practice, to which I now turn. When judges sentence people, they follow the official understanding, but those tasked with bringing subjects to trial follow the widespread parole of the law. I want to show that Ghanaian NGO workers and civil servants were initially enthusiastic about law enforcement but came to reject it precisely because of their opposition to punitive rationality.

You can go and visit her. Take her some bread. And some soap. She will not have those in the prison.

I believe you are going to ask me "why was the cut girl not prosecuted" because in law if somebody willingly offers herself up for a criminal activity to take place, then that person can be said to be abetting the crime, and this is a complex issue that has come up in the course of our work in the FGM on the enforcement of the law.

I was rather thinking maybe you petitioned because I saw her released. Or it could be CENSUDI? I don't know whether CENSUDI did it.

Come and work here. Will you come and work here, in Ghana?

7

Against Sovereign Violence

"The Law Against FGM Is Imprisonment," proclaimed a poster carried by students marching on the streets of Bolgatanga in May 2004 to mark Ghana's first celebration of Zero Tolerance to Female Genital Mutilation Day, inaugurated the year before by the IAC. This march was not a public protest but an orchestrated show of support that GAWW organized in collaboration with regional government officials and schoolteachers. The teachers had hastily drawn the posters in the wee hours of the night and distributed them to students, who were to serve as the youthful public voices of opposition to cutting.

The double meaning of the poster proclaiming, "The Law against FGM Is Imprisonment" fascinated me: I knew that the poster was intended to convey that the penalty for FGM is incarceration and that was how it would have been understood. Yet if we were to read that statement literally, we would find a poetic construction that takes the law as its object: the law *itself* is imprisonment. This would constitute a metaphorical critique declaring the law violent and questioning the state's use of force. In actuality no one would have read the poster this way: few Ghanaians openly opposed the legislation against cutting, and even fewer did so in public. As I showed in the previous chapter, the effort to increase punishment and incarceration would win the day in Ghana's parliament in 2007, and those who opposed the reform had little say in it. Yet this poster's unintended slippage between the governmental injunction to respect the law because of its force and the critique of this very force foreshadowed an unexpected change in regional understandings of the value of punishment and social order secured by the rule of law.

The shift occurred in the aftermath of the prison sentences handed to two circumcisers: Fefe Dari, from the Wa District in the Upper West Region, and

85

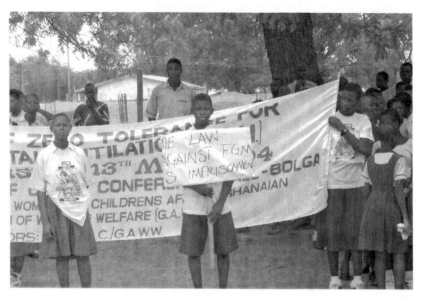

FIGURE 19. "The law against FGM is imprisonment": Students ready for an anti-FGM march.

Abampoka Mbawini, from Bawku in the Upper East, both of whom were sentenced several months before the march and three years before Parliament agreed to revise the law. Newspapers and radio widely reported the punishments of Dari and Abampoka, and some observers expected that these much publicized events would bring on a series of arrests. But punitive enforcement of the law ended just as the punitive rationality gathered steam in Parliament. As MPs were starting to articulate arguments for more stringent punishment, civil servants and NGO workers tasked with law enforcement in the Upper East began to question the violence inherent in the existing law. The imprisonment of the elderly circumciser did not sit well with them, although they were enthusiastic about law's potential to end cutting and proud of their participation.

Although these were not the first cases of Ghanaian circumcisers' being sentenced to prison, they have been the last.[1] In my fieldwork I witnessed the aftermath of these last arrests of circumcisers and saw opposition to law enforcement gradually building. Parliament would decide the legislative fate of the law against cutting, but NGOs and regional civil servants determined its social life. Both determinations were made away from the public eye, where much government action takes place, but ultimately were no secret. As I will make evident, NGO workers and civil servants at first embraced the subject positions of citizen–law enforcers but later turned against the punitive rationality of law.

In Ghana the zero tolerance paradigm led to passage of the reforms but was also challenged, albeit not in the form of public debate. The events I describe here unfolded outside of public deliberations about appropriate measures to end cutting. The challenges to punitive rationality resulted from civil servants' practice and deep involvement in law enforcement. For regional governmental workers, the trials and imprisonment of Dari and Abampoka revealed the pitfalls of the langue of law, or formal understandings of law enforcement, and altered the contours of what was morally thinkable and desirable. NGO campaigns had initially drawn regional workers into the orbit of law enforcement, and they enthusiastically participated in the networks of surveillance and in the arrest and prosecution of the circumcisers. While in formal understandings, law enforcement is defined by punishment—one must pursue not the spirit but the letter of the law, the law "by the book"—the Ghanaian public understands deterrence as operating according to the logic of discipline: bringing people "to the book" and summoning them before the law is sufficient. Thus those who had to reckon with the practical consequences of punishment and imprisonment of circumcisers reversed their positions. Two years after her imprisonment, Abampoka received a presidential pardon, and Dari was released from jail early. No one else has been prosecuted, despite occasional reports about instances of cutting and despite—or perhaps because of—the enactment of the more stringent legislation in 2007.

In this chapter I describe this reversal of punitive rationality by closely attending to the experiences of regional civil servants and NGO workers and their shifting perspectives on law and justice. My goal is to explore and contextualize the *instability* of the punitive rationality, showing that it is contested even when it seemingly wins the day. The following ethnography traces how the law was enforced by way of an NGO-fueled collaboration with the police and shows why the initial enthusiasm about the law morphed into a tacit rejection of sovereign violence, leading governmental workers to disidentify with the dominant social order. It is important to note that this opposition was gradual and quiet. It did not take the form of public protests, debates, or organized campaigns. It gathered force from sensibilities not easily located in stable ideologies, public discourses, or discrete cultural formations. Rather, these sensibilities were formed at the interstices of governmental logic and a number of principles on which society is built—the ethics of relational personhood, mutual accountability, and the logics of discipline, which postulate that people should be brought "to the book" but not punished "by the book." Although the governmental ideology of law and order is a palpable force in the lives of governmental workers, it is not the only one, and much of what transpires in their collaborative exercises of law enforcement at the margins of the state is experimental and unpredictable. The law meets and makes its subjects here, and here it faces contestation. This is where NGO workers and civil servants start to question the violence that is enacted through law enforcement and begin to ask, paraphrasing Benjamin, what law "does to the victim" as well as what it does to "the doer" (1986: 299).

EARS ON THE GROUND: CITIZENS IN PARAFORMAL LAW ENFORCEMENT

Abampoka Mbawini and Fefe Dari were arrested and tried as a result of the mobilization of NGO-created watchdog committees that created new kinds of citizen enforcers. Watchdog committees were initially established in the late 1980s to instill the spirit of communal supervision and self-discipline in rural areas of northern Ghana and in the Muslim and migrant *zongos* (neighborhoods) in the South. After the enactment of the 1994 law, the committees were meant to extend its reach and ensure its continuous presence; the intended effect of the committees was to prevent cutting by spreading surveillance throughout the capillaries of society. Like other aspects of NGO work, watchdog committees were sporadic but consequential, as they were responsible for all the circumcisers arrested and prosecuted, as well as for some preventative interventions.

Except for RHI, Dr. Adjei's NGO in Bolgatanga, most NGOs had watchdog committees, but not all were created equal. The community-based NGOs, such as Muslim Family Counseling Services (MFCS) in Nima and the Programme for Rural Integrated Development (PRIDE) in Bongo, never pursued any arrests. Both organizations saw trust coupled with authority as the basis of their work and said that the very existence of the watchdog committees prevented the occurrence of cutting.

MFCS-created watchdog committees consisted of young men who were the NGO's "ears on the ground" and whose only aim was to forestall cutting.

Mr. Yahaya from MFCS emphasized that the purpose of the watchdog committees was not to report cutting to the police but to prevent it from happening in the first place:

> The watchdog committees, they are members of the community. They
> could be young men or young women, but mostly we had young men
> participating. And they knew about all the impending marriages, you
> know, or they kept an eye on the adolescent females, who they thought
> could be victims of this thing, and they monitored the families. So any
> time they got wind of an impending circumcision, they quickly went
> to the families and warned them that if they carried it out, you will be
> reported. Yeah, to the, the police. You know, the security services. Yeah.
> And that helped to actually reduce the prevalence, yeah, and eventually, in
> some communities, it died out completely. Yeah. Because they knew that
> if they did it in that community, they were liable to being prosecuted.

For Mr. Yahaya the watchdog committees were a "good practice" because they prevented cutting from occurring by promoting self-surveillance within the group. Charged with monitoring, the committees combined semiformal surveillance with the institutional backing of law. After the U.S. Embassy sponsored an MFCS project in Jasikan, a migrant town in the South, cutting was indeed prevented.

These committees brought new subjects into being: young men were mobilized to monitor the desires of young women and families for cutting. These men were encouraged to think of themselves as an informal police force but one that would report to the NGOs rather than the state. Like the "boys" organized by political parties (Nugent 1995), young men on the watchdog committees were afforded social and political agency and thus materialized as political actors. In Bongo, young women volunteers such as Cecilia also participated and experienced a sense of power and pleasure. She told me that she was trained to report any instance of cutting and that she was sure she would know if cutting were to happen, although she did not expect it to. According to Cecilia, no one could escape from surveillance because word spreads in the village. On her face was a smile and in her voice a tinge of satisfaction and perhaps even pride.

GAWW created more extensive, but loose and circumstantial, committees that, at least on paper, involved a variety of people and institutions: from village-based health volunteers and youth leaders to community nurses, NGO workers, and local government officials. They were seen as performing a preventative role, and GAWW defined them as "a body or group of people who have come together to render local security services to their respective communities for the protection of life and properties." In practice, these were people who GAWW hoped would condemn the practice during community functions and wear t-shirts with anticutting messages. Because GAWW workers were not in touch with the committee members, the NGO did not have much trust in their efficacy. When Edna began to praise GAWW's groups, Mrs. Mahama interrupted her, self-critically assessing the NGO's failure to keep a close tab on the groups.

> MRS. MAHAMA: Don't talk of the watchdog committee because they are not watching.
>
> EDNA: In fact we have set up a lot of them, but the problem is monitoring because you need to have funding. But they are helping because we can also cite the arrest case. Was it not through a watchdog committee?
>
> MRS. MAHAMA: The so-called watchdog committees—are they working?
>
> EDNA: They are not working again because we don't visit them again.
>
> MRS. MAHAMA: We just do this once, say that "oh, you talk, watch, do this," and then?

Mrs. Mahama thought the watchdog committees were "not watching" because the NGO was not watching them. Consistently self-critical, and in keeping with her habitual practice of emphasizing failure, Mrs. Mahama did not want to portray the committees as more successful than she thought they were. Edna wanted to portray GAWW as more successful and pointed out that although the groups were not sufficiently motivated, they did contribute to the arrest of Fefe Dari. They agreed that for the committees to surveil and monitor cutting, they needed to be subjected to surveillance by GAWW and that the NGO should offer the committees further incentives and tangible benefits such as gifts or cash. Otherwise, Edna added, laughing, "they also have their priorities, we can't complain," suggesting that committee members had to spend their time earning money, rather than volunteering for the NGO.

Mrs. Mahama told me about her surprise when one GAWW committee lived on despite the NGO's lack of engagement with it. She took a donor official from Equality Now on a monitoring visit to one of the project sites in the Northern Region, all the while worrying that the group would turn out to be nonexistent. She was quite relieved when the group revealed itself to be fully functioning:

MRS. MAHAMA: I was very, very, very delighted, you know, in Walewale. They all came, and they had stories to tell about what they were doing. You see, in fact I was really very glad. I thought that, oh, we will just be disgraced, and then this thing, but they came.

EDNA: Because is a long time [since] we visited them.

MRS. MAHAMA: A long time. But they came, and then they told their stories and this thing. Even the t-shirts we gave to these women; the women, they still wore their t-shirts.

EDNA: T-shirts. Anytime [we go, we are told,] "Look, we are keeping them." Right now, if we go to organize a program somewhere and they are the women's groups with those t-shirts, they normally wear the t-shirts.

The group's existence was evidenced by the objects and narratives through which they performed their NGO-ized identity: they wore GAWW t-shirts and had "stories" to tell—about preventing cutting and about educating other villagers. With this evidence in hand GAWW was able to prove to its donors—who were performing yet another level of monitoring and surveillance—that the village-level surveillance system was functional.

GAWW's discourse of "underground resistance" leaves little room to explain such enthusiasm for self-surveillance. In practice recruits regularly reported instances of cutting and tried to prevent them. Musa was particularly proud of one such prevention. A volunteer whom he had recently trained, and who lived in a village near Bawku, contacted Musa to report an impending cutting, and Musa traveled to the village to hold an impromptu workshop:

I was in Tamale. So Madam [Mrs. Mahama] sent me the money, then I hired a pickup, straight to Bawku. So I got there, then we had a community durbar. You know, we have this projector, GAWW bought a projector. We have a projector, then what we do is we use a laptop, then show a film. You know this, our devastating film. We show it and explain to the people, especially the youth, the effects of FGM. That day they were very sorry at the school; they said they never knew this was what was going on. I told them this was the implication, but we got the information that this is what is happening in your community. They said, "Yes, is true," and they even pointed [out] the houses of the people who wanted to do it. So they went there—the youth mobilized, went there. And I gave them copies of the law . . . to study. So they went and told them [people considering cutting], "If you are caught now, it is not three years, it is five years"—you know it has been increased. And that it is not only the perpetrator but all those who consent to it [who] are all involved because you will all be sentenced. Yes, so they are scared.

The stories Musa most liked to tell were stories of prevention, as GAWW had never intended the law to facilitate arrests or imprisonment. But he and Mrs. Mahama were involved in the arrest of Fefe Dari, which they later regretted. Equally important, GAWW had no sovereignty over how the laws it had helped pass would be enforced. Although GAWW wanted the law to prod and compel, rather than punish, other activists had different visions in mind. The appearance of a new NGO that wanted to enforce the law according to its langue, or, as Ghanaians put it, "by the book," was central to the circumcisers' arrests.

LAW BY THE BOOK: THE ERADICATION COMMITTEES

In 2003 the German Embassy in Accra sent out a call for proposals for projects related to female genital cutting. GAWW's application for educational workshops did not succeed, and funding went to a Tamale-based organization called the Center for Human Rights Education and Advocacy, an NGO that had never worked on cutting. It was directed by Mr. Alhassan, a lawyer in training and a longtime human rights activist who had returned to Ghana after many years of studying in Ukraine and England. While abroad he was an organizer of the Amnesty International chapter at his university, and he was involved with the Eastern European Human Rights Network, which, he said, fought the resurgence of xenophobia directed at Africans and other foreigners. When I met him, Alhassan was completing his certification to practice law in Ghana and was working with the NGO dedicated to human rights education. The German Embassy program was an opportunity to tap into a new source of funding and expand the reach of his NGO.

One reason his NGO received funding, he thought, was because it emphasized what he called "a firm approach to law enforcement." Its proposal was to strengthen law enforcement by way of arrests and punishment:

> The difference between our work and that of other NGOs involved in the
> FGM project is that we took up the issue of making sure that the law
> was enforced. We wanted to see to it that the main stakeholders who were
> to make the law work are aware of the existence of the law and also the
> communities get to know that the law needs to work. Anybody who
> perpetuates that offense of circumcising or excising women will be punished
> as defined in the law. And that is the difference between us and other NGOs
> in the area. We seem to be more concerned about enforcement of the law.

Alhassan's paradigm shift in law enforcement spoke to the donor's emphasis on "good governance" and "rule of law." He wanted the law against cutting to be enforced not by way of education or prevention but by arrests and imprisonment, as defined in the letter of the law. Alhassan proudly told me that his NGO's work had indeed "produced very good results" and that "the committees on the ground have also performed very creditably" by arresting Abampoka Mbawini and Fefe Dari. Their imprisonment was the indicator of project success that could be shown to the donors.

The committees to which Alhassan referred were the District FGM Eradication Committees, their very name suggestive of the tougher line he wanted to convey—they were not just to monitor and watch (like the watchdog committees that were still in operation) but to *eradicate*. He described the eradication committees as a structure that would supplement the existing law enforcement apparatus, given that, as he put it, "we don't have a state structure that will want to ensure that the practice is stopped." He sounded like Jane, the feminist lawyer, but he did not think that enforcement would flow from the letter of the law:

> In Ghana there is no state structure. [Cutting] has been criminalized in
> Parliament [but] there is no state structure or institution that has the
> responsibility of ensuring that the practice stops. So, I mean, this really
> creates a vacuum which allows people to carry on the practice.

In 2003 he filled this vacuum with the eradication committees, which he described as an alternative structure comprising "the health workers, the police, the district assemblies, the gender desk officers, the chiefs, the assembly people, and then human rights workers." This NGO-organized formation was imagined as an integrated chain of information: "So the community people will report to a member of the committee, then the member will also pass on the information to us, then we will inform the police. This is how it's done." In practice, as I will show, getting results from this structure—arrests and trials—took much more than passing on the information.

Alhassan thought that the committees would cultivate an enforcement-oriented sensibility in civil servants because their participation would remind them of the law's regulatory power and hold them accountable to one another. He also reasoned that in a state without a structure, those who go beyond the call of duty need a pat on the back:

We also tried to put into place a kind of recognition of all those who will be able to help us apprehend perpetrators. So the letter that you saw with the district, the circuit court, was like a commendation, which is our practice in any place that people perform well in ensuring that somebody who carries out FGM is arrested, prosecuted, and convicted. We try to show our commendation to these institutions and the personalities involved. We think that that is basically to motivate people to let them also know that the work that they are doing, they are not alone in it, that they have other partners. And I can say comfortably that the police in the Upper West Region have expressed an appreciation to us for sending them a letter of commendation after the arrest of Dari.

Alhassan understood the national mood of state employees as a form of loneliness and hoped to move them to action by way of individual and collective recognition and appreciation. In his vision the eradication committees would form a new kind of legal sociality that supplemented and exceeded existing forms of citizenship.

Histories of Policing and Paraformal Law Enforcement

Watchdog and eradication committees are new to Ghana, but paraformal law enforcement is not. Forces outside formal institutions have long maintained state and social orders. In precolonial times mutual surveillance and accountability enforced social order, colonialism institutionalized legal pluralism, and, more recently, J. J. Rawlings's military regime (1981–2001) mobilized paramilitary forces and so-called vigilante groups. The NGOs' establishment of watchdog committees and faith in their efficacy should therefore not be read as either a simple imposition of a neoliberal paradigm or an expression of indigenous sensibilities but as an assemblage of social and governmental techniques of law and order that have long mixed formal and informal mechanisms.

Precolonial Ghanaian societies did not secure order by way of policing or professionalized institutions and "did not have a specialised group of people specially vested with the responsibility of day-to-day maintenance of law and order" (Tankebe 2008: 68). The maintenance of order was a social and collective responsibility that relied on watchful attention and mutual surveillance. Social order was backed by force, much like law, but the force that threatened those who transgressed it was only partly of the present world. Ancestral punishment was the primary mechanism of securing order, and it was seen as immediate, inescapable, and severe.

When the British instituted the penal system and policing under colonialism, their force was palpable but seen as illegitimate, since the police served the colonizers' interests. Described as paramilitary forces (Defflem 1994: 52) that exercised "wide-ranging discretionary powers without accountability" (Tankebe 2008: 75), the colonial police abused their power in the name of the rule of law. Policing bore the imprint of indirect rule in that it distinguished between the unarmed Native Authority Forces, whose duty was to enforce newly codified customary laws, and the centralized police forces that safeguarded the colonial enterprise by surveying "the European owned mining infrastructures, agricultural production areas, and the transportation of goods" (Defflem 1994: 52).

After independence, paramilitary policing continued, as did police repression (Nugent 1995). Police forces were involved in political affairs, such as the overthrow of the first president, Kwame Nkrumah; the detention and abuse of political prisoners; and renewed formation of paraformal militias. Under the Rawlings regime, law enforcement was widely dispersed among the citizenry: he instituted the countrywide Civil Defence Organisation, known as the militia, as well as the Committees for the Defence of the Revolution, or CDRs. Inspired by their Cuban, Libyan, and Burkinabe namesakes, these committees were meant to spread and secure the spirit of revolutionary vigilance and class struggle across society and to serve as extensions of the state's reach. Like the subsequent watchdog committees, they were referred to as "ears on the ground" (Nugent 1995). Mostly comprised of men, the committees were empowered to directly mete out punishment. However, they should not be imagined as fully realized panopticons—in practice, their work was uneven and haphazard, and they had least impact in rural areas (Nugent 1995).

In the 1980s GAWW collaborated with the Committees for the Defence of the Revolution. Before the passage of legislation against cutting, GAWW had persuaded chiefs and several district assemblies in northern Ghana to pass bylaws that criminalized the practice. Bylaws are regional laws that chiefs and district assemblies are authorized to pass but can enforce only informally. To that end district assemblies vowed to form "vigilante groups" consisting of chiefs, assemblymen, and CDR members who would be alerted "whenever a girl is circumcised or an identified circumcisor [sic] refuses to stop the practice"; they were also to mete out punishment.[2] With these collaborations, GAWW instituted a form of aspirational parastatal governmentality that was seamlessly fused with the fervor of the military regime. In practice the vigilante groups are not known to have meted out punishment for cutting, but they served as precursors to, and overlapped with, the subsequently formed watchdog committees.

The name of paraformal law enforcement has shifted from vigilante groups to watchdog committees, and so has the ideology. What was, in the Rawlings era, a safeguarding of "the spirit of the revolution" became, after the transition to democracy, "monitoring the rule of law." But while the systems of governance and their ideologies were changing, the people they relied upon were often the same. Paul is one of the men who belonged to the CDR and later became an NGO volunteer in Bongo affiliated with Dr. Adjei's NGO as well as with the Red Cross and the Ghana Health Service. He remembers that his CDR was tasked with intervening against circumcision, but that its members rarely did.

The watchdog committees are one of several NGO formations that blend the old and the new in exercising power. In contrast to theorizations of NGOs as the first conduits of dispersed governance instituted by neoliberal ideology and practice, the history of GAWW's involvement in law enforcement by way of collaboration with the CDRs is evidence of more complex genealogies, including one rooted in the Rawlings-era postrevolutionary socialist practices of outsourcing paramilitary and paraformal sovereign violence.

The contemporary NGO watchdog committees' mobility and infiltration of the capillaries of the state supplement the otherwise inert law enforcement apparatus. In Ghana the police do not chase, hunt, track, surveil, or infiltrate; at most they catch their prey at roadblocks. They do not perform encompassment (Ferguson and Gupta 2002). They justify immobility by performing incapacity: "We don't even have fuel to go and investigate reported incidents" highlights the material limits they face—the police are indeed without gas at times—but the statement also serves as a legitimated excuse (Hodžić 2011).

Although Ghana has a long history of granting police and watchdog committees informal and semiformal powers of law enforcement, Ghanaians often view trials and imprisonment as inadequate. Comparatively speaking, Ghana has few prisoners; its thirteen thousand prisoners put it near the bottom on the list of global incarceration rates (it ranks 191 out of 218 countries), with fifty-six prisoners per 100,000 people.[3] (The United States leads the world with 730 prisoners per 100,000 people.) The Ghanaian cultural logics of discipline and punishment are grounded in history that predates the institutionalization of police and prisons but are also informed by the governmental habit, from colonialism to today, of suspending the rule of law and outsourcing the enforcement of extralegal sovereign violence.

FUELING THE POLICE: WHEN NGOs ENFORCE THE LAW BY THE BOOK

Police inertia is a social constant, and the eradication committees enforced law by the book only when impelled by NGOs. Both circumcisers' arrests, to which I now turn, were circumstantial, haphazard, and depended on NGOs that were physically present in the districts where cutting occurred. Both arrests occurred in the immediate aftermath of NGO projects: Fefe Dari and Abampoka Mbawini were arrested and tried in the aftermath of not one but two NGO campaigns.

Fefe Dari: Protecting the Circumciser

Fefe Dari was arrested with direct participation from GAWW and a few weeks after Alhassan's formation of the Wa District eradication committees. A villager who remains anonymous reported to the nurse at the nearby health center that three children had been cut. The nurse traveled to the district capital, Wa, where she reported to district health authorities what the villager had said. Coincidentally, GAWW was offering a series of workshops for health workers in the Upper West Region at the time, and the NGO was visiting the district health office when the nurse arrived. Mrs. Mahama told me about the unfolding of the subsequent events: "We happened to be at the public health office, the district health office, . . . [when] the nurse came in to report it. The director of health said, 'Ah, this is your case.'" With that statement the state performed incapacity and outsourced "the case" to GAWW (this also occurred in Accra, where the Ministry of Women and Children's Affairs sent people who reported incipient cutting to GAWW for assistance). Mrs. Mahama and Musa went to the Women and Juvenile Unit of the police service and traveled with the police to the health center, where they were told to come back the following day, as night was approaching and Dari's house was far away. They doubted they would be able to find Dari or that she would willingly come to the health center the following day, but the greater problem proved to be police inertia.

When Mrs. Mahama and Musa arrived at the police station the next morning, the police said they were unable to travel to the village. As Mrs.

Mahama put it, "It's somehow difficult for them to [make] any arrest." The police, she said, made excuses: "That they didn't have fuel in their car, and then the car was, this thing, for [dispatched] somewhere, something else, so what what what." If rural women are bereft of energy because they are depleted of blood, the same is true for police who lack gasoline, or so they constantly claim. Although she was not convinced by the excuses offered by the police, Mrs. Mahama told them, "'Okay, we could use my pickup.'"

The police, Mrs. Mahama, and Musa traveled together in the pickup truck, but when they were ten kilometers from the village, the truck got stuck in the riverbed, and they had to complete the journey on foot. As Mrs. Mahama tells the story, the difficulty of getting to the village plays an important role. To get the vehicle out of the riverbed, she and Musa needed help from village youth, who were unaware that Dari was to be arrested. These youth later came to embody Mrs. Mahama's discomfort with Dari's arrest.

To Mrs. Mahama's surprise, Dari was waiting for them at the health center as summoned by the nurses the night before and then took GAWW and the police to the three circumcised children and their mother. Mrs. Mahama took about thirty pictures of the children, their cut genitals, and of Dari sitting surrounded by the children. All then went back to Wa and took the children to the hospital, where they were examined. In the hospital, according to Mrs. Mahama, Dari confessed: "She accepted it, she said she did it." Because of the confession, "we said, 'Okay then, it is fair'" that she be taken into custody.

The following day Mrs. Mahama and Musa went to Tumu, a town at the other end of the region, to conduct another workshop. They stressed that they had nothing to do with Dari's trial: "By the time we came back from Tumu, the case had already been this thing [closed], and then the woman was sent straight to prison in Tamale." Dari was sentenced to five years of hard labor. Crucial to GAWW's subsequent representation of the limits of its responsibility is that Mrs. Mahama and Musa were absent from Dari's sentencing—they brought Dari to the attention of the authorities, as was their duty, and that was where their involvement ended.

In contrast Alhassan happily took credit for Dari's sentence, because the people involved in the arrest and trial were members of the eradication committee he had organized:

> The people who were so instrumental in the arrest and prosecution were people that we have used in our workshop in Wa: the Woman and Juvenile Unit of the Ghana Police Service, and the prosecutor [who] was our resource person, he spoke on the enforcement of the law—abolishing

FGM in that district in the Wa Municipal Area. And the other stake-holders who did so well were the health workers and then some people from the community.

Thus the arrest required both the "structure" that Alhassan had established and the presence of GAWW at the scene. But after Alhassan publicly took the credit for Dari's arrest and sent letters to the Wa District congratulating its committee on a job well done, he became the target of Mrs. Mahama's ire. "We told him our piece of mind," she told me. "'You don't claim credit where it is not due.'" Mrs. Mahama found herself caught between feeling ambivalent about her involvement and wanting GAWW to be recognized for Dari's arrest. I could sense her conflicted feelings in the way she alternated between expressing and withholding empathy for Dari:

> I really felt sorry for her. Because she may not have actually known what she was doing, but it's an offense, anyway. She said she didn't even know that there was a law. But she certainly knew. They all know about the law, or else they wouldn't be hiding somewhere, doing it. Yeah, they all know about it.

Here Mrs. Mahama worked out her ambivalence about the incarceration sentence by sentence. Over time this discomfort only grew. When I saw Mrs. Mahama in 2009, she brought up Dari's sentence several times, and in the midst of one conversation I had with her and Edna, she blurted out that Dari's was a false confession:

> She said that "Oh, somebody else did it." And we said, "Okay, then, get that person for us. Tell us where to find her." [She said] that at the moment she cannot find the woman. They were giving stories. So we said, "Okay, if you are able to find the one who did it, then we will leave you." But she accepted [responsibility]. Later on I got to know that she didn't do it herself. One old lady she went and brought. So, in fact, she was protecting the old lady.

Dari confessed to protect the actual circumciser. When Mrs. Mahama first heard this, she did not trust it but changed her mind later after someone else from the district confirmed the truth of Dari's statements.

In retrospect the false confession explains why so many things seemed wrong with the picture GAWW originally painted. I was in Accra when Mrs. Mahama returned from Wa and showed me the pictures of Dari and the children. Dari was in her late forties, decades younger than any other circumciser I had ever met or heard about. Mrs. Mahama also told me that the circumcised children were Dari's granddaughter, who was a baby, and two nieces, aged one and a half and five. It seemed strange that Dari would have cut girls of such different ages at the same time; if she had been a circumciser, she would have cut each of them at the appropriate age. I knew that one reason why, during the last half century, people paid less attention to the precise age of cutting is that circumcisers were less available, and families started bundling girls of various ages, having them cut at the same time when the opportunity arose. Mrs. Mahama was not interested in asking too many questions until another villager confirmed that Dari was not the culprit, which forced Mrs. Mahama to reckon with her role in the arrest.

To participate in an arrest of a circumciser is one thing, but to contribute to the arrest of a grandmother who is protecting a circumciser is another. In both GAWW's and globally dominant depictions, circumcisers and grandmothers are portrayed as the ultimate villains, stubborn keepers of a tradition they impose on unsuspecting youth. Mrs. Mahama's encounter with a grandmother who had sacrificed herself for the benefit of another called this monolithic depiction into question.

Both Mrs. Mahama and Edna were torn by Dari's sentence and had difficulty reconciling their regrets and their aspirations for ending cutting. Their accounts of their role in the arrest attest to deep-seated internal conflicts. After Mrs. Mahama told me that the confession was false, Edna placed Dari in the context of cutting, thus imbuing her with responsibility for it, and said, "So she helped the old lady, I am sure she held the children, and the old lady did the cutting." If Dari had held the children while they were being cut, to Edna this meant Dari was culpable. Mrs. Mahama, in turn, said that Dari was not "aware of the law" but then exclaimed, in unison with Edna, "But ignorance of the law is no excuse! You see, ignorance of the law is no excuse!" This common statement represents the government's official stance and was something to hold on to.

The young people who had helped GAWW drag the pickup out of the riverbed and thus unwittingly contributed to Dari's arrest were the focal point of Mrs. Mahama's regret. Unable or unwilling to verbalize her own remorse, she projected it onto them, imagining that they felt betrayed by GAWW:

> You see, they thought that we were just going to pull the woman's ear and then leave her. You see? She then had to go to prison for all those years,

and they felt very bad about it. And since then we haven't been to the village again. We say we are not going there and stick a foot there.

Imagining the youth's bad feelings was Mrs. Mahama's way of reckoning with her own, as "pulling the woman's ear" is seen as adequate punishment, but a prison sentence is not. The youth also represented people to whom she would be accountable, were she to return to Dari's village. On many occasions Mrs. Mahama told me that she intended to visit Dari, but she never did. To visit someone is to show care and concern and to pay one's respects. Mrs. Mahama was afraid to return to the scene of the arrest, as she knew that she would have been remembered, and the youth came to materialize the potential retribution she feared.

As I listened to Mrs. Mahama, I was trying to make sense of her NGO's advocacy for reforming the law. The stricter law, which extended culpability to parents and guardians, had not been passed when Dari was sentenced but took effect two years before these conversations in 2009. According to the new law, Dari would have been imprisoned, not because of a false confession but because of her involvement in getting her granddaughter cut. I asked Mrs. Mahama and Edna how they would have felt if the law had already been in force when Dari was sentenced. "But it wasn't!" they said. There was nothing to discuss. Mrs. Mahama and Edna had no time for questions about the inherent dilemmas in enforcing the new law or for moral nuances of this stricter legislation.

Musa, however, thought that the new law would have spared Dari, saying: "She would have been punished anyway, but it wouldn't have been severe." He considered the revised law more just because he thought that it appropriately distributed sanctions among those who shared culpability, circumcisers and parents:

But the actual fact is that, if you don't invite the circumciser, he cannot just come to your house and get hold of a girl and start circumcising. So that it is not the circumciser who is seen as the bad person, but the parents of the child or the guardians who send the children for circumcision must be punished as well.

In subsequent conversation I learned that he had only a vague understanding of the length of the sentences approved by Parliament. In time I would discover that this view was shared by most NGO workers and civil servants, including those who had lobbied for the legislation; they thought that the reform had only redistributed culpability, not increased the punishment. When I told Musa that the minimum sentence was now five years' imprisonment, for both parents and circumcisers, he shrugged his shoulders and said that he did not think that it would ever come to that. And historically speaking, he was right—the new law has never been enforced by the book.

How do we understand Musa's equanimity and Mrs. Mahama's and Edna's ambivalence? The combination of Dari's false confession and GAWW's direct involvement in her arrest generated unusual emotional responses, but these responses tell a larger story about NGOs' experimentation with legal advocacy. Mrs. Mahama, Edna, Musa, and others had not envisioned the consequences of enforcing the law by the book. Together with feminist advocates, they designed an experimental system of governance that they thought would unfold in accordance with the parole of law enforcement, but they never paused to consider that actual people might be imprisoned.

Mrs. Mahama thought there were both right and wrong reasons to be disturbed by the prison sentences and that only some people had the right to question them. She was particularly opposed to international opposition to the arrests, which she and Edna both characterized as "nonsense." They were upset when their office received calls from an international human rights organization inquiring about the arrests and asking whether Dari had legal representation during her trial. Mrs. Mahama found moral doubts acceptable if expressed in a private domain but not if the legality or justice of the arrest was publicly questioned. She saw the international concern as misplaced and wrongheaded, and disparaged a newspaper article written by an American woman that raised questions about the arrest. Her outrage—in the form of the exclamation "Nonsense!"—also sums up her attitude regarding the public character of Western qualms about anticutting campaigns. Whereas in liberal multicultural democracies of the global North, objecting to cutting requires a public performance of cultural sensitivity, even for those whose private thoughts and feelings are less nuanced, in Ghana public discourses require taking a tough stance and keeping complex sentiments to oneself. Ghana has no public discourse that can overtly object to existing laws and campaigns.

But international human rights organizations are far from being the only ones raising questions of injustice. After Abampoka Mbawini was arrested and sentenced with the help of members of the regional eradication committee, the committee members began questioning the injustice and violence of law, using language that both included and exceeded liberal parameters of fair trial and due process.

The Beginning of the End

In January 2004 the Bawku Circuit Court sentenced Abampoka Abane Mbawini to five years in prison for cutting seven girls. Like Fefe Dari, Abampoka was arrested in the wake of two NGO projects: two months after Alhassan's Center for Human Rights Education and Advocacy held a workshop in Bawku and formed an FGM eradication committee, and one month after another NGO from the region, ZOVFA (Zouri Organic Vegetable Farmers Association), held a sensitization program in the village itself. Alhassan's presence at the trial, and the understanding that he was a "human rights lawyer," were crucial to the unfolding of the trial and the imposition of the maximum sentence. The judge's official explanation for why he gave Abampoka the maximum sentence cited her knowledge of the criminality of her act and the deterrent effect of the punishment:

> I was tempted to take the advanced age of the accused into consideration in passing sentence and would have imposed on her the minimum sentence prescribed by law. However, the accused has admitted that she is well aware that what she did was a criminal act yet she went ahead to do it. Under these circumstances I think she deserves an exemplary sentence as punishment to her and deterrent to others. Accused is accordingly sentenced to five (5) years of imprisonment to be served at the Tamale female prisons. (Police Bawku Case RO N.O. 27/04)

Although the public record will archive only this official narrative of exemplary punishment that should serve as a deterrent, Abampoka's sentence provoked critical responses in the region. Almost everyone who was involved in the case and who contributed to her arrest and punishment was conflicted: all wanted cutting to end and the law to work as a deterrent, but they did not agree on what this meant. Over time their ambivalence about punishment turned into its rejection. In pages that follow I detail how this shift occurred from the perspectives of two civil servants, a nurse and a gender desk officer, who were key to Abampoka's arrest.

"Human as We Are"

Imagine you are a nurse assigned to the Bawku District Health Administration. You may or may not receive your salary regularly. The villagers for whom you are responsible are supposed to have universal health care but cannot afford to pay for it, and there are not enough health care providers. Your job is to support public health outreach in rural areas, which at times consists of being paid by NGOs as a "resource person" to give talks. You are also invited to NGO and state workshops where you are supposed to enhance your knowledge about harmful traditional practices and where you are impelled to identify not with the women and men for whom you are responsible but with discourses that see rural subjects as undeserving of care. You are offered a better position in the Ghanaian polity if you accept the role of a modernizing agent who mediates between tradition and modernity, law and order. You are invited to become a member of an FGM eradication committee and are asked to help enforce the law. You are told that you can help end cutting, strengthen the rule of law, make the state strong. You are excited.

Angela, a public health nurse, had attended Alhassan's workshop in the autumn of 2003 and became a member of the eradication committee. She was employed at the district health office and had intimate knowledge of the villages around Bawku, where she had given presentations about the health effects of cutting at NGO-organized events. When in January 2004 word reached her that Abampoka had cut seven girls in the village of Yelego, Angela knew exactly what to do. She contacted Esther, the gender desk officer at the seat of the district government, who was also a member of the FGM eradication committee.

Esther asked the police to investigate, but the police were "making delay tactics," she said. I asked Esther why they did that. The standard GAWW answer is that the police are not educated about the law, while feminist lawyers complain about masculinist and patriarchal police, but Esther had a different explanation: "You know, human as we are, they, a bit of things come in, and then they don't want . . . because they believe that it is traditional practice."

For the police cutting was outside the realm of criminality, and Esther succeeded only when a police officer trained by Alhassan got involved. They did not have an arrest warrant, but they all (Esther, Angela, and the police) traveled to the village and apprehended Abampoka in her house. They then asked the local assemblyman to tell them where the cut girls lived, but he refused and said the circumciser should show them the way, which she did. What happened next is somewhat murky. According to the assemblyman, they took one cut girl, a seventeen-year-old from Kumasi who was visiting her natal home, as well as her parents, to the police station. According to Esther, they also encountered the other girls who had been cut and took pictures of them. According to Angela, the girl's mother "dodged" when she saw the police and escaped arrest. What is clear is that Abampoka was brought to the

Bawku police station, where she admitted that she had performed cutting, and was then released on bail, paid for by a civil servant from the village. Only the seventeen-year-old from Kumasi was examined in the hospital and asked to serve as a witness at the trial; other girls and their parents ran away to Burkina, it was said.

After Esther notified Alhassan about Abampoka's arrest, he came to Bawku to ensure that she was tried and sentenced. When she did not arrive for her scheduled court appearance, Alhassan pressured the police to pursue the case and persisted when they refused. At this time Esther agreed with Alhassan and was invested in having Abampoka arrested, so, like Mrs. Mahama in Wa, she provided the police with a vehicle: "But the police were making delay tactics again for the culprit to go away. Then I stood on the police. They said they had no car, I got a car for them. So we went there in the night. They delayed and we got there in the night." When I interviewed Alhassan several months after the arrest, he was still surprised by the resistance he encountered not only from the villagers but also from the police. For him, a long-time activist who had spent many of his formative years outside the country, the discourse of human rights violations was closer to home than the opposition to incarceration:

> But let me also say that even after she was arrested, she was granted bail and it was like nothing—it seemed nothing was going to happen to her. Because the day that they were supposed to bring her back to the police, the person who stood in and granted the bail did not turn up with her. So it took us, we spent one full day, went to her place in the village and tried to locate the surety before they realized that, "No, it's something more serious" than they anticipated. And all this time we were also on the police. So the police realized that; we even made them aware that it was even wrong in the first place for them to have granted her bail under the circumstances. Because the village where she carried out the circumcision is about five kilometers from the border with Burkina Faso. And the experience was that even some of the victims had crossed the border into Burkina Faso. So what was the assurance or guarantee that she herself wouldn't abscond? So we were quite worried and then, fortunately, we were able to, they brought her back to the police.

In his account of the arrest Alhassan placed himself in and out of the narrative, much like Mrs. Mahama in her account of Dari's arrest. "*We* spent one full day," he says, but "*they* realized" that the resistance was more serious than anticipated. "*The police* realized," he also begins, but then switches to "*we* even made them aware" that granting the bail was wrong. My sense was that, for Alhassan, these turns of phrase are less a sign of a moral ambiguity than of code switching between his participation in the punitive power of the state and the ideal-typic role of the NGO, which is supposed to do its work by applying pressure but not by merging with the state.

All this time Abampoka was at home, waiting to be tried. The problem, then, was not that the circumciser had fled across the border, as Alhassan and others feared, but that she had support from the police, other villagers, and the civil servant who did not want to surrender her.

Esther described the opposition to the arrest more dramatically, saying that she, Alhassan, and the police were "nearly lynched" by a mob. This depiction of threatening grievous violence stands in sharp contrast to the disciplinary violence that Abampoka and the cut girl experienced after their arraignment. Like other cut girls taken to hospitals and police stations, they were subjected to the gazes of the authorities. Everyone recorded them in pictures and audio interviews: Angela, the nurse, photographed Abampoka and the cut girls; Alhassan also took pictures and interviewed them. He said he wanted to "understand," not unlike an anthropologist, and the girls were unable to refuse him. For an NGO, taking pictures is an important means of documenting its presence at the scene of an arrest and thus demonstrating efficacy to donors and other remote audiences.

Esther told me that in court, Abampoka was read the charge and admitted her guilt. But she was also confused and "was telling a lot of stories." Esther hoped that Abampoka would say something to redeem herself but instead she told the truth, not knowing that "the truth was getting her into trouble":

> I was thinking she will prove innocent, maybe to be ignorant about the whole thing, the harmful effects, but she never did. She spoke about how she was trained by an NGO. ZOVFA trained her and told her the harmful effects of the this thing and gave her seed money as a living. And according to her, she actually stopped it and went down south. Then, when she came back, people from Yelego came and pricked her to perform on those girls. She told them that it is not allowed because the chiefs have banned it, but they said they were going to keep it a secret. So she performed on those ladies. Actually she said she was sitting in her house. She—it wasn't her intention to do that. Because she knows that it is very harmful, but they pleaded with her and she did it.

Abampoka's declaration that she performed cutting only because she was asked to do so by the girls' families had no legal weight in the eyes of the judge.

The many stories she told—about having been told about the harmful effects of cutting, about her poverty, and about knowing that the "chiefs had banned it"—served only to underscore her guilt. As Angela put it, because Abampoka "accepted knowing about the ban," the judge could not show any mercy.

Both Angela and Esther were disturbed that Abampoka did not have a lawyer. Esther told me: "You know, if it had been a different person, they would have coached her... "Don't say this, don't say this," but because of her age, she said the truth. She thought she was saying the truth to come out, so she told the judge everything."

In principle the Constitution of Ghana requires that "a person charged with a criminal offence shall... be given adequate time and facilities for the preparation of his defence" and "be permitted to defend himself before the court in person or by a lawyer of his choice" (Article 19). In practice not everyone has legal representation. "Some people have lawyers, others don't," I was told by a man with whom I struck up a conversation while waiting outside the court building and who, as a hobby, regularly attended the Bawku court proceedings. Moreover, few of those charged with criminal offenses are given adequate time and facilities to prepare their defense. Trials are swift: the records I obtained from the Tamale Female Prison show that the circumcisers were tried within several days of their initial arrest.

Angela agreed with Esther that Abampoka was incapable of defending herself and that a lawyer would have found a way to defend her. When I first met Angela, she, too, thought that it was not too late to get Abampoka a lawyer who would "shorten the time for her." Abampoka was bereft not only of legal representation but also of social support, as she did not have time to summon her children. The children were themselves poor labor migrants and probably could not have done much for her, but they could have mobilized help from others. When I stopped by Abampoka's house several months after her arrest, a man was working on the adjacent farm. He was her son, he told me, and he did not know how to assist his mother or how she was faring in prison. "Now that you are asking of her, perhaps you can help?" he inquired. I told him all I could do was try to visit her soon.

Abampoka's lack of legal representation stood in contrast to the NGO's legal intervention, represented by the figure of Alhassan. He stayed in Bawku to observe Abampoka's trial, and his presence was crucial to its unfolding; in effect, he was monitoring the court proceedings and had inserted himself as a third interested party. The registrar at the Bawku court told me that precisely because "the human rights activist was there," the judge had to sentence

Abampoka to what was then the maximum sentence, five years in prison. Esther and Angela also told me that the presence of a "human rights lawyer" put pressure on the police and the judge: "Because he was around, they made the whole thing to go fast," Angela said. Alhassan represented the rule of law itself and human rights, principles that are higher than any particular law or its application.

Danilyn Rutherford argues that sovereignty is always dependent on and inflected by an audience; in the absence of witnesses, proclaiming sovereign acts would have little meaning or legitimacy (2012). The constitution of sovereignty thus depends on *whose* eyes are watching. But also important here is the work spectators do. When Alhassan observes the court proceedings and Mrs. Mahama lends her car to the police, they are not simply witnessing acts of the state but are compelling, fueling, and daring state actors to act. The extensive recordings of the arrests in the form of pictures and audio interviews are also both a promise and a threat of another audience, farther away, in the nation's capital and across the borders of the country. For Judge Jacob Boon this included the national reporters who would relay Abampoka's punishment to the public so that the "exemplary sentence" would serve as a "punishment to her and deterrent to others."

In private, however, the judge "felt remorse" and was troubled by Abampoka's sentence, the registrar told me. The judge had sought the registrar out after handing down the sentence:

> He came into my office and told me about the case at 4 P.M. I was in my office right next to the courtroom, but I wasn't aware of it. I had just seen an old lady shivering, but I thought she was there for her son, I didn't know it was her who was charged. So I was surprised when the judge told me about the case, and I said, "Ah, in this court?" I asked the judge why he gave her such a long sentence, and he said that he himself wasn't happy about it but that he couldn't do otherwise, since she said she knew about the law. And FGM is inhuman, he said.

Like others, the judge calibrated his regret and did so by weighing cutting against the "inhumanity of FGM." At stake here are two competing frameworks of humanity and their corollary understandings of values. Is it inhuman to cut girls, as the judge and Alhassan asserted and as NGOs often claim? Or is it inhuman to imprison an elderly circumciser and enforce the law by the book, as implied by the police and civil servants who felt ambivalent about the arrest? In Bolgatanga, gender activists who supported the campaigns against cutting were disturbed by the punishment and used the language of human rights to question it. When I told Elizabeth about my research on Abampoka's arrest, Elizabeth asked me if anyone had visited her in prison: "We need to look into the human rights situation, you know," she said. Elizabeth supported GAWW and Dr. Adjei, but she mobilized the discourse of human rights to question the imprisonment of the elderly circumciser. The language of humanity had become not only a counterdiscourse to sovereign violence but also a terrain of contestation about its legitimacy.

The opposition to Abampoka's imprisonment is not surprising in the context of the Ghanaian penal system, as her gender, age, and the nature of her offense made her an unlikely prisoner. The cultural and institutional logics that guide how and whom the state prosecutes make a young man the public face of criminality, and the offenses associated with it are theft and robbery. Therefore, when the court registrar saw Abampoka, his first thought was that she was there for her son. Theft by young men is the proper subject of policing and of popular outrage. When Esther told me, somewhat approvingly, that the government pardons some prisoners who were sentenced for "minor reasons," she drew the line at theft: "Not a thief, no. If you are a thief, no. Not a criminal." In contrast, when in 2011 the news media reported that a ninety-one-year-old woman had been charged with swindling, Ghanaian cyberspace lit up in debate; not everyone agreed that she was innocent, but her age was the reason many took issue with the criminal charges. Ghana has few women prisoners (1.8 percent of the prison population) and virtually none of them is old.

Indeed, Fefe Dari and Abampoka Mbawini were the only prisoners in the Tamale Female Prison for a time. When they were released, the prison guards missed them, they said, because the guards "had no other companions and people to chat to." Not only Angela and Esther had feelings for Abampoka—the punishing authorities had them too. The guards expressed relationality in the language of friendship, which was meant to ameliorate the prison conditions. They told Musa, who spoke with them on my behalf (as a foreigner, I was not allowed into the prison), that they had befriended Abampoka and other circumcisers. "We used to talk to them, we got used to them," the guards told him, enchanting him with their account. "They were not maltreating them, because they felt they were women like them," said Musa, who was inclined to accept the guards' reports that the prisoners "had the best time there."

WHEN RIGHTS FEEL WRONG: CORPOREAL SENSIBILITY

I have not found the mouth to tell my story.

AMA ATA AIDOO

The ethnographic description of the turmoil felt by almost everyone involved in the arrest and sentencing of Abampoka barely hints at the obstacles I encountered as I tried to understand it. While some people used the discourse of human rights, most civil servants had no readily available language for their ambivalence about punishment. They certainly needed time to trust me, but even when they came to do so, they had no idioms of dissent for objecting to law enforcement by the book. Given the public discourse about the state's failures and the value of the rule of law, punishment was something they could not *not* desire.

I first began to understand this fraught relationship to punishment by noticing the discrepancy between their words and their body language, which signaled their ambivalence about what they perceived as excesses of legal power. Angela and Esther bore the brunt of the work of enforcing the law at its frontiers; in contrast to those of us who discuss the limits of law in classrooms or NGO conference rooms, they faced these limits daily. Even several months after Abampoka's trial, Angela and Esther both looked ill at ease when discussing it, but the first thing they said was that they were proud of their surveillance role and their participation in the arrest.

Angela, whose role in the arrest embodied the nodal point between the village and the state, was visibly disturbed by the arrest and her role in it. When I began to interview her, she seemed so ill at ease that I considered not proceeding and decided to address her discomfort directly:

SAIDA: So I can ask you about it [the arrest]?

Five seconds pass, then Angela utters a barely audible sound and makes a slight head movement.

SAIDA: Um, does that mean yes or no?

Three seconds pass. Angela laughs.

ANGELA (IN A MORE ANIMATED VOICE): I say it's okay.

Three seconds pass.

SAIDA (HESITANTLY): Sometimes people say things, but their bodies tell me a different story.

ANGELA: Oooh.

SAIDA: And your body is telling me a different story. So that's why I want to make sure. I don't want to—

Angela laughs with what sounds like a mixture of nervousness and relief.

SAIDA: A yes is a yes, a no is a no, and there are lots of things in between, so that's why I'm asking again? [Six seconds pass.] I am just a student, and this is for my research. Any benefit to knowledge is not worth causing any person any kind of difficulty. So, I don't want to—

ANGELA: No problem, you go ahead.

In retrospect, it is not clear to me that Angela considered saying no an option. I was introduced to her by her superior, a doctor in charge of the District Health Administration who had flamboyantly welcomed me in Russian (like Alhassan, he had studied in the former Soviet Union) and allowed me to interview Angela. The line between the director's permission and order is a thin one, and Angela had a strong sense of duty. I had spent much time thinking through the ethical implications of my research but had not anticipated that an interview with a civil servant would be one of the most difficult moments. "How will you interview the village women?" I was often asked. "What about the power relations between you and the illiterate women?" "How will you talk to the women who were cut?" I knew enough about violence to understand that cut women may or may not have difficulty talking about it—the act of cutting was for the most part not experienced as violent or traumatic. However, I was not prepared for the suffering of a nurse who did not have "the mouth to tell" her wounds.

For much of the interview Angela's speech was punctuated by pauses, gasps, and uncomfortable laughter. Both she and Esther averted their gazes, and their gestures were stiff. Their bodies were slumped in the chairs or nearly frozen in space. When I asked Angela how she felt about the arrest, she stepped outside her own thoughts and affects and discussed the logic behind the arrest:

SAIDA: Were you in favor of the arrest, did you want the woman to be arrested or not?

ANGELA: Well, the woman being arrested was to put some fears into others who would have heard that this is what has happened, and then so she

herself would be scared from doing it again. Aha. So this was the
intention: we just wanted to put some fears into the people.

By using a passive construction, Angela shifted the conversation toward the
purpose behind the arrest: it "was to put some fears into others." In so doing,
she indicated that intent was what mattered and that what was intended dif-
fered from the eventual outcome. In her view the logic of deterrence legitimized
the arrest, as its purpose was not to punish Abampoka but to send a message to
others. At this moment Angela located herself in the collective *we* of the logic
of arrest as a threat: "We just wanted to put some fears into the people."

One problem she articulated was that "the woman didn't know what
would happen to her." It soon became clear that Angela had not known what
would happen to Abampoka either and that, given the reluctance of police to
enforce the law, the very notion of state sovereignty over the exercise of legal
violence was in question:

SAIDA: Did you think that the case would be taken to court?

ANGELA: Well, the case going to court or not going to court, that one was . . .
We weren't to determine that! We weren't to determine that. Aha.

SAIDA: Who was to determine it? The police, or—?

ANGELA: Yes, the police and the, the, the . . . I don't know. Because, some
of these things, you can even do the arrest, and it can get to the police
station, and it will end there. It wasn't the first time we did the arrest and
it ended nowhere.

What state policies say about the responsibilities of various governmental
offices mattered little in this context. In ordinary circumstances Abampoka's
arrest may have ended with the initial report to Esther or the police. As
Angela put it, "Because certain times, when I hear of it and then come to tell
her [Esther], before we can take any other, any action, we don't get the head
and tail of it." Nor did Angela expect Abampoka to be sentenced:

Well, in actual fact, going to court does not necessarily mean prosecution.
You can go to court, but if you're able to explain yourself, you can be,
this thing, discharged. My opinion was, um, we just wanted to deter the
people, aha, from doing it, so this was our main aim of handling the issue.

I understood that Angela could not reconcile her belief in the productive
power of arrests with their unforeseen consequences—that the elderly circumciser would be imprisoned rather than merely arrested and disciplined.

Meanwhile Angela's own standing in the community shifted after the arrest, and she broke down while talking about her disrupted relationships with the Yelogo villagers. They chastised her during the arrest, calling her a traitor.

> Even when we went to do the arrest, they were telling me, they were calling me, saying that they know me, so what was I [doing]? I said, "You know me, but I am doing my work as a health worker. So it's because I'm working with you people, so that's why I've come with people, so you know the importance of the, the issue."

She did not think she was trusted anymore, she said, shedding tears that she quickly wiped away. Only after she said this did she relax.

Angela did not have a ready-made language for critiquing the law, objecting to experimentations with its enforcement, or expressing the sorrow she felt as a result of her participation. As a civil servant she did not see herself in a position to object to the law or the state. Indeed, none of the regional midlevel civil servants did.

In his ethnography of East German journalists whose knowledge was considered inadequate by the postunification regime dominated by the West, Dominic Boyer argues that the journalists repeatedly expressed their objections to the discourse about their inadequacy through gestures and bodily comportment. Boyer noticed that when the topic of East German deficiency came up, the conversation with his interviewees "would reach a strange and awkward pause" (2005: 257) marked by quickened breathing and retraction into "a position of defensive readiness." The journalists would fidget, tremble, or open their mouths without saying anything. When they did speak, however, they brushed off the critique and rejected it as irrelevant to their circumstances.

Boyer reads the halting speech and the "gestural grammar" of his interlocutors as a form of knowledge that he calls corporeal expertise. Angela's gestures and the micropractices of her body operate in a slightly different register. They are forms not of knowledge but of complex, embodied sentiments that entail ambivalence toward the penal system as well as traces of damage from participating in the networks of surveillance. As a result of experiments with the langue of law, circumcisers were sentenced, but those mobilized to enforce the law also were exposed to harm. Angela's corporeality is an index of this unspeakable harm, one that had no discursive legitimation. Instantiating the rule of law and an effective state was something that Angela and others could not *not* want, yet the legal practices that were meant to curb what is understood as harmful traditional practices violated their ethical dispositions. In the face of this conflict, all they could tell me was that Abampoka's imprisonment did not feel right.

Angela and Esther frequently told me that they "feel for" Abampoka. Abampoka, they said, did not have her children by her. Nobody brought her food in jail. She was alone. They narrated stories of visiting her in the Bawku jail and taking her food and soap, neither of which is adequately provided for. Angela realized that Abampoka was in effect abandoned. Angela also encouraged me to buy some bread and soap for Abampoka when I went to Tamale. Alhassan also took her food when he visited her, for despite his self-professed "firm approach," he wanted to demonstrate care and concern. He told me that even though she knew about the law, "she never thought she would be arrested," and she had promised never to do it again.

Like Mrs. Mahama, Angela and Esther oscillated between expressing their empathy and insisting on Abampoka's culpability, often switching between these two positions in one breath. Esther told me: "I am feeling it that she is seventy years, but I felt she should have proved at least a bit innocent. When I told her anytime the ladies are bleeding, how she feels, [she said] that is normal." Esther's empathy was tempered by the circumciser's coldblooded and unresponsive attitude to the suffering of girls who had lost blood.

Angela and Esther tried to reconcile their ambivalence by convincing themselves that all they had done was their duty; they told me that they did not see themselves in any way responsible for Abampoka's sentence because they were just "doing their work." This bifurcated conception of duty and personal attachment is widely shared in Ghana, Jennifer Hasty found in her study of the government's anticorruption unit (2005a). Those working for the Serious Fraud Office see themselves as only doing their duty; to resolve a case and elicit a confession, they sidestep "the issue of guilt altogether and establish a more humanistic interpersonal relation" (290). But for those involved in Abampoka's arrest, sidestepping the issue of personal responsibility was not sustainable. In the long run, for Angela, Esther, and others, the most difficult thing was not convincing villagers and others that they had acted righteously but convincing themselves.

One thing that greatly troubled them was law's systemic injustice. For them justice meant recognizing collective responsibility for the act of cutting rather than imprisoning a single individual. Struggling to find words to describe her sense of injustice, Angela pointed out the paradox of the cut girl's agency in "giving herself" to cutting and then serving as a witness for the prosecution:

> But now, if you talk about only the one who does the act, even the one who gave herself for the . . . [cutting], that person is rather used as a, a, a— what? A witness, on the other side! Meanwhile, if she hadn't given herself, the thing wouldn't have taken place. Which is not, I mean, it's not correct.

Angela saw Abampoka as one of many people responsible for the act of cutting and was incensed by legal definitions of victimhood and culpability. It was simply "not correct" to imprison a circumciser and use the girl who had requested her services as a witness. By using this popular phrase to express moral wrongfulness, Angela found the law wanting. To be clear, Angela did not question the criminalization of cutting as such but its bifurcation of victims and perpetrators.

Angela was not alone in expressing these sentiments. The regional director for the Commission on Human Rights and Administrative Justice in the Upper East Region told me that the police were particularly reluctant to enforce this law precisely because the girls wanted to be cut: "So [the police said]: 'Where do you expect me to go and see and catch this person who, you know, is doing it in some hidden room somewhere, with the tacit support of the victim? So it is some kind of collusion, how am I going to get them?'"

Angela's feelings of empathy for Abampoka were not those of humanitarian compassion toward an innocent, pure, and morally deserving victim of suffering (see Ticktin [2011]). Nonetheless, agency emerged as the terrain on which she articulated this critique. Angela's emphasis on the girl's agency, on her voluntary submission to cutting, resonates with the argument of the feminists who pushed for making cut girls subject to imprisonment, as I discussed in chapter 6. These momentary recognitions of cut girls' agency are restricted to the legal realm and stand in sharp contrast to common discourses about girls being "brainwashed" into accepting cutting. Alhassan put it more neutrally, telling me that the cut seventeen-year-old who had testified at Abampoka's trial "was not forced" to get cut but that "her grandmother and the other women gave her a kind of counseling and other things, and then built up her courage and then morale to go for it, which she did." Angela's reference to the girl who "gave herself" underscored both the structures of power that produce and regulate cutting and the girl's agency in voluntarily submitting, or giving herself, to it. In this rendering there are no pure victims or culprits; rather, people are compelled to act by complex forces.

According to Angela, the desire for cutting and the responsibility for its execution operate on a compounded terrain: Abampoka did not want to cut the girls but was "lured" into it by the girls' parents. The parents are as responsible as Abampoka because they pleaded with her to perform cutting: they "called her to come and assist them to get out of that shame"—of having uncut daughters—and she therefore "had to do it." The girls, meanwhile, "gave themselves." Everyone was compelled toward the act of cutting and was therefore equally responsible. But because the law separates victims from perpetrators, the circumciser was punished while those who compelled her to cut walked free and even served as witnesses at the trial.

Angela's protest against the "incorrectness" of law enforcement was informed by NGO advocacy, as she mentioned that "adding that clause" (by which she meant the proposed reforms) would remedy the law's injustice. When I said that the reform would lead to more, rather than fewer, prison sentences, Angela disagreed:

> No, no, no. The thing is, it's not necessarily imprisoning them but bringing them to book. You see, their fellow people, their colleagues, would hear and say, "Ay, this is for when they did this, the other time, it was this and that, so don't do it!" If they hear of someone intending to do it, they'll say, "Hey, if you do it, you'll face consequences." So it will help to scare the people.

Angela thought that the revised law would bring more people *to* book but that it would not be enforced *by* the book. Rather, cut girls would be charged "in a way," she told me, and their parents would face "some small consequences." The law would not punish but would inform arrestees about the seriousness of their offense, mete out some consequences, and then release them. Nobody should be imprisoned, but everyone should feel the force of the law and feel subject to legal authority. For Angela this promised a morally appropriate legal framework with an effective structure of deterrence.

Angela believed that once girls understood that they were subject to arrest, they would discipline themselves accordingly and decide to forgo cutting. But girls already thought themselves subject to arrest. In the village where Abampoka was arrested, distrust of the law and legal authorities was acute. Of the seven girls cut by Abampoka, six had fled when the police had come to the village. When, months later, I visited their village with a teacher who was their assemblyman, I was not able to meet the girls—people were still afraid of strangers who were inquiring about cutting. "Three of them got married in Burkina," I was told, and "three of them died of pneumonia." The girls were off-limits, either in death or across the border. These idioms, usually used by NGOs to draw attention to the harms of cutting, were now appropriated as idioms of protection.

GOVERNMENTALITY AGAINST ITSELF: HALTING SOVEREIGN VIOLENCE

In 2009, five years after Abampoka's incarceration, she should have been released from prison. I was in Ghana for follow-up fieldwork and quickly learned that Abampoka had been released much earlier. As I traveled from Accra to Bolga, Bawku, and Tamale, I realized that all NGO workers and civil servants knew that and had their own theory about how it happened.

I eventually found the answers I was looking for at the Tamale Legal Aid office. The workers told me that they had received a request to represent Abampoka from her son-in-law, a teacher who worked in Tamale, as well as from the local Department of Social Welfare. At their request the Legal Aid office requested and won a presidential pardon for Abampoka. But then came a surprise: the lawyer who represented her, they said, was Alhassan—the very man who was instrumental in getting her imprisoned and sentenced in the first place. I could speak with him if I waited for him to finish his session with a client, they added. I was grateful for this gift of time, and as I sat in their office and chatted with the workers, my mind was desperately trying to reconcile how the man who had served as an informal coprosecutor had become Abampoka's defense lawyer.

After receiving his Ghanaian law degree, I learned, Alhassan was posted to Tamale's Legal Aid office and found himself on the other side of the law: seeking, rather than enforcing, justice. He was still interested in making law work and moving it from paper to the courtroom, but was now doing so in the service of those accused. He was as principled as ever, I realized after talking to him, but the legal principles he was upholding were no longer the same. In addition to working on Abampoka's pardon, Legal Aid had secured an early release for Fefe Dari; she was freed after serving two years of her five-year sentence, which was the earliest allowed by law.

That Alhassan himself was the one who worked for Abampoka's pardon is perhaps an accident of fate, yet the story of her sentencing and pardon reveals shifts in the value of punishment and law enforcement "by the book." The initial enthusiasm for enforcing the law generated an immanent critique of sovereign violence.

In Bawku, where cutting was still practiced, I learned that Abampoka's sentence was the last one given to a circumciser. This was not for lack of reports about cutting or arrests of circumcisers but because NGOs and eradication committees no longer fueled law enforcement. In the years since Abampoka and Dari were sentenced, instances of cutting had been reported to both GAWW and to Esther, the gender desk officer in Bawku, but neither was interested in enforcing the law by the book. I gleaned this from the way in which they discussed their inability to prosecute. Esther told me that some circumcisers had been apprehended but not sent to court "because of the conflict"—the political violence that flared up from time to time. The police had as little interest in prosecuting circumcisers as ever, but Esther no longer prodded them. In 2007 she had received a report about cutting from a health volunteer and informed the police who were to travel and apprehend the circumciser, but the plan was called off. Rather than urging the police to arrest the circumciser as she had done in Abampoka's case, Esther now stopped pushing. Whereas five years earlier she fueled the police by lending them her vehicle and alerting Alhassan, she now aligned herself with the police officers' reasoning: everyone agreed that they could not arrest the circumciser on the day of an important festival and that searching for the circumciser later would be futile. In the aftermath of Abampoka's sentence, Esther had learned that arrests lead to punishment and that law enforcement by the book could be avoided only if no arrests took place. To be clear, her opposition to the arrest took the form of letting the police let the circumciser go.

While haunted by Abampoka's fate, Esther continued to feel ambivalent about the circumciser's imprisonment. Esther had stopped by Abampoka's house once and saw workers repairing the roof; this was after catastrophic flooding, when Abampoka and many others received humanitarian aid in the form of housing reconstruction. Glad that Abampoka had been released and was receiving assistance, Esther surmised that she had been well cared for in the prison:

> I know she was being taken good care of because I was relating. Because she was old, they made her to sit down, they were feeding her. Oh, when she

came out, she was very plump and very nice. Better than—because in the house, she was struggling to eat herself.

Esther concluded that prison officers treated Abampoka well, since that is what she would have done in their situation—she was relating to guards relating to Abampoka. Abampoka's plump body was an index of the care she received in prison, which was "better than—." Here, she stopped herself, not allowing herself to quite say what first came to mind—that Abampoka was better fed in the prison than at home.

Writing about hunger in the Brazilian Northeast, Nancy Scheper-Hughes identified the concentration camp as an "unsettling metaphor" (1993: 32) whose relevance to the lives of the people with whom she worked was more than metaphorical. In the wake of theorizations of the camp as a paradigm of modernity (Agamben 1998), anthropologists are quicker to reach for this metaphor, but Scheper-Hughes meant something more specific. The nutritional value of food and the average daily intake of calories in the Brazilian Northeast were similar to those of prisoners held in the German concentration camps in World War II. They could survive but just barely and only if they tightly held on to life. Esther's quick decision not to complete her sentence ("better than") reveals her disquiet at the comparison of prison and home. Although intended as a testament to humane prison conditions, her statement contained an implicit indictment of the scarcity and deprivation women like Abampoka experience in their everyday lives.

Remarkably, Esther's narrative of Abampoka's release from the prison mirrors the narrative of cut girls' release from cutting. "When she came out, she was very plump and very nice" is something said about cut girls who have healed. Abundant nurturing during the time of healing was recognition not only of the increased need for nourishment in order to build blood but also of the ordeal of cutting itself. Looking plump means looking beautiful and was meant to make up, in some small measure, for the suffering caused by cutting. For Esther, Abampoka's plump body was meant to make up for her suffering in the prison.

When I saw Abampoka in 2009, she was frail and wore old, torn clothes. I sat down at a small bench inside her compound but did not talk to her for long and did not interview her. I had arrived by car, with an NGO worker and a Red Cross volunteer, and Abampoka seemed scared of us. After greeting us, she asked, "Will you take me away?" The young girls who were working with her on her field ran away when they saw us approaching. As we were leaving, Abampoka made a begging gesture, putting her fingers close to her mouth and then stretching her hand toward me. She was hungry and needed money, she said.

Praying for Arrests

Esther was not alone in her refusal to lobby for arrests, for despite the organization's enormous efforts to reform the law, GAWW was also reluctant. Unlike Alhassan, GAWW leaders never intended for the law to be enforced by punitive means, but neither could they publicly state that they were opposed to arrests and punishment. They worked out their dilemma through practice: rather than getting involved in arrests, they were now praying for the law to be enforced.

Mrs. Mahama told me about two occasions when they chose not to advocate for arrests and trials. In 2008 an elderly man was arrested in Bole for having circumcised an infant girl five years earlier. Newspapers reported that the child's mother had paid for the circumcision but later died and that the aunt who was raising the girl reported the circumciser to the police. The police were debating whether to charge him and others with a criminal offence. GAWW considered urging the police to press charges, but Mrs. Mahama said that something came up and they were not able to do so.

When I was in Accra in the summer of 2009, they had just received notice that cutting had occurred in the Brong Ahafo Region, where a father had allegedly coerced his daughters to get cut. GAWW wanted to get involved, Mrs. Mahama told me, but during our conversation it became clear that they were not planning to do so. She and Edna talked about it unison:

EDNA: This BA case, if we are able to follow, definitely the father would not escape.

MRS. MAHAMA: The father would not escape.

EDNA: And because he would not like to be punished alone, I am sure he would voice out where the circumciser is. So we are using the new law now, to take action.

MRS. MAHAMA: We are even praying that at least we should be able to arrest one or two people, the parents. I mean we are just praying for, and if we get this man, believe you me—

EDNA: If we get this man, and this man is punished, that is a very good message for us. So they will then know that the persons, too, are not safe if they do it.

If in 2003 Mrs. Mahama lent her car to the police to arrest Dari, by 2009 Mrs. Mahama was praying for arrests. She and Edna thought that imprisoning the parents would serve as an exemplary punishment, and would communicate the revised law's main objective, which is that no parents are safe if their children are cut. But GAWW leaders no longer wanted to be actively involved in arrests or trials and did not fuel the enforcement apparatus. Their prayers testify to their waning desire to actively engage with law enforcement and express a shifting sense of responsibility: the NGO no longer wanted to partake in the exercise of sovereign violence. Mrs. Mahama's embrace of Christianity likely shaped her language, as well as her views, about justice being in God's hands—she, too, was now "praying for justice" (Greenhouse 1989). The power of the Christian God, unlike the power of ancestral gods, is separate from the material realm of the living, and in this way Mrs. Mahama could exculpate herself: justice was in God's hands alone.

The Subjects of Punishment

For Mrs. Mahama, Angela, Esther, and others, participation in arrests transformed how they relate to subjects of campaigns. In public and NGO discourses, the subjects of anticutting laws are nameless and exist largely as pronouns: *she, he,* and *they.* These pronouns reflect who counts as morally deserving of protection and care and who is punishable and bereft of moral worth:

The circumcisers are a *they:* anonymous, homogenized subjects. *They* refers not to a collection of individual people but to an amorphous group that should be managed, administered, and regulated.

The parents and the grandmothers are also an undifferentiated and undeserving *they,* seen as culprits who force or brainwash their daughters and granddaughters and who therefore must be punished so that the girls are protected.

Young women who willingly submit themselves to cutting are also a culpable *they* who are to be punished so that they can be protected from their own desires. At times they are referred to as a *she* or by name; they are subjects of both protection and punishment.

A "little girl" is an anonymous but deserving figure, a *she* who is innocent and in need of protection.

They, I have shown, is a frequent pronoun in Ghanaian NGO work. NGO governmentality takes the third person plural as its object: it constructs a *they* or a *them* as an objectified population that needs to be known and administered. By constructing *them* as objects of concern, governmental workers secure maximal distance from rural Ghanaians. Encountering a circumciser (Abampoka), a grandmother (Fefe Dari), and a cut girl (the witness at Abampoka's trial) and witnessing their legal fate meant that NGO workers and civil servants had to use names rather than pronouns. They became interested in their fate, offered them care, and began to feel responsible for their imprisonment.

This shift from imagining an undifferentiated population to relating to specific people triggered a realignment of governmental workers with the subjects they govern. NGO workers and civil servants who formerly discussed the ignorance and "intractable customs" of *them* now encountered specific people who had more than a figurative existence. The undifferentiated *they* was replaced by a specific person, a *she* with a name, a face, a presence, and a possibility of relationality—*"I feel for her."* The recognition of Abampoka's personhood also entailed a recognition of a shared social field in which people are mutually accountable and indebted to each other. Governmental workers saw themselves as implicated not only in the arrest but in the social relations that govern everyday life. On that day in 2004 when we heard that Abampoka had been sentenced to five years, and Musa asked Hope, "Could *you* send *your mother* to prison like that?" he was demanding that Hope imagine herself in relation to Abampoka and in a web of mutual accountability and responsibility. Musa was linking Abampoka to relations that were both his and hers.

Patriarchal Excuses or Critique of Punitive Rationality?

When Ghanaians and those familiar with Ghana hear my analysis of how NGOs advocated for a stricter, more punitive law but eventually opposed punishment, they often become uncomfortable. In the Upper East Region the eventual refusal of civil servants to participate in sovereign violence closely resembles the modus operandi of the police: immobility, insolence, and refusal to enforce laws, including those widely considered just, necessary, and appropriate. To those familiar with Ghanaian women's struggle to claim their rights, the refusal to enforce the law against cutting also looks antifeminist, as both the police and government officials frequently declare that violence against women is a private matter outside their domain (Hodžić 2009). How do we understand the opposition to a particular punitive rationality in this context?

The rejection of enforcing the anticutting law may be seen as politically suspect, as it parallels government's opposition to the objectives of other women's rights legislation. To undermine feminist advocacy for the women's rights–based Domestic Violence Bill, the government mobilized an amalgam of discourses, including the right to privacy, the primacy of adjudication by kin and chiefs, the ineptitude of law as a tool for social change, and the impossibility of enforcing laws in a weak state. This was another instance in which the government was performing its own weakness and incapacity. Regional NGO workers and civil servants opposing the Domestic Violence Bill also often referred to material incapacity, bringing up the poor prison conditions and the irony that women would have to bring food to their husbands who were imprisoned for violating them.

As a result of this recent history, the line between opposing law enforcement and opposing feminist advocacy in Ghana is perilously thin. The statements made in both cases are indeed the same, and their meanings can be derived only from the contexts in which they are uttered. Only a contextualized analysis can reveal the extent to which the desire for appropriate sanctions and justice is grounded in underlying norms of equality and harmony (Greenhouse 1989) or the exercise of power by way of "harmony ideology" (Nader 1990).

The question "Is opposition to women's rights laws antifeminist?" has only a contextual answer: in Ghana, yes, at times but not always. Whereas the opposition to criminalizing domestic violence *was* indeed antifeminist in tenor and practice, the critique of punishing circumcisers, which I analyzed in this chapter, was not.[4] The regional civil servants in question were enthusiastic about ending cutting and intent on enforcing the law; they were not a priori opposed to it. They developed a profound ambivalence about punishment *after* getting deeply involved with prosecutions and confronting the limits of the law for securing justice. I understand the civil servants' eventual refusal to enforce the law by the book not as a rejection of the law's objectives but of its means. Although they aimed for a cessation of cutting and hoped that the law could contribute to this goal, they did not want to participate in the exercise of its punitive force, which they saw as excessive and unjust.

Indeed, given these civil servants' location at the margins of the state, they had much to gain from participating in law enforcement. They initially welcomed the opportunity to combat the notion of northern Ghana as ungovernable, especially given how cutting marks the region as the nation's Other. They could remake themselves as citizen-enforcers who fully belonged to the nation-state by upholding the value of law and order that was said to make the state accomplished and effective. Alhassan told me that he had an eye on an even more remote, global audience: he wanted to revise the public idea of not just northern Ghana but of Africa. His aim was to contribute to the kind of active governance that proves Africans to be not only victims but historical agents. This impulse is one that anthropologists understand well.

However, civil servants like Angela and Esther could not reconcile their notions of appropriate punishment and of the disciplinary force of law with practices of incarceration. Their performance of incapacity was not a modus operandi, as it was for the police, but a consequence of an intimate encounter with the injustice of law and their critical reflection about it. So, I hope to have shown, behind what might appear to be antifeminism and inertia is a complex web of shifting attitudes toward punishment, as well as attempts to reconcile law, ethics, and justice.

Feminist theorists insist on the right to critique the infatuation with law in order to defend, and strengthen, feminist practice. Regional civil servants may or may not recognize themselves in theoretical debates, but their critique of punishment is equally geared toward a vision of a more just society, rather than one that would uphold masculinist privilege.

However, patriarchal arguments at times spilled over to arguments against punishment of cutting. The regional director for the Ghana National Commission on Children, for instance, endorsed the notion that chiefs are the proper custodians of law. She told me that cutting should be outlawed by chiefs, and enforced by them, not by the state. In practice, however, chiefs were the informants who notified the watchdog committees and requested their intervention in several arrests of circumcisers. So the imaginary of a competition between chiefs and the police has little to do with their actual dispositions; although elders and chiefs are continually constructed as symbols of indigenous law and order, free from state intervention, as elsewhere on the continent, they "use the coercive power of the modern state" (Perry 2009: 34).

Two male civil servants also told me that they opposed the criminalization of domestic violence and were ambivalent about the criminalization of cutting for the same reasons. As one put it, he had personally "always kicked against the law," given that in Ghana "implementation is always a problem," and laws cannot be enforced. For these men the state's weakness appeared to be not only an explanation but an excuse.

My Mother, the Circumciser

In 2009 I got to know Francis, a high-ranking politician who had served as a regional minister for the Upper East and whose critique of punitive rationality was explicit and unusual. Francis had spent much of his life in southern Ghana as a child of migrants, and he had also studied abroad yet maintained a home base in a village close to Bolga. Unlike most Ghanaians, he was openly sympathetic to the experiences of the circumcisers who found themselves jailed "for no fault of theirs" and for "their spiritual practices." He thought that culturally meaningful practices should not be countered by legal means. Like Dr. Adjei, he viewed reorientation as both more effective and more appropriate:

> And they have their beliefs, and reasons for those beliefs. And so all you needed to do was to identify those beliefs and be able to reorientate them to see those beliefs differently. And that works well. All we need to do is sit with them, reorient them, and let them see the other side of the coin. And then they themselves can be the good lawmakers and implementers and enforcers. Okay, because if we have to force, it is like, because we have power, so we are forcing [them] to deal with it, but it is no fault of theirs. What they are doing, they have a good reason, they've done it all over the years. Let us now let them see that that good reason no longer works.

Unlike Dr. Adjei and other NGO workers and civil servants who are impelled to operationalize civilizing discourse, Francis wanted to convey that the reasons for cutting were once valuable. Reorientation did not entail overcoming ostensible rural ignorance but changing beliefs that were no longer supported by "good reasons." Nonetheless he shared the NGOs' modernist paradigm, which construes knowledge about *beliefs* as a building block of interventions: the goal was "to identify those beliefs and be able to reorientate them to see those beliefs differently." Recall that understanding "the good reasons" was the paradigm that Elizabeth tried to put into effect and that backfired. When governmental workers were unable to identify the original reasons for cutting, they turned to contemporary patriarchal explanations.

Yet Francis's notion that cutting was once good is notably similar to rural women's articulation of the value of cutting. As we saw in chapter 5, these women insist on the historical value of cutting while simultaneously embracing change. They would agree with Francis that "the good reason no longer works" but not why that is the case. The problem they see is not that they are outside modern values but that they are outside the material benefits of modernity.

Francis directly aligned himself with rural women by referring to them as his mothers. We know the thinking of our "own mothers at home," he said. This was not an antifeminist stance, he told me, saying that Olivia, a well-known women's rights advocate from Bolga, agreed with him: "The way her mother thinks here is the same way that my old lady also would think. Because the cultural things, they flow on the same latitude and longitude."

This professed intimacy with rural women and the shift in alignment are made possible by the power relations that subtend them—it is easier for a cosmopolitan Ghanaian politician to align himself with rural women and men than it would be for ordinary NGO workers and civil servants. The latter possess authority in part by defining themselves in opposition to rural subjects, and they are charged with maintaining order at the state's margins. In contrast this cosmopolitan politician could plausibly express his affinities in terms of kinship with rural women and object to punitive intent of law on the same grounds.

Musa was another governmental worker who used the languages of kinship and intimacy to articulate his opposition to punishment. I sat with him in the garden of Bolgatanga's Comme Çi Comme Ça hotel in the summer of 2009. In the years since I first met him, he had become less closely affiliated with GAWW; he was focused on completing his master's studies but was also disappointed by the NGO's refusal to distribute resources fairly among its workers.

As we discussed Abampoka's release, I reminded Musa that many years before, when he had first heard about her sentence, he had challenged Hope's views by asking her, "Could you send your mother to prison like that?" He remembered challenging Hope to see Abampoka as a person who is related and relatable, rather than a mere cipher, and still felt the same, he told me. Musa had been implicated in Dari's arrest and felt uneasy about the sentences that both women received. In a lengthy explanation that followed, he outlined for me the contours of an ethical framework of relatedness, mutual entanglements, and the powerful force of social sanctions that precede and exceed the law:

Let me just say, I am coming from the North, and the North comprises the three regions. So our traditions and cultures are almost the same. So we know that the older person in your house or in another person's house should be treated or given the same treatment like your own grandmother. You understand what I am trying to say? At first, when you go out and you see an old lady and you don't greet her, she has the right to come to your house and tell your parents that you met her and you didn't greet, or she was carrying a load and if you never helped her, you would be punished for that. So those kinds of values actually would let you know that when somebody is within a particular age . . . So you see, because of these values, sometimes [when] you sit down and then you look at somebody, [that person] doesn't merit so much punishment. A little would even deter the person. They are such that when a small thing frightens them, [it] would live with them forever. That is how they are, and then when you do that, they have their own ways of saying . . . So we know the person might go home to curse you because of what he has undergone or he or she has undergone, and it works. Once you believe in it, it works. So these are some of the things that I always consider. But Hope, she comes from an urban place—Accra is urban. And they are mostly with this nuclear family system, but we practice the extended family system so much. So probably my sister or my auntie is somewhere married to another family, and if you traced [my genealogy] you would come to see that I have a relationship or a relation in that particular house.

Musa's was a "relational empathy," as Bornstein puts it, "that turns strangers into kin (2012: 22). Although Musa was from the Northern Region, and Abampoka from the Upper East, he saw a regional affinity and a potential for relatedness. In an ethical framework that values mutual entanglements, the scope of relatedness extends beyond ethnic identity or easily traceable biological kinship. Musa likened Abampoka to a mother because she may well be a relative, given that everyone is related if one looks hard enough.[5] Abampoka's age facilitated this conversion, as every elderly woman had to be both feared and treated well. The cursing he mentioned points to his belief in the power of women's words and their potential for witchcraft, which works "once you believe in it." An elderly woman was to be respected and feared, or else one would face a threat of social sanctions as well as of witchcraft.

In Musa's view one reason Hope was unable to envision a lesser punishment for Abampoka was the limitations that an Accra urbanite would feel regarding extended kin. I did not have to ask whether this was the only relevant factor, or whether what also mattered was the public discourse that defines northern Ghana as the country's Other and its people as not fully belonging to the nation-state, for Musa had some things to say about this on his own. In Accra, he said, "they look at the North as a curse." I asked him to explain.

> I remember, in a class, a colleague gave an example that the North was just like hell, meanwhile you have never traveled to the North. That the North was hot. Just talking about the North being hot, being what and what, "the people are not civilized," he said it in the lecture hall. So I turned to look at my colleagues from the North who were in the lecture hall with me and they were older than me. I was expecting a response from them but like they were quiet so I raised my hand and then I reacted. I reacted, I reacted, and had a heated argument with the lecturer who was in front of me, and I said he shouldn't have allowed the boy make that statement.

Musa does not talk about this kind of discrimination in public nor do other northern Ghanaians who live in Accra. But many have acutely felt the effects of living in a state that marks them as the nation's Others. The public and legal understanding that people who practice cutting are unrelatable and therefore not full people also sees them as being so far outside legality that they need particularly harsh punishment.

Musa contested punishment not on the basis of an ethnic identity but affinity. For Musa, being from northern Ghana provides the possibility of situating Abampoka within the field of a mutually accountable collective that has the power to discipline as well as punish in ways that exceed those of the law. Not everyone who opposed the punitive character of the anticutting law was northern Ghanaian. Dr. Adjei is a well-educated southern Ghanaian who seemingly has little in common with the rural people of the Upper East Region. But they were his patients of thirty years as well as his NGO's target population, and he felt accountable to them. Thus proximity—rather than identity—and concomitant notions of responsibility shaped his opposition to criminalization, which he expressed in pragmatic terms ("You don't need law"). The language of motherhood used by Musa and Francis is rare, but the ethical disposition and value of proximity it expresses is at the core of the widespread rejection of sovereign violence.

I do not mean to extol proximity or universalize it as an ethical framework, but I want to highlight its conditions of possibility and its political ramifications.[6] In the context of a hegemonic ideology that bifurcates the primitive and the civilized, the traditional and the modern, the rural and the urban, the southern and the northern, claiming intimacy and kinship is a political act with radical consequences. By distancing themselves from values that accord law and order primacy over justice, and by constructing the circumcisers as relatable, NGO workers and civil servants disidentified with the dominant order. Disidentification, again, means working on and against an oppressive order, not from the outside but from within (Muñoz 1999).

This final point is especially important in reference to the "zero tolerance to FGM" campaigns in the global North, where the punitive rationale of treating migrants as suspect citizens goes largely unopposed. Unlike their Ghanaian counterparts, civil servants and others in the global North who are charged with surveilling Africans identify with the state order, not with the migrants.

CONCLUSION

And one cannot emphasize too strongly the fact that it is precisely in order to exorcise the possibility of that kind of law—the law that establishes and guarantees inequality—that primitive law functions as it does; it stands opposed to the law of the State. Archaic societies, societies of the mark, are societies without a State, *societies against the State*. The mark on the body, on all bodies alike, declares: *You will not have the desire for power, you will not have the desire for submission*. And that non-separate law can only have for its inscription a space that is not separate: that space is the body itself.

PIERRE CLASTRES

What was it like before the white man?
I don't know mate I never been there.

ELIZABETH A. POVINELLI

In his essay "Of Torture in Primitive Societies," Pierre Clastres (1989) poses a memorable challenge to the notion of stateless and lawless societies, as well as the analytics of "lack" that had long dominated anthropology. He argues that these putative stateless societies do not lack a state; rather, they are against it. They do not lack law—their law is inscribed on bodies through the pain and torture of initiation. Initiation *is* the law. This is the social law of membership and equality. The law of initiation says, "You are one of us. Each one of you is like us; each one of you is like the others. . . . None of you is less than us; none of you is more than us. And you will never be able to forget it" (185). The law marked on the initiated bodies permanently communicates: "You are worth no more than anyone else; you are worth no less than anyone else" (186). These laws hold the group together, and make everyone a full member of the community, *"nothing more, nothing less"* (185; the emphasis is Clastres's).

While Clastres's language of a "primitive" society is both modernist and racist, his argument about initiation as a means of securing membership and social belonging resonates with what I understand about historical practices of female genital cutting in the Upper East Region. Here I am interested in Clastres's claim that the law of initiation not only guarantees equality but also prohibits inequality, which would inevitably arrive with the advent of the state and its law. As he writes, "The law, inscribed on bodies, expresses primitive society's refusal to run the risk of division, the risk of a power separate from society itself, a power that would escape its control" (186). By binding its members together, initiation integrates law into the social body and inscribes it on individual bodies. While Clastres does not minimize the pain of initiation, and refers to it as torture, his sympathies are clear: if the law of initiation is a "terrible cruelty," the law of the state is a "more terrifying cruelty" (188). State law is a "harsh, separate law, the law that imposes the power of the few on all others in a divided society" (186). This despotic law "establishes and guarantees inequality" (188)—an argument echoed by Benjamin, Foucault, and others. Societies that mark the bodies of their members through initiation resist this law of the state and the inequality and division it would bring. They are therefore not stateless but against the state, against state law.

If we accept Clastres's argument, initiation is the law of equality and membership. But campaigns against cutting have the same goal, although they articulate it in different registers. When Nkrumah condemned tribal marks and circumcision, he did so in the name of equality and national unity. Now that the political unit was a nation, tribal marks and circumcision meant separation and division; they were markers of difference, not sameness. Today Ghanaian campaigns against FGM take place in the name of gender equality. Ghanaian societies that cut girls did not circumcise boys, but NGO workers emphasize that cutting women's external genitals is not the same as cutting off the tip of the foreskin but more akin to complete castration. In Bongo and elsewhere in the Upper East, men now get circumcised, as a result of labor migration. Giggling with the pleasure of performing liberation, Asibi, my hosts' elderly neighbor, told me, "Now it is the men who are cut, not us. We have tricked them."

Cutting no longer safeguards the law of equality (in Clastres's sense), if it ever did. But neither does state law. My analysis attests to the resonance of Clastres's argument about the social value of egalitarian justice as a form of law. However, I have tried to show that the social value of justice ultimately opposes the value of punishment not from outside the state but from within. The civil servants and NGO workers who eventually opposed punishment did so after they became intimately involved in the exercise of law's power. What we see here is not a society against the state; rather, the social and the governmental are entwined. Arrests of circumcisers came to an end because of opposition within the state. The punitive excesses of state law are contested by governmental workers themselves—civil servants and others who make up the state and whose bodies bear its traces. They wielded the law of social accountability and ethical relations to oppose the law of the state from within: the Legal Aid office sought presidential pardons, advocates for law reform now pray for arrests, and civil servants allow the police to let the circumcisers go. The discourses that animate their opposition are both governmental and *of* the state, such as the right to a lawyer and due process, and an assemblage of sentiments and historically inflected notions of properly distributed punishment and an ethics of care and mutual accountability. Earlier, I showed that rural women also use an assemblage of governmental and historical understandings of blood to contest biopolitical notions of harm and make claims on the state by using its languages of the census and democracy.

Today, Clastres's literal positing of a prior time (Povinelli 2011b) seems wrong, but I suggest that the notion of society against the state, or the idea that there is an outside to governance that can escape its reach and desires to do so, still informs anthropological imagination. Biehl responds to this by taking Clastres specifically to task in reference to capitalism, writing:

> What about life inside capitalism? Why this investment in a counter-ideology to capitalism that rests on the imaginary of a capital's outside? How to make sense of contemporary realities of society inside the State and people who mobilize to use the state, forging novel, tenuous links between themselves, the state, and the market place? (2013: 589)

These are the questions I want to conclude with. But rather than locating society inside the state in "ordinary people" whose knowledge is subjugated, as Biehl does (582), I have shown that governmental agents and targets alike were equally transformed by their confrontations with governmental power and sovereign violence.[7] Rather than separating governmental work and ordinary life, I have pointed to their intersections, arguing that Ghanaian opposition to law enforcement by the book is a form of governmentality against itself.

The power that works upon subjectivity and possibility of regional affinity bears traces of colonialism and is constituted by ongoing imperial formations. I have suggested that problematizations of cutting have shaped both subjects and governance and their co-constitution, that knowledge has multiple layers of authority, and that disidentification with dominant orders derives from already fractured social worlds of governmental agents and targets. The "ethical relation" (Spivak 1999: 6) at stake here is not single but multiple: the effects of anticutting campaigns that matter are not only the "native informants" produced by global forces but also the commencement of different ethical relations among Ghanaians themselves.

Epilogue

In July 2015 Barack Obama gave a speech at the African Union Headquarters in Addis Ababa, a first for a U.S. president. He highlighted the inequality of African women as an obstacle to the continent's progress in the twenty-first century and its partnership with the United States. Obama emphasized girls' education but then mentioned cutting, as he had a few days earlier in Kenya, saying, "When African girls are subjected to the mutilation of their bodies, or forced into marriage at the ages of 9 or 10 or 11—that sets us back. That's not a good tradition. That needs to end."[1] Earlier in the year the White House had issued a statement in support of the Zero Tolerance for Female Genital Mutilation/Cutting Day, but Obama's prominent speech to the African Union lent greater weight to anticutting discourses. His words were received with applause, from both the African delegates and the international media.

The *Guardian*—the liberal British newspaper with a dedicated End FGM Global Media Campaign—was cautious about the import of the speech. A reporter wrote that "activists are concerned his [Obama's] message did not reach the people who needed to hear it the most in remote, traditional villages where circumcision continues."[2] Despite the transformations that have taken place in these regions since 2006, here, too, the discourse about underground cutting prevailed, and the article stressed the limits of interventions. The *Guardian* quoted an activist sheikh as saying, "There are people still doing it in hiding. They go to that area to escape the law and after circumcising their children, they bring them back." The article ended with the words of Jaha Dukureh, the *Guardian*-sponsored activist who is the face of the underground discourse in the United States.

Who is it that cannot let go of FGM? And why is it that when cutting is on the wane, the discourse about the intractability of the threat of FGM is the rise? I hope I have shown that there is too much talk about why Africans, as Kenyatta wrote long ago, "cling to this custom" (1965: 129–30) and too little understanding of its endings. The governmental politics of ending cutting is imbued with translocal discourses that deny the practices are waning. These discourses simultaneously disavow the violence that cut and uncut women face—the violence of extractive and sensitizing governance and the liberal love of law. Women and men who have ended cutting have no nostalgia for it, but they do want to enter into the kind of reciprocal relationship with the state and NGOs that they had with the gods: one of giving and taking, attention, care, and accountability. That this type of governance remains elusive makes Ghana both an important node in an evolving global present and a harbinger of a future in the making.

The real concern today is not the ostensible underground persistence of cutting but the global North's gesture of looking to Africa for hope and solutions while designing punitive zero tolerance policies against African migrants. While Ghanaian governmental workers ultimately disidentify with sovereign violence on the basis of immanent critique, those who govern the lives of African migrants in the global North do not. They share the Euro-American enthusiasm for security and punitive rationality that is legitimized in the name of empowering immigrant girls. Because this discourse deploys native informants, it elides feminist critique. I hope that by illuminating the here-and-there and then-and-now of anticutting campaigns, this book offers tools for critical thought and practice alike. I know that my work does not end with these pages.

ACKNOWLEDGMENTS

The rewards would not be much. Hardly anything. . . . Most of
the time, it will be plain old verbal "thank-you" very timidly said,
and in silence, a blessing of the womb that bore you.

AMA ATA AIDOO

How do we give thanks meaningfully? The answer to this question is culturally
mediated and formed somewhere in the substratum of the ethical core that structures all social relations. I feel my difference most intensely when I am thanked with
loud words of gratitude, rather than simple gestures.

Ethnography is the stuff of life. The making of this book has brought me closer
to many people who have invited me into their lives and homes, shared intimate and
difficult moments, encouraged me, supported me, challenged me, and made me
think and feel differently. I thank you all, and you will know it as our lives are
intertwined in big and small ways.

The research and writing of this book have been supported financially by the
Rocca Scholar program of the Center for African Studies at the University of
California, Berkeley, and the Human Rights Center Research Award; fellowships
from the Graduate Division of the University of California, San Francisco; a George
Mason University Faculty Research and Development Award; a research grant from
the Harry Frank Guggenheim Foundation; a fellowship from the Institute for the
Social Sciences of Cornell University; grants from Cornell's Office of Faculty
Development and Diversity; and a Faculty Fellowship from Cornell's Society for the
Humanities. The publishing of this book has been supported by the Hull Memorial
Publication Fund of Cornell University.

ACRONYMS

CDR	Committee for the Defence of the Revolution
CENSUDI	Centre for Sustainable Development Initiatives
CHRAJ	Commission on Human Rights and Administrative Justice
FGC	Female Genital Cutting
FGM	Female Genital Mutilation
FGM/C	Female Genital Mutilation/Cutting
GAWW	Ghana Association for Women's Welfare
GNCC	Ghana National Commission on Children
IAC	Inter-African Committee on Harmful Traditional Practices Affecting the Health of Women and Children
IFAD	International Fund for Agricultural Development
IMF	International Monetary Fund
MFCS	Muslim Family Counseling Services
NCWD	National Council on Women and Development
NDC	National Democratic Congress
PRIDE	Programme for Rural Integrated Development
RHI	Rural Help Integrated
UNFPA	United Nations Population Fund
UNICEF	United Nations Children's Fund
WHO	World Health Organization
ZOVFA	Zouri Organic Vegetable Farmers Association

NOTES

1. Ethnographic journal articles and book chapters available to me at that time provided cultural descriptions of various practices of cutting and discussed it as pivotal to social and symbolic orders (Kenyatta [1938] 1965; Griaule 1970; Hayes 1975; Boddy 1982, 1989; Talle 1993; Kratz 1993; Gruenbaum 1996).

2. This does not mean that anthropologists have not participated in public debates; I soon came to understand the extent to which, even when they did so, their participation was readily misconstrued. I refer to a historically situated experience, as well as my sense that the forms and modalities of anthropological analyses and engagements should have pushed further, both politically and theoretically. While anthropologists debated cutting in liberal terms, whether by endorsing or critiquing mainstream liberal positions, few engaged in an ethnography *of* liberalism that would question liberalism's very terms or analyze debates about cutting as constitutive of liberal governance.

3. Many, such as Rogaia Abusharaf, Fuambai Ahmadu, Claudie Gosselin, and Ylva Hernlund, have left the (North American) academy.

4. One diasporic African activist who lived in London and represented the Foundation for Women's Health, Research and Development was at the conference. Coincidentally, I was her host, and I learned from her about the difficulties she encountered when advocating simultaneously against cutting and against tacit feminist racism.

5. *Duldung* (toleration, sufferance) was the legal policy framework for the temporary suspension of deportation granted to Bosnian refugees for the duration of the war in Bosnia.

6. Wanjiru Kamau-Rutenberg, "Someone Is Listening!! Good News from the Challenging Clitoraid Campaign," *Can? We? Save? Africa?,* April 9, 2010, https://savingafrica.wordpress.com/page/8/.

7. Spivak borrows the term *native informant* from ethnography but repurposes it to reveal the conditions of this subject position, which is both called for and

needed by the West as well as foreclosed by it. Denied autobiography and normativity, the native informant structures the (im)possibility of the ethical relation: "I think of the 'native informant' as a name for that mark of expulsion from the name of Man—a mark crossing out the impossibility of the ethical relation" (1999: 6). Denied the name of Man, the native informant is denied humanity.

INTRODUCTION

1. I use pseudonyms for all people with whom I conducted formal ethnographic research and who I befriended. I also use pseudonyms for public figures and scholars I quote but did not formally interview, since they may have understood their statements as private. I do not use pseudonyms for people about whom I learned only from archival materials, newspaper articles, or public debates. This includes widely known public figures I met on several occasions, but with whom I did not conduct ethnographic research and did not formally interview: the early leaders of the Ghana Association of Women's Welfare (GAWW), Gloria Aryee, Marjorie Bulley, and Emma Banga, and the former circumciser Abampoka Mbawini.

After much deliberation, I have decided against using pseudonyms for the NGOs I write about. In my earlier work I assigned NGOs pseudonyms, because identifying an organization is tantamount to identifying those who run it. However, the pseudonyms did not protect anybody—given the prominence of the NGOs and my detailed description of their work, Ghanaians and scholars who study Ghana knew the organizations to which I was referring. The NGO pseudonyms were also jarring to my ears, as they lent an aura of trivial and unwelcome fiction. Although using pseudonyms might have benefited my work by pointing to the constructed character of ethnographic knowledge, again, only Ghanaians and those who study Ghana would have noticed the fictions. Before reaching my decision to identify the NGOs, I discussed this question with the leaders of Rural Help Integrated (RHI) and GAWW, as well as directors of other NGOs. GAWW leaders wanted the NGO to be named, and RHI officials told me to follow ethnographic conventions. This did not solve my problem, as there are no established conventions. In the end I concluded that the benefits of using the NGOs' real names outweighed the drawbacks. I see one of this book's contributions as its enrichment of the historical archive about a place and people who are largely misunderstood and who might one day benefit from knowing the real names of the organizations described in this book.

2. By *governmental* I mean the practices and agents of governmentality, understood in Foucauldian terms as exceeding the state. Thus "governmental workers" include both NGO workers and government-employed civil servants. Governmental knowledge includes both applied knowledge produced for specific and immediate purposes of governance (baseline surveys, evaluation reports, and so on), as well as knowledge that underwrites and organizes the rationality of governance (such as ethnographic knowledge of ethnic groups and cultural values, social science

knowledge about poverty, epidemiological and statistical knowledge about health and population, and so on).

3. Neither cutting nor debates about it and efforts to end it are limited to Africa and Africans. Cutting used to be mapped onto global blackness (in Africa, indigenous Australia, South America) and is now mapped onto Islam. As I began this project, many asked me why I was going all the way to Africa when I could do the same research at home in Bosnia, where rumors had it that Wahabi Islamization had given rise to female genital cutting.

4. Throughout the book I use the term *governance* in place of the common Foucauldian term *government* in order to avoid confusing the latter and the concrete entity of the government of Ghana. In doing so, I retain the theoretical meaning of Foucauldian government—the "more or less calculated and systematic ways of thinking and acting that aim to shape, regulate, or manage the comportment of others" (Inda 2005b: 1).

5. This theorizing itself is gendered. It is likely not coincidental that those who have analyzed, and at times glorified, the condition of being against and separate (against the state, against the law, not governed) are men (J. Scott 2014; Chatterjee 2004; Clastres 1989), whereas a generation of feminist anthropologists has theorized "partial connections" (Strathern 1991), friction that emerges from touch (Tsing 2005), and multiplicity (Mol 2002).

6. Peter Baker, "Obama Will Travel to Ghana," *New York Times,* May 16, 2009, http://thecaucus.blogs.nytimes.com/2009/05/16/obama-chooses-ghana-for-first-africa-trip/?_r=0.

7. "We Are Not Savages—Chief Nana Kwa Bonko V," *GhanaWeb,* January 13, 2003, www.ghanaweb.com/GhanaHomePage/NewsArchive/We-Are-Not-Savages-Chief-Nana-Kwa-Bonko-V-31766.

8. This internal dynamic went unremarked by anthropological commentators such as Kratz (2007) but is meticulously explored by Bayo Holsey, who noticed how cutting serves as a marker of northern savagery while she was conducting research on a different topic altogether (2008).

9. In contrast to the directors of large international NGOs situated in Accra who emphasize their political identities and leftist upbringings in the student movement (Yarrow 2008a), directors of women's NGOs in the Upper East legitimize their work not in reference to their formerly state-sanctioned leftist ideological commitments but to personal experiences of gendered forms of oppression, exclusion, and violence.

10. In my course on cutting, students who try to articulate a critique of Western voices of reason also notice that they feel this imperative. Consider the following paper excerpt: "Like some of the authors we have read, I now feel it is my obligation, in order to legitimize myself, to say that this last paragraph does not mean that I support FGC. But I also feel that it is strange, and almost counter-productive, that I have to state that." See "Passions for Ending Cutting: 'Civilizing Women,'" Anthropology, FGM, and Human Rights, October 7, 2013, https://anthropologicalreflections.wordpress.com/2013/10/07/key-points-from-boddys-civilizing-women/.

11. Scholars have examined this conflict and its sociopolitical consequences in detail (L. Thomas 2003; Kanogo 2005; Boddy 2007; Hetherington 1998).

12. A particularly illustrative example of collaborative claims is the 2009 film *Africa Rising: The Grassroots Movement to End Female Genital Mutilation,* produced by a global feminist NGO called Equality Now and directed by Paula Heredia.

13. By *decolonial,* I mean an analysis that actively fights the effects of colonialism on thinking, practice, and the senses.

14. Frederick Douglass made a similar argument in his speech "What to the Slave Is the Fourth of July?" in 1852, arguing against the white American call for slaves to "prove that we are men" and that slavery is wrong. Needed was not light but fire, he wrote. The full text of the speech can be found at http://teachingamericanhistory .org/library/document/what-to-the-slave-is-the-fourth-of-july/.

15. Nivedita Menon, "Unintended Consequences of Feminist Action: Prabha Kotiswaran," *Kafila,* February 18, 2013, http://kafila.org/2013/02/18/unintended-consequences-of-feminist-action-prabha-kotiswaran/.

16. "Immanent critique" uses the tools of that which it critiques in its critique.

17. Exceptions include anthropological *historiographies* of colonialism (Lentz 1999; MacGaffey 2010), as well as studies of migration from, but not *in,* the region (Schildkrout 1970; Lobnibe 2008; Behrends and Lentz 2012) .

18. I understand "materialization" as a process that is more substantive than "construction" and that points to effects of power on bodies, subjects, and institutions. Power is materialized by "constituting an object domain, a field of intelligibility, as a taken-for-granted ontology" (Butler 1993: 35).

19. Dorkenoo referred to the African Charter for Human Rights, which explicitly opposes cutting, and touted Burkina Faso as an example of success in ending cutting. www.theguardian.com/global-development-professionals-network/2013 /apr/22/female-genital-mutilation-africa.

20. Helene Michaud, "Dutch Government: 'Say No to Female Genital Mutilation,'" The Female Genital Cutting Educational and Networking Project, March 12, 2009, www.fgmnetwork.org/gonews.php?subaction =showfull&id =1259862630&ucat =18. The liberal term *reverse development cooperation* unwittingly reveals the pretenses of horizontality and egalitarianism in typical, that is, nonreverse, cooperation. For despite the professing of mutuality, development cooperation ascribes knowledge, rationality, and reason to the global North that are to be transferred to the South in the form of "capacity building."

21. Speech given on October 3, 2009. See "Koenders at the International Conference on Violence against the Girl Child," Government of the Netherlands, October 3, 2009, www.government.nl/documents-and-publications/speeches /2009/03/10/koenders-at-the-international-conference-on-violence-against-the-girl-child.html.

22. "Woman Bailed over 'FGM Conspiracy' Following Heathrow Arrest," *BBC News,* February 9, 2016, www.bbc.com/news/uk-england-northamptonshire-31311848.

1. The translation of this hadith is from the Muslim Women's League, which states that it "is found in only one of the six undisputed, authentic hadith collections, that is in the Sunan of Abu Dawud (Chapter 1888)"; "Female Genital Cutting," Muslim Women's League, January 1999, www.mwlusa.org/topics/violence &harrassment/fgm.html. I have also heard the translations "If you must, cut a little," and "Reduce, but do not destroy." Another translation is "Circumcise but do not go too far, for this is better for appearance and gives more pleasure to the husband" (Fluehr-Lobban 2013: 97). Gruenbaum (2001: 64) gives a range of additional translations.

2. These debates have been held by African migrants in the global North (Johns-dotter and Essén 2004), British colonial officials governing Sudan (Boddy 2007), as well as religious figures, and scholars (Abusharaf 2006b).

3. My emphasis on colonialism is also circumscribed by the lack of available literature about the precolonial history of northern Ghana; especially lacking is attention to gendered social and governmental histories.

4. The Raëlian movement's racist campaign is an obvious target of criticism, as not only its motto but also its effort, credibility, and motives were questionable. Some critics wondered whether the money raised was indeed spent on the hospital, and others pointed out that Clitoraid was not collaborating with local organizations and existing hospitals. A closer look at the Raëlian organization reveals that its members believe in UFOs, do not otherwise engage in humanitarianism, and started their project in a Muslim-majority country despite overtly despising Islam.

5. For examples of critical voices in the blogosphere, see "IDAHO: Africa," *Gukira,* May 9, 2010, http://gukira.wordpress.com/2010/05/09/idaho-africa/, and the postings on the website africasacountry.com.

6. Wanjiru Kamau-Rutenberg, "Clitoraid, or Why You Shouldn't Try to Adopt African Women's Genitalia!" *Can? We? Save? Africa?,* n.d., https://savingafrica .wordpress.com/clitoraid/.

7. Keguro Macharia, "Queer Genealogies (Critical Notes)," *Bullybloggers,* January 13, 2013, https://bullybloggers.wordpress.com/2013/01/13/queer-genealogies-provisional-notes/.

8. Analyzing Wa Thiong'o's novel, Keguro Macharia highlights how circumcision tied girls to the land and how *existence* in a variety of Bantu languages always includes an adverb for place, because being and personhood are expressed as being-in-place (2012: 7).

9. Protestant missions in Kenya began expressing opposition to circumcision in 1906, and those concerns escalated into a national crisis by the late 1920s; in contrast the Catholic Church tolerated circumcision (Kanogo 2005: 73), as it did in the Northern Territories as well.

10. Colonial Office, Female Circumcision: Parliamentary Questions, December 1929–January 1930, CO 533/392/11, Kew Archives, London.

11. Acting colonial secretary to the chief commissioner of Northern Territories, Tamale, August 16, 1930, No. 2566/S.S.Misc. of 8/3/1930, NT 1627, Ghana National Archives—Tamale, Tamale, Ghana.

12. Acting colonial secretary to the chief commissioner of Northern Territories, Tamale, August 16, 1930.

13. Provisional Commissioner's Office, Navrongo, "Excision of Girls," September 1, 1930, 868/48/1922, Ghana National Archives—Tamale.

14. By *pakuguga* they meant circumciser; the correct term today is *pokubego*.

15. Chief Commissioner's Office, Tamale, "Female Circumcision and Status of Women in Tanganyika Territory," June 15, 1931, 827/128/1930, Ghana National Archives—Tamale.

16. P. E. Mitchell, "Female Circumcision and Status of Women in Tanganyika Territory," April 26, 1930, 827/128/1930, Ghana National Archives—Tamale.

17. Provisional Commissioner's Office, "Excision of Girls."

18. Assistant District Commissioner, "Extract from Bawku District Informal Diary," January 5, 1933, Case 63–32, Ghana National Archives—Tamale.

19. Provisional Commissioner's Office, "Excision of Girls."

20. District Commissioner's Office, Wa, Report on clitoridectomy in Wa, March 18, 1933, NT 588, Ghana National Archives—Tamale.

21. Chief Commissioner's Office, Tamale, Report on female excision, September 8, 1930, 1208/128/1930, Ghana National Archives—Tamale.

22. Provisional Commissioner's Office, "Excision of Girls."

23. Chief Commissioner's Office, Tamale, Report on female excision, September 8, 1930.

24. Acting colonial secretary to the chief commissioner of Northern Territories, Tamale, August 16, 1930.

25. Acting colonial secretary to the chief commissioner of Northern Territories, Tamale, August 16, 1930.

26. Chief Commissioner's Office, Tamale, Report on female excision, September 8, 1930.

27. Provisional Commissioner's Office, "Excision of Girls."

28. District Commissioner's Office, Wa, Report on clitoridectomy in Wa.

29. Chief Commissioner's Office, Tamale, "Female Circumcision and Status of Women in Tanganyika Territory."

30. Secretary for Native Affairs Office, Report from the Acting Director of Medical and Sanitary Services with enclosures, November 27, 1930, 735/S.N.A.40/1930, NT 2344, Ghana National Archives—Tamale.

31. Colonial Secretary's Office, Accra, letter requesting a report on the discontinuation of clitoridectomy, December 19, 1932, NT 3400, Ghana National Archives—Tamale.

32. District Commissioner's Office, Gambaga, Report on Clitoridectomy in Gambaga, January 10, 1933, No. 15/28/22, NT 116, Ghana National Archives—Tamale.

33. District Commissioner's Office, Wa, Report on clitoridectomy in Wa.

34. District Commissioner's Office, Bawku, Report on clitoridectomy in Bawku, March 18, 1933, NT 595, Ghana National Archives—Tamale.

35. Acting Chief Commissioner of the Northern Territories, Report on clitoridectomy in the Gold Coast, March 16, 1949, 106/128/1930, Ghana National Archives—Tamale.

36. "Extract from Navrongo District Informal Diary," August 1931, Case 38, Ghana National Archives—Tamale.

37. Another discourse is emerging on the fringes of Ghanaian public discourses: an assertion that those taken as slaves would have helped develop the country and that the nation continues to suffer the effects of their loss.

38. Societies described as stateless or acephalous, such as the Tallensi, were at times integrated into and subservient to the Mamprusi kingdom (Skinner 1964). Fortes knew this but ignored it for purposes of theorizing the Tallensi political structure as outside state incorporation (Allman and Parker 2005). I have found that genealogies of one of the clans in Bongo include stories of their Mamprusi ancestry. See also Lentz (2006) on ethnic formation in the wider region.

39. These schemes were geared toward creating agricultural surplus in order to foster local and regional trade (Whitehead 2006; Chalfin 2004).

40. The specific contours of colonial governance that resulted in disenfranchisement of northern Ghana have long been documented by historians and are increasingly discussed by anthropologists.

41. Many have argued that the British associated Westernization with the germinating anticolonial political dissent that was antithetical to their interests and that they wanted to prevent it from taking hold in northern Ghana (Grischow 2006; Hawkins 2002). As MacGaffey writes, "British officials deliberately sought to limit the exposure of northerners to 'progressive' ideas that might discipline them to subservience" (2010: 431).

CHAPTER 2: MAKING HARMFUL TRADITIONAL PRACTICES

1. The reclassification of ethnicity is a living and dynamic process. The Bongo District government now claims that people who live there are not Frafras but Bosis and highlights the distinctiveness of local rituals and language. See "Bongo," ghanadistricts.com, 2006, www.ghanadistricts.com/District.aspx?Bongo&r=150.

2. Kofi Akosah-Sarpong, "Northern Ghana: Engaging Cultural Inhibitions," *New Statesman*, August 30, 2007, www.thestatesmanonline.com/pages/news _detail.php?newsid=4602&section=9.

3. UN Economic and Social Council, "The Implementation of the Human Rights of Women: Traditional Practices affecting the Health of Women and the Girl Child," UN Office of the High Commissioner for Human Rights, July 9, 1999, E/ CN.4/Sub.2/1999/14, http://ap.ohchr.org/documents/alldocs.aspx?doc_id=7060.

4. Hernlund describes Gambian NGOs with a similar strategy (2000: 245).

5. Dr. Adjei, report on eliminating FGM in Ghana, October 15, 2003, document in possession of the author.

6. Article 272 (c) of the 1992 Constitution.

7. Fati Paul, report on FGM in Ghana, November 1990; document in possession of the author.

8. Nawal Nour's clinic and advocacy for African women in Boston are the exception. Nour, a Sudanese American physician, founded the clinic herself, not in conjunction with anticutting organizations.

9. Vaginal fistulas are injuries that leave a woman incontinent. For many years WHO and others attributed fistula formation to cutting but have retracted these claims in recent years.

10. By 2010 in the three northern regions, "less than 50 percent of the population 11 and older" were literate (Ghana Statistical Service 2012: 6). The lack of schools often gets lost in governmental debates about cultural reasons for poor school attendance. One ethnographic moment stands out to me: an NGO-sponsored event at which the results of educational "mapping" were presented by the regional minister. NGO workers had solicited various cultural reasons for why children, especially girls, were not in school, but the map inadvertently illuminated an underlying problem: in the village that had a primary school, most children were enrolled, whereas the village that lacked a school suffered from low enrollment.

11. In a rare case of UN-sponsored critiques of the World Bank's policies in Ghana, a reporter for a UN magazine interviewed the Ghanaian geographer John Nabila, who shed light on how economic liberalization policies contribute to regional inequality and exacerbated scarcity: "Policies promoted by the Bank led to the removal of government subsidies for agricultural inputs, irrigation schemes and farm extension services. Meanwhile, tariffs on imported rice were also cut, flooding the domestic market with cheaper rice from Asia. Unable to compete, nearly half a million rice farmers, many of them in the north, were driven out of business, and domestic rice production fell drastically" (Harsch 2008: 4).

12. The governmental discourse of subsistence farming is so prevalent that the north-south migration is predominantly described as seasonal—because they are farmers, the story goes, northerners travel south for work during the dry season and return home in time for the harvest or for rituals. In actuality, migration is discontinuous and far less stable. Households in rural Bongo were bereft of most of their members even during the farming season. Some villagers told me how they spent entire periods of their lives in southern Ghana, while others spent a year or two and then returned. Some never return and instead start new families in the South (Lobnibe 2008). Others experience misfortune, like Atampoka's husband and brother, whose caskets arrived in Bongo without explanation. Furthermore, the rituals for which northerners return are not funerals or female genital cutting—neither of which they can afford, they say—but census taking and voting, which often require them to be present in their place of birth.

13. "Fact Files," Ghana NSEM, www.ghanansem.org/index.php?option=com _content&task=view&id=22&Itemid=63.

14. In 2010 the International Organization for Migration (IOM) confirmed the continuing outmigration of Ghanaian health-care professionals, showing that 56 percent of the doctors and 24 percent of the nurses trained in Ghana work abroad. The United States alone is home to nearly eleven thousand medical doctors from sub-Saharan Africa.

15. As I discuss in subsequent chapters, we should understand these statistics not as hard evidence but as revealing the trends and contours of scarcity.

16. Anthropologists also invoke the notion of the "harsh environment" in the Upper East but without the implication that the people themselves are to blame for it: "The harsh environment and insufficient medical care and nutrition of pregnant women account for frequent miscarriages, stillbirths and a high infant mortality rate" (Meier 1999: 91); "geographically, the low soil fertility and harsh climate of the savannah, marked by pronounced seasonality, a short growing season and periodic drought, are in profound contrast with the abundant natural fertility and rainfall of much of the south" (Whitehead 2006: 279).

17. International Fund for Agricultural Development, "Rural Poverty in Ghana," Rural Poverty Portal, n.d., www.ruralpovertyportal.org/web/guest/country /home/tags/ghana#.

18. Intergovernmental, state, and NGO accounts of poverty have long borrowed from one another. Contemporary explanations of northern Ghanaian poverty were also applied to other African states where development discourses shape governance and justify dispossession and expropriation (Ferguson 1994; Hodgson 2001; Mitchell 2002).

19. This discourse no longer holds complete sway when neoliberal financial interests trump development. Financial institutions have reevaluated African population growth in the wake of the "Africa Rising" paradigm and its construction of the continent as an investment opportunity. For investors population growth means more consumers and is therefore a positive trend.

20. The edited collection *Producing African Futures* (Weiss 2004) offers a range of anthropological framings of specific ways in which neoliberalism shapes contemporary crises of social and economic reproduction.

21. Apusigah contrasts the Ghanaian government and World Bank's prioritization of economic indicators with "community perspectives" on poverty, which are both more social and more specific: "Members of diverse communities talk of poverty as a fact of their lived realities. They explain the circumstances, situations, challenges and difficulties they live through on a daily basis" (2005: 5).

22. Robert wears many hats—he cofounded PRIDE and is a local politician who represents his village in the district assembly, but his paid job is with the government's development agency. He would describe all his efforts as geared toward "development," therefore I also refer to him as a development worker.

23. They also invoked numbers to convey the abysmal schooling conditions and to establish that it was the government that was failing the students. The entire village seemed to be aware that the best student had earned only fifteen of thirty points on a state-administered exam.

1. The direct quotes in the discussion that follows come from scores of interviews and conversations with various Ghanaian NGO workers and government officials.

2. Dr. Adjei directed the Ghanaian portion of the World Health Organization study on the obstetric consequences of cutting (WHO Study Group on Female Genital Mutilation and Obstetric Outcome 2006). A total of 6,413 women were interviewed and underwent gynecological examinations by trained midwives and nurses, who noted, among other things, whether the women were cut and their precise "type of FGM."

3. In addition to contributing to the WHO study, Dr. Adjei analyzed the Ghanaian data in more detail, referring specifically to the Upper East Region. These documents are in possession of the author and are left uncited to preserve Dr. Adjei's confidentiality.

4. While Michelle Johnson emphasizes the continuation of cutting among some West African immigrants in Portugal (2007), others who have studied this question have systematically shown that cutting in Europe is rare (Johnsdotter and Essén 2015), although public and governmental paranoia persists (Johnsdotter 2004).

5. Beenish Ahmed, "The Shocking Rise of Female Genital Mutilation in the United States," Thinkprogress, March 18, 2013, http://thinkprogress.org/world /2015/03/18/3635252/fgm-america/D; Nina Strochlich, "The U.S. Female Genital Mutilation Crisis," *Daily Beast,* February 5, 2015, www.thedailybeast.com /articles/2015/02/06/female-genital-mutilation-skyrockets-in-the-u-s.html; Nina Strochlich, "America's Underground Female Genital Mutilation Crisis," *Daily Beast,* June 11, 2014, www.thedailybeast.com/articles/2014/06/11/america-s-underground-female-genital-mutilation-crisis.html.

6. British Council, "The Interaction Leadership Programme," 2005, www .britishcouncil.org/cameroon-governance-interaction.htm.

7. Document in possession of the author.

8. This is also how Cassiman describes Kasena marriage: "In reference to their customary marriage, Kasena say that marriage used to start with the excision of the young girls. As part of the ritual, the girls' hair is shaven to mark the pattern of a cross as a sign of maturity. They can then wander through the market and people are made to acknowledge their mature state. They are left to roam around in small groups as newly excised girls, who are about ready for marriage" (2000: 109).

9. While Christianity dominates these debates both in the Upper East Region and in national public discourse, Islam is mobilized for the same purposes; this was made evident during recent antigay demonstrations that united Christians and Muslims against homosexuality.

10. Scholars use the term *diviner* (Allman and Parker 2005; Fortes and Mayer 1966), but Ghanaians refer to them as soothsayers.

11. Gods are materialized in objects. By "the thing," Azure might mean either the soothsayer's stick, which mediates the power of ancestral gods, or the thing, that is, god, of cutting.

CHAPTER 4: MISTAKEN BY DESIGN

1. The volunteer training sessions occur regularly; RHI replaces any volunteer who moves away, and since many leave for southern Ghana in search of work, RHI must continually enlist new volunteers. However, those volunteers who stop participating or fail to show up for quarterly meetings are not replaced; RHI considers those who remain in the area to be members of the organization, regardless of their level of interest or involvement.

2. Watkins and Swidler (2013) argue that public health interventions work even when they fail because everyone profits from them, including volunteers. In Ghana volunteers and villagers profit least of all, as benefits of NGO-ization are supposed to trickle down but do not.

3. If coercion is the only way to hold the participants' attention, the character of the organizers' self-perceived authority will be tenuous and unstable. Nevertheless, this form of containment is commonplace and is likely to be familiar to any traveler departing from Accra's Kotoka International Airport. In contrast to their practices elsewhere in the world, international airlines departing from Accra demand that passengers arrive three to four hours before departure, and check-in is closed two hours before the flight. Although air passengers everywhere are contained inside a terminal, in postcolonial Ghana the period of containment is lengthened to maximize crowd management.

4. The stages in parentheses are WHO labels that have been adopted by Ghanaian NGOs.

5. In Gurene women refer to their cutting in the active voice, saying, "I cut," not "I got cut."

6. That powerful knowledge is not on the surface of things is evident not only in traditional cosmology and oratory practice but also in the mundane worlds of NGO and state bureaucracies. Information is closely guarded and not readily shared. Funding forms, brochures, and reports are distributed with great care along the lines of existing investments in personal relations, professional networks, or surprising gestures of goodwill.

7. Hasty (2005b) makes a similar argument in her discussion of Ghanaian journalists' oratorical style.

8. RHI second quarter report for 2004, in possession of the author.

9. When, on the second day of the workshop, Mrs. Mahama asked the nurses to narrate their own experiences with FGM as health-care providers, she faced silence. The nurses had been taught that knowing FGM does not mean knowing it intimately, so they were not ready to talk about their experiences and drew instead on a

common repertoire of general statements, such as "80 percent of them do it" and "they have tearing problems."

CHAPTER 5: BLOOD LOSS AND SLOW HARM IN TIMES OF SCARCITY

1. Widows are vulnerable because rights to such resources such as land and housing reside with men and the patrilineal family. Most families do not respond to scarcity and adversity by starving widows of resources, accusing them of witchcraft, or banishing them, but enough do that they inspired local feminist and Christian groups—loosely defined, the NGO Nitu worked for was both—to advocate for the widows.

2. Recent ethnographies of development, HIV/AIDS, and orphan care in Africa (Bornstein 2001; Nguyen 2010) have noted contestations of resources and social authority between NGOs and families.

3. The relevance of blood to conceptualizations of health is not limited to West Africa. As Scheper-Hughes and Lock write, blood "is a nearly universal symbol of human life, and some peoples, both ancient and contemporary, have taken the quality of the blood, pulse, and circulation as the diagnostic sign of health or illness" (1987: 18). Janice Boddy has also examined references to blood and health in Sudanese practices of cutting (2007: 109–27).

4. Of the nearly four thousand people who donated blood in Bolgatanga during a four-year period, 95 percent were men (Amidu et al. 2010).

5. Neither is it "simulacrum" (Mbembe 1992) nor "hypernormalization"—the adoption of the form and content propagated by governing authorities (Boyer and Yurchak 2010). While hypernormalization deftly masks the underlying opposition to the dominant framework, Bongo women's proximity to NGO discourses is not a performative strategy of subversion. They are not overidentifying with NGOs to hide their actual views but draw on a different set of shared frameworks to critique the processes by which political economy shapes body and society.

6. On food production see Madeleine Bunting, "How Can Africa Grow More Food," *Guardian,* December 3, 2010, www.theguardian.com/global-development /poverty-matters/2010/dec/03/africa-agriculture-food-boost-production.

7. "Koforidua Regional Hospital in Acute Shortage of Blood," *News Ghana,* April 5, 2016, https://www.newsghana.com.gh/koforidua-regional-hospital-in-acute-shortage-of-blood/; "Patients in Danger as Korle Bu Blood Bank Dries Up," *Joy Online,* December 19, 2012, http://edition.myjoyonline.com/pages/news/201212/98941 .php; "National Blood Bank Empty," *Modern Ghana,* December 16, 2007, www .modernghana.com/news/367338/1/national-blood-bank-empty.html.

8. "Kessben Foundation, KATH Realize 205 Pints of Blood," *Joy Online,* August 30, 2007, http://lifestyle.myjoyonline.com/pages/health/200712/11861.php; "Record Blood Donor Gives Prize to Charity as Luv FM Rounds Up 2015 Blood Drive," *Joy Online,* December 12, 2015, www.myjoyonline.com/news/2015

/December-12th/record-blood-donor-give-prize-to-charity-as-luv-fm-rounds-up-2015-blood-drive.php.

9. "Korle-Bu Blood Bank Besieged by Blood Contractors," *GhanaWeb,* May 6, 2011, www.ghanaweb.com/GhanaHomePage/NewsArchive/Korle-Bu-Blood-Bank-Besieged-By-Blood-Contractors-208127.

10. The National Blood Service is an agency located in the Ministry of Health and is responsible for "ensuring a coordinated national approach to the provision of safe, adequate and efficacious, blood and blood products, making it timely, accessible and affordable to all patients requiring blood transfusion therapy in both public and private health care institutions in the country." See "About Us," National Blood Service, Ghana, n.d., http://nbsghana.org/sample/sub-page-11.

11. Before the introduction of structural adjustment programs, health care was relatively affordable but inaccessible to many in the Upper East Region. After structural adjustment, the government instituted a "cash and carry" policy demanding payment for health services. The National Health Insurance Scheme was an effort to combine neoliberal principles of market-rate insurance with humanitarian responsiveness to the health care crisis. In 2003, I attended meetings of the Ministry of Health and its donors, who were encouraging Ghana to adopt so-called smart insurance models that would not deplete state coffers; the National Health Insurance Scheme was a solution they designed together. In 2013 Ghanaian media announced that the insurance scheme was insolvent: hospitals were no longer accepting insurance cards and were asking patients to pay for prescription drugs. Also, the hospitals were bereft of supplies because the National Health Insurance Authority had not reimbursed them for expenses incurred; see "Ghana: Rejection of NHIS Cards at Hospitals," *allAfrica,* January 25, 2013, http://allafrica.com/stories/201301251639.html.

12. In Ghana blood was historically figured as a substance that can recalibrate an individual's social standing as well as the values of the larger social body. The Asante are said to have used human blood to blacken their stools and thereby enhance their power (Rathbone 1989: 448). During colonialism the label "ritual murders" was applied to cases in which people were sacrificed for ritual "medicine"—blood and body organs were used in rituals aimed at securing wealth and political power (Gocking 2000: 198) and in grief killings that marked the passing of a powerful king (Rathbone 1989).

13. "Strange Killings Hits [sic] Twifo Praso," *Ghana Web,* June 1, 2016, www.ghanaweb.com/GhanaHomePage/crime/Strange-killings-hits-Twifo-Praso-443693.

14. I borrow the pebbles metaphor from Fischer (2010) and Biehl (2013).

15. These movies tend to figure traditional medicine and spirituality as evil and products of the devil; see Comaroff and Comaroff on how the invocations of the devil add global and contemporary dimensions to the blood idiom (1999a: 292). Christianity is also increasingly important in the context of artistic production that depicts salvation in the blood of Jesus (Gilbert 2006: 349).

16. Rather than narrowly assessing risk of potential harm to my research subjects, this and other health administrators and representatives of ethics boards

unofficially expand their mission, taking it upon themselves to evaluate potential research-based extraction. They are motivated by worries about the lack of reciprocity in research projects as well as the history of researchers' extracting raw data from Ghana without sharing the resulting knowledge. Blood is but the most visceral symbol of this body politics and its larger ethics of exchange. For example, this official asked me to demonstrate how my research would directly benefit Ghanaians before granting me his preliminary approval.

17. Fairhead, Leach, and Small (2006) describe a similar situation in the Gambia.

18. Leah Elingwood, "What's a Little Blood Worth," *Students for Development Blog*, August 11, 2010, www.sfdblog.ca/fr/whats-a-little-blood-worth/.

19. The scholarship on scarcity in northern Ghana has something to learn from this critique. Scholars need to reckon with Agnes's complaints about scarcity and inequality at the threshold of life; when they are analyzing malnutrition and food shortages, they celebrate local agency by asserting that "Africans adapted to nutritional deficits in significant and creative ways" (Curtin 1983: 371). Destombes (2006), among others, provides a salutary analysis of the fact that northern Ghanaians' malnutrition does not prevent them from working. Agnes's desire for a fair share, rather than a life of prolonged minimal existence, should raise questions about any easy affirmation of agency and creativity. Agnes and others are well aware of their ability to circumvent scarcity, but they insist on pointing out the injustice of suffering from it. Having seen how others profit from their labor and their votes, they would like their agency and creativity to be directed beyond mere survival.

20. I thank Gracia Clark for this formulation.

21. While global health paradigms often isolate so-called local determinants of health, anthropologists insist that a myriad of historical and contemporary global factors condition health and survival in the global South. These include histories of exploitation; politics of trade; and politics of finance, security, border control, migration, and development, as well as neoliberal governance, restructuring, and privatization of the state.

22. Sherine Hamdy argues that "poor Egyptian kidney-disease patients understand and experience their illness in terms of Egypt's larger social, economic, and political ills," which, in the case of her research, "implicate corrupt institutions, polluted water, the mismanagement of toxic waste, and unsafe food"; she calls these explanations of disease "political etiologies" (2008: 53). Nordstrom (2009) extends this argument by noting that Angolan street children have a *better* understanding of how the violence of geopolitics, and extralegal trade in particular, shapes their lives and especially their health.

23. I borrow this phrase from Lawrence Cohen (1999), who points to the stakes of ethical and analytical claims about which wounds hurt most.

24. Women in Bongo do not refrain from judging and blaming individuals, but they hold them accountable for their individual acts, not for larger social ills. When news arrived that a young migrant from the village had murdered her infant child, she was vilified. No one asked who fathered the child or inquired further into her

circumstances, but neither did anyone turn her story into a case of a larger problem of loose, immoral northern girls in the South.

CHAPTER 6: THE FEMINIST FETISH

1. Riles and Miyazaki (2005) take a different analytical angle, pointing to the epistemological equivalences in understandings of failure of knowledge between anthropologists and financial traders, but these authors also reference the actual failure of markets.

2. The term *fetish* is not free of colonial, Eurocentric notions of African spiritual objects and animist practices as flawed and improperly sacred. The associated objection is that the fetish makes something out of nothing, that it attributes *too much* power to a worldly object. For my purposes this objection constitutes a question: How do Ghanaians judge when law becomes improperly sacred and too powerful?

3. For Foucault law is primarily a set of commands and prohibitions that exemplify the juridical, negative conception of power tied to sovereign rule. This reductive definition of law is rhetorically strategic on his part: to draw attention to the importance of disciplinary and productive power, he minimizes law's regulatory power. This is particularly evident in his writings in *History of Sexuality, Vol. 1* (1990). Law, he writes, is "utterly incongruous with the new methods of power" that are "not ensured by right but by technique, not by law but by normalization, not by punishment but by control" (89). And, to understand modern power properly, "we shall try to rid ourselves of a juridical and negative representation of power, and cease to conceive of it in terms of law, prohibition, liberty and sovereignty" (90–91). This location of power outside the juridical means that law is equated with sovereignty, repression, and coercion. Scholars sometimes contend that these matters should be explored in light of other aspects of Foucault's work that suggest a "more interesting view of law as, in some important sense, constitutive of the new forms of modern power," meaning productive power (Hunt and Wickham 1994: 48). Foucault himself does not take this route, although he concedes that law is "increasingly incorporated into a continuum of apparatuses (medical, administrative, and so on) whose functions are for the most part regulatory" (1990: 144).

4. The ICC is an example of how the dialectic of order and disorder affects Africa specifically: charged with prosecuting genocide, crimes against humanity, and war crimes in signatory countries, the ICC has targeted only African states. This selective focus on Africa has been challenged both within and outside the ICC. As Kamari Clarke writes, the geopolitically uneven distribution of ICC jurisdiction was built into its mandate: the codification of the ICC charge was a result of political struggles about which crimes count as the most serious and worthy of prosecution. (See Clarke's contribution to the "Africa Question" at http://iccforum.com/africa.)

5. Queer theory is also concerned with the shift from antinormative to normative aspirations and practices and often interprets this trend in temporal terms as well.

6. Historians and anthropologists focus on the operations of legal fetishism across postcolonial contexts, but the center-periphery axis is difficult to ignore.

7. The rich critical literature on women's rights raises parallel questions but is less attuned to questions of punishment and criminalization and is therefore not my primary frame of reference here.

8. Administrators for the Domestic Violence and Victim Support Unit (known by its former acronym, WAJU) are mandated to assist victims but are rarely able to investigate. Their work largely consists of gathering reports and providing statistics to the national government, to be circulated in documents for the United Nations (Hodžić 2011). Like other police forces, they cite material conditions such as the lack of vehicles and fuel as reasons for their inability to assist beyond taking reports.

9. GAWW 1994 Annual Report for the IAC; GAWW correspondence with the IAC, 1993–94, p. 1, all documents in possession of the author.

10. GAWW report to the embassy of the United States, 2002; document in possession of the author.

11. *Trokosi*, enshrined in law as customary servitude, refers to an Ewe practice of giving girls to shrines in atonement, mostly to perform labor. Ghanaian public debates about trokosi are similar in tenor and focus to those about cutting, but unlike cutting trokosi has its public proponents.

12. "Dial SOS Circumcision and Stop Girls Being Cut," *IRIN,* March 18, 2005, www.irinnews.org/report/53474/burkina-faso-dial-sos-circumcision-and-stop-girls-being-cut.

13. A few years later, in 2006, the IAC lobbied the WHO to retain the term *FGM* by presenting letters from dozens of member organizations and affiliates. Although Kouyate despised the "semantics battle field," he wrote an impassioned five-page statement demanding the term *female genital mutilation.* He wrote: "Out of respect for the millions of girls and women in Africa suffering in their flesh, let us stop this dance with words around Female Genital Mutilation" (document in possession of the author).

14. In the end the legal experts did not take the suggestion to explicitly extend culpability to cut girls and women but did use language that would allow their prosecution. The memorandum sent to the attorney general left room for the interpretation that no one is exempt from prosecution; this implication is even clearer in the final bill passed by Parliament (Criminal Code [Amendment] Bill, GPC/Assembly Press, Accra, GPCI AIJ 4/300/2/2006).

15. My suggestion is not that everyone should be consulted about proposed laws, as this imperative can be used to oppose legislation that the state considers challenging; I have written elsewhere that the Ghanaian government opposed feminist advocacy for the Domestic Violence Bill by arguing that it was counter to popular, majority opinion (Hodžić 2009). Rather, my point is that GAWW and feminist lawyers continually spoke in the name of cut women without ever being guided by

their desires; the activists impelled northern Ghanaians to speak but ignored their voices.

16. GAWW report to the U.S. Embassy, 2002; document in possession of the author.

17. "FGM Now a Big Crime," *Accra Mail,* June 15, 2007.

18. Cynthia Boakye, "MPs Divided over Sentences for FGM," *Statesman* (Accra), July 6, 2007.

19. "FGM Now a Big Crime."

20. I found only one public objection: an editorial (*Mirror,* June 30, 2007) that relativized harm by comparing FGM to FSM and FHM—the author's neologisms for skin bleaching (female skin mutilation) and hair straightening (female hair mutilation).

21. *Public Agenda,* June 11, 2007.

22. More recently Ghanaian journalists have written scathing reports about these matters, and Ghana also has been visited by a UN Special Rapporteur on Torture. As a result prison conditions have become yet another issue that is framed as a source of Ghana's shame and one that could "harm Ghana's international reputation" ("UN Official: Ghana's Jails Cruel and Inhuman," *Al Jazeera,* November 15, 2013, www.aljazeera.com/news/africa/2013/11/un-official-ghana-jails-cruel-inhuman-2013111564627505652.html).

CHAPTER 7: AGAINST SOVEREIGN VIOLENCE

CENSUDI (Center for Sustainable Development Initiatives).

1. NGOs and civil servants knew of no additional trials since 2004, and none has been reported by the media, NGOs, or foreign agencies, such as the U.S. State Department and the Canadian Immigration and Refugee Board, which monitor Ghana's law enforcement activities.

2. IAC Evaluation of GAWW, 1993, p. 3; document in possession of the author.

3. "Ghana," World Prison Brief, June 2016, www.prisonstudies.org/country /ghana; "Highest to Lowest: Prison Population Rate," World Prison Brief, n.d., www.prisonstudies.org/highest-to-lowest/prison_population_rate?field_region_ taxonomy_tid=All.

4. As I discuss in earlier chapters, the antifeminism generated in relation to the question of cutting is articulated not by questioning the law but in debates about virginity and in the nostalgia for the patriarchal marital social order that cutting ostensibly safeguarded.

5. Claiming kinship is just as ambivalent as opposition to law: it can be a radical or a conservative act that entrenches the existing social order. References to kinship can be used to oppose feminist advocacy, as was the case in the government's opposition to the Domestic Violence Bill. In Indian family courts, Srimati Basu has also shown, judges invoke kinship metaphors to signal proximity, care, and informality

but do so in a way that reproduces patriarchy: "the court becomes a space where familiar expectations about gender norms may prevail" (2012: 482).

6. Proximity can also lead to violence—as Sartre said long ago in reference to anti-Semitism, it was the neighbor who was hated and killed. I know this all too well from Bosnia, but we also see it in Ghana, where the intimacy of violence is revealed by the Bawku conflict, which pits entangled groups against one another.

7. Feldman (2008) and Sharma (2008) also show that a variety of people are compelled to participate in the governance of self and others.

EPILOGUE

1. Office of the Press Secretary, "Remarks by President Obama to the People of Africa," Whitehouse.gov, July 28, 2015, https://www.whitehouse.gov/the-press-office/2015/07/28/remarks-president-obama-people-africa.

2. David Smith, "Obama's Call to End Female Genital Mutilation Yet to Reach Ethiopia's Villages," *Guardian,* August 1, 2015, www.theguardian.com/world/2015/aug/01/ethiopia-barack-obama-female-genital-mutiliation-villages.

REFERENCES

Abusharaf, Rogaia Mustafa. 1998. "Unmasking Tradition." *Sciences* 38 (2): 22–27.

Abusharaf, Rogaia Mustafa, ed. 2006a. *Female Circumcision: Multicultural Perspectives*. Philadelphia: University of Pennsylvania Press.

Abusharaf, Rogaia Mustafa. 2006b. "'We Have Supped So Deep in Horrors': Understanding Colonialist Emotionality and British Responses to Female Circumcision in Northern Sudan." *History & Anthropology* 17 (3): 209–28.

Agamben, Giorgio. 1998. *Homo sacer: Sovereign Power and Bare Life*. Stanford, CA: Stanford University Press.

Ahmed, Sara. 2010. *The Promise of Happiness*. Durham, NC: Duke University Press.

Aidoo, Ama Ata. 1977. *Our Sister Killjoy: Or, Reflections from a Black-eyed Squint*. London: Longman.

Ako, Matilda Aberese, and Patricia Akweongo. 2009. "The Limited Effectiveness of Legislation against Female Genital Mutilation and the Role of Community Beliefs in Upper East Region, Ghana." *Reproductive Health Matters* 17 (34): 47–54.

Akyeampong, Emmanuel, Allan G. Hill, and Arthur Kleinman, eds. 2015. *The Culture of Mental Illness and Psychiatric Practice in Africa*. Bloomington: Indiana University Press.

Allman, Jean, and John Parker. 2005. *Tongnaab: The History of a West African God*. Bloomington: Indiana University Press.

Amadiume, Ifi. 1997. *Re-inventing Africa: Matriarchy, Religion, and Culture*. London: Zed Books.

Amidu, N., W.B.K.A. Owiredu, O. Addai-Mensah, A. Alhassan, L. Quaye, and B. Batong. 2010. "Seroprevalence and Risk Factors for Human Immunodeficiency Virus, Hepatitis B and C Viruses Infections among Blood Donors at the Bolgatanga Regional Hospital in Bolgatanga, Ghana." *Journal of the Ghana Science Association* 12 (1): 77–88.

Apter, Andrew. 2005. "Griaule's Legacy: Rethinking 'la parole claire' in Dogon Studies." *Cahiers d'études africaines* 177 (1): 95–129.

Apusigah, Agnes Atia. 2005. "Diagnosing Poverty in Northern Ghana: Institutional Versus Community Views." *Ghana Journal of Development Studies* 2 (2): 2–11.

Asad, Talal. 2003. *Formations of the Secular: Christianity, Islam, Modernity.* Stanford, CA: Stanford University Press.

Awedoba, A. K. 2008. *Cultural Sensitivity and Programming: The Case of Government of Ghana—UFPA 5th country programme 2006–1010.* Accra: Chasglo Print Services.

Awedoba, Albert K., and Aaron R. Denham. 2012–13. "The Perception of Abnormality in Kasena and Nankani Infants: Clarifying Infanticide in Northern Ghana." *Ghana Studies:* 41–67.

Bacchi, Carol. 2012. "Why Study Problematizations? Making Politics Visible." *Open Journal of Political Science* 2 (1): 1–8.

Banga, Emma Hellen, Yvon Yangyuoru, Alimatu Mahama, and Boniface Gambila. 1999. Unpublished draft report on the Study of the Effect of Legislative Abolition of Female Genital Mutilation. Legon.

Banga, Emma Hellen, Yvon Yangyuoru, Alimatu Mahama, and Boniface Gambila. 2001. A Study on the Effect of Legislative Abolition of Female Genital Mutilation (FGM). Unpublished report. Legon.

Basu, Srimati. 2012. "Judges of Normality: Mediating Marriage in the Family Courts of Kolkata, India." *Signs* 37 (2): 469–92.

Bayart, Jean-François. 1993. *The State in Africa: The Politics of the Belly.* London: Longman.

Behrends, Andrea, and Carola Lentz. 2012. "Education, Careers, and Home Ties: The Ethnography of an Emerging Middle Class from Northern Ghana." *Zeitschrift fuer Ethnologie:*139–64.

Benda-Beckmann, Franz von, Keebet von Benda-Beckmann, and Anne Griffiths, eds. 2009. *The Power of Law in a Transnational World: Anthropological Enquiries.* New York: Berghahn.

Benjamin, Walter. 1986. *Reflections: Essays, Aphorisms, Autobiographical Writing.* New York: Shocken.

Benning, Raymond. 1975. "Colonial Development Policy in Northern Ghana, 1898–1950." *Bulletin of the Ghana Geographical Association* 17:65–79.

Berlant, Lauren. 2011. *Cruel Optimism.* Durham, NC: Duke University Press.

Bernstein, Elizabeth. 2014. "Militarized Humanitarianism Meets Carceral Feminism: The Politics of Sex, Rights, and Freedom in Contemporary Antitrafficking Campaigns." *Signs* 36 (1): 45–71.

Biehl, João. 2013. "Ethnography in the Way of Theory." *Cultural Anthropology* 28 (4): 573–97.

Bledsoe, Caroline H. 1980. *Women and Marriage in Kpelle Society.* Stanford, CA: Stanford University Press.

Bledsoe, Caroline H. 2002. *Contingent Lives: Fertility, Time, and Aging in West Africa.* Chicago: University of Chicago Press.

Bledsoe, Caroline, Fatoumatta Banja, and Allan G. Hill. 1998. "Reproductive Mishaps and Western Contraception: An African Challenge to Fertility Theory." *Population and Development Review* 24 (1): 15–57.

Boddy, Janice. 1982. "Womb as Oasis: The Symbolic Context of Pharaonic Circumcision in Rural Northern Sudan." *American Ethnologist* 9 (4): 682–98.

Boddy, Janice. 1989. *Wombs and Alien Spirits: Women, Men, and the Zar Cult in Northern Sudan.* Madison: University of Wisconsin Press.

Boddy, Janice. 2007. *Civilizing Women: British Crusades in Colonial Sudan.* Princeton, NJ: Princeton University Press.

Bornstein, Erica. 2001. "Child Sponsorship, Evangelism, and Belonging in the Work of World Vision Zimbabwe." *American Ethnologist* 28 (3): 595–622.

Bornstein, Erica. 2012. *Disquieting Gifts: Humanitarianism in New Delhi.* Stanford, CA: Stanford University Press.

Boyer, Dominic. 2005. "The Corporeality of Expertise." *Ethnos* 70 (2): 243–66.

Boyer, Dominic, and Alexei Yurchak. 2010. "American Stiob: Or, What Late-Socialist Aesthetics of Parody Reveal about Contemporary Political Culture in the West." *Cultural Anthropology* 25 (2): 179–221.

Brada, Betsey Behr. 2013. "How to Do Things to Children with Words: Language, Ritual, and Apocalypse in Pediatric HIV Treatment in Botswana." *American Ethnologist* 40 (3): 437–51.

Brown, Wendy. 1997. "The Impossibility of Women's Studies." *differences: A Journal of Feminist Cultural Studies* 9 (3):79–102.

Brown, Wendy. 2003. "Neo-liberalism and the End of Liberal Democracy." *Theory & Event* 7 (1): n.p.

Brown, Wendy, and Janet Halley. 2002a. Introduction to Brown and Halley 2002b, 1–37. Durham, NC: Duke University Press.

Brown, Wendy, and Janet Halley. 2002b. *Left Legalism/Left Critique.* Durham, NC: Duke University Press.

Brown, Wendy, Christina Colegate, John Dalton, Timothy Rayner, and Cate Thill. 2006. "Learning to Love Again: An Interview with Wendy Brown." *Contretemps* 6:25–42.

Butler, Judith. 1993. *Bodies That Matter: On the Discursive Limits of Sex.* New York: Routledge.

Cardinall, Allan Wolsey. (1920) 2012. *The Natives of the Northern Territories of the Gold Coast: Their Customs, Religion and Folklore.* London: Forgotten Books.

Cassiman, Ann. 2000. "A Woman Is Someone's Child: Women's Social and Domestic Space among the Kassena." In *Bonds and Boundaries in Northern Ghana and Southern Burkina Faso,* edited by Alexis B. Tengan and Sten Hagberg, 105–31. Uppsala Studies in Cultural Anthropology. Vol. 30. Uppsala, Sweden: Uppsala University Press.

Cassiman, Ann. 2010. "Home Call: Absence, Presence and Migration in Rural Northern Ghana." *African Identities* 8 (1): 21–40.

Chalfin, Brenda. 2001. "Border Zone Trade and the Economic Boundaries of the State in North-east Ghana." *Africa: Journal of the International African Institute* 71 (2): 202–24.

Chalfin, Brenda. 2004. *Shea Butter Republic: State Power, Global Markets, and the Making of an Indigenous Commodity.* New York: Routledge.

Chalfin, Brenda. 2010. *Neoliberal Frontiers: An Ethnography of Sovereignty in West Africa.* Chicago: University of Chicago Press.

Chatterjee, Partha. 1989. "Colonialism, Nationalism, and Colonialized Women: The Contest in India." *American Ethnologist* 16 (4): 622–33.

Chatterjee, Partha. 2004. *The Politics of the Governed: Reflections on Popular Politics in Most of the World.* New York: Columbia University Press.

Chen, Nancy N. 1992. "'Speaking Nearby': A Conversation with Trinh T. Minh-ha." *Visual Anthropology Review* 8 (1): 82–91.

Choy, Timothy K. 2005. "Articulated Knowledges: Environmental Forms after Universality's Demise." *American Anthropologist* 107 (1): 5–18.

Clarke, Kamari Maxine. 2011. "The Rule of Law through Its Economies of Appearances: The Making of the African Warlord." *Indiana Journal of Global Legal Studies* 18 (1): 7–40.

Clastres, Pierre. 1989. *Society against the State: Essays in Political Anthropology.* New York: Zone Books.

Cohen, Lawrence. 1999. "Where It Hurts: Indian Material for an Ethics of Organ Transplantation." *Daedalus* 128 (4): 135–65.

Comaroff, Jean. 2007. "Beyond Bare Life: AIDS, (Bio)Politics, and the Neoliberal Order." *Public Culture* 19 (1): 197–219.

Comaroff, Jean, and John Comaroff. 1991. *Of Revelation and Revolution.* Chicago: University of Chicago Press.

Comaroff, John, and Jean Comaroff. 1999a. *Civil Society and the Political Imagination in Africa: Critical Perspectives.* Chicago: University of Chicago Press.

Comaroff, Jean, and John Comaroff. 1999b. "Occult Economies and the Violence of Abstraction: Notes from the South African Postcolony." *American Ethnologist* 26 (2): 279–303.

Comaroff, Jean, and John Comaroff. 2003. "Ethnography on an Awkward Scale: Postcolonial Anthropology and the Violence of Abstraction." *Ethnography* 4 (2): 147–79.

Comaroff, Jean, and John Comaroff. 2006a. Introduction to Comaroff and Comaroff 2006b, 1–56.

Comaroff, Jean, and John Comaroff, eds. 2006b. *Law and Disorder in the Postcolony.* Chicago: University of Chicago Press.

Comaroff, Jean, and John Comaroff. 2006c. Preface to Comaroff and Comaroff 2006b, vii–x.

Comaroff, Jean, and John Comaroff. 2012. *Theory from the South, Or, How Euro-America Is Evolving toward Africa.* Boulder, CO: Paradigm Publishers.

Couso, Javier, Alexandra Huneeus, and Rachel Sieder, eds. 2010. *Cultures of Legality: Judicialization and Political Activism in Latin America*. Cambridge: Cambridge University Press.

Crampton, Alexandra. 2013. "No Peace in the House: Witchcraft Accusations as an 'Old Woman's Problem' in Ghana." *Anthropology & Aging Quarterly* 34 (2): 199–212.

Curtin, Philip D. 1983. "Nutrition in African History." *Journal of Interdisciplinary History* 14 (2): 371–82.

Defflem, Mathieu. 1994. "Law Enforcement in British Colonial Africa." *Police Studies* 17 (1): 45–68.

Der, Benedict G. 1998. *The Slave Trade in Northern Ghana*. Accra: Woeli Publishing.

Der, Benedict G. 2001. "Christian Missions and the Expansion of Western Education in Northern Ghana, 1906–1975." In Saaka 2001, 107–38.

Destombes, Jerome. 2006. "From Long-Term Patterns of Seasonal Hunger to Changing Experiences of Everyday Poverty: Northeastern Ghana c. 1930–2000." *Journal of African History* 47:181–205.

Dietz, Ton, and David Millar, eds. 1999. *Coping with Climate Change in Dryland Ghana: The Case of Bolgatanga*. Amsterdam: Netherlands Research Programme on Climate Change.

Dietz, Ton, David Millar, Saa Dittoh, Francis Obeng, and Edward Ofori-Sarpong. 2004. "Climate and Livelihood Change in North East Ghana." In *Impact of Climate Change on Drylands,* edited by A. J. Dietz, R. Ruben, and J. Verhagen, 149–72. Norwell, MA: Kluwer.

Dorkenoo, Efua. 1994. *Cutting the Rose: Female Genital Mutilation, the Practice and Its Prevention*. London: Minority Rights.

Dorkenoo, Efua, and Scilla Elworthy. 1992. "Female Genital Mutilation: Proposals for Change." *Minority Rights Group International Report*. Vol. 92/3. London: Minority Rights Group.

Droney, Damien. 2013. "Ironies of Laboratory Work during Ghana's Second Age of Optimism." *Cultural Anthropology* 29 (2): 363–84.

Dumett, Raymond, and Marion Johnson. 1988. "Britain and the Suppression of Slavery in the Gold Coast Colony, Ashanti, and the Northern Territories." In *The End of Slavery in Africa,* edited by Suzanne Miers and Richard Roberts, 71–116. Madison: University of Wisconsin Press.

Elyachar, Julia. 2002. "Empowerment Money: The World Bank, Non-Governmental Organizations, and the Value of Culture in Egypt." *Public Culture* 14 (3): 493–513.

Elyachar, Julia. 2006. "Best Practices: Research, Finance, and NGOs in Cairo." *American Ethnologist* 33 (3): 413–26.

Engle, Karen. 1991. "Female Subjects of Public International Law: Human Rights and the Exotic Other Female." *New England Law Review* 26:1509–26.

Escobar, Arturo. 1995. *Encountering Development: The Making and Unmaking of the Third World*. Princeton, NJ: Princeton University Press.

Fabian, Johannes. 1983. *Time and the Other: How Anthropology Makes Its Object.* New York: Columbia University Press.

Fairhead, James, and Melissa Leach. 1996. *Misreading the African Landscape: Society and Ecology in a Forest-Savanna Mosaic.* Cambridge: Cambridge University Press.

Fairhead, James, and Melissa Leach. 2003. *Science, Society and Power: Environmental Knowledge and Policy in West Africa and the Caribbean.* Cambridge: Cambridge University Press.

Fairhead, James, Melissa Leach, and Mary Small. 2006. "Where Techno-Science Meets Poverty: Medical Research and the Economy of Blood in The Gambia, West Africa." *Social Science and Medicine* 63 (4): 1109–20.

Fanon, Frantz. 1967. *A Dying Colonialism.* New York: Grove.

Farquhar, Judith. 2009. "The Park Pass: Peopling and Civilizing a New Old Beijing." *Public Culture* 21 (3): 551–76.

Fassin, Didier. 2012. *Humanitarian Reason: A Moral History of the Present.* Berkeley: University of California Press.

Feld, Steven. 2012. *Jazz Cosmopolitanism in Accra: Five Musical Years in Ghana.* Durham, NC: Duke University Press.

Feldman, Ilana. 2008. *Governing Gaza: Bureaucracy, Authority, and the Work of Rule, 1917–1967.* Durham, NC: Duke University Press.

Ferguson, James. 1994. *The Anti-Politics Machine: 'Development,' Depoliticization, and Bureaucratic Power in Lesotho.* Minneapolis: University of Minnesota Press.

Ferguson, James. 1997. "Anthropology and Its Evil Twin: 'Development' in the Constitution of the Discipline." In *International Development and the Social Sciences,* edited by Frederick Cooper and Randall M. Packard, 150–75. Berkeley: University of California Press.

Ferguson, James. 2006. *Global Shadows: Africa in the Neoliberal World Order.* Durham, NC: Duke University Press.

Ferguson, James, and Akhil Gupta. 2002. "Spatializing States: Toward an Ethnography of Neoliberal Governmentality." *American Ethnologist* 29 (4): 981–1002.

Ferme, Mariane. 2001. *The Underneath of Things: Violence, History, and the Everyday in Sierra Leone.* Berkeley: University of California Press.

Fischer, Michael M.J. 2010. "Comment on João Biehl and Peter Locke's Article 'Deleuze and the Anthropology of Becoming.'" *Current Anthropology* 51 (3): 337–38.

Fluehr-Lobban, Carolyn. 2013. *Islamic Law and Society in the Sudan.* New York: Routledge.

Fortes, Meyer. 1965. "Ancestor Worship." In *African Systems of Thought,* edited by Meyer Fortes and G. Dieterlen, 16–20. London: Oxford University Press.

Fortes, Meyer. 1970. *Time and Social Structure and Other Essays.* New York: Humanities Press.

Fortes, Meyer, and Doris Y. Mayer. 1966. "Psychosis and Social Change among the Tallensi of Northern Ghana." *Cahiers d'études africaines* 6 (21): 5–40.

Fortun, Kim. 2001. *Advocacy after Bhopal: Environmentalism, Disaster, New Global Orders.* Chicago: University of Chicago Press.

Foucault, Michel. 1984. *The Foucault Reader.* Edited by Paul Rabinow. New York: Pantheon.

Foucault, Michel. 1990. *The History of Sexuality, Vol. 1: An Introduction..* New York: Vintage.

Foucault, Michel, and Paul Rabinow. 1997. *Essential Works of Foucault, Vol. 1: Ethics, Subjectivity and Truth.* New York: New Press.

Fricker, Miranda. 2007. *Epistemic Injustice: Power and the Ethics of Knowing.* Oxford: Oxford University Press.

Gabiam, Nell. 2012. "When 'Humanitarianism' Becomes 'Development': The Politics of International Aid in Syria's Palestinian Refugee Camps." *American Anthropologist* 114 (1): 95–107.

Gaines, Kevin K. 2006. *African-Americans in Ghana: Black Expatriates and the Civil Rights Era.* Chapel Hill: University of North Carolina Press.

Garritano, Carmela. 2012. "Blood Money, Big Men and Zombies: Understanding Africa's Occult Narratives in the Context of Neoliberal Capitalism." *manycinemas* 3:50–65.

Geertz, Clifford. 1973. *The Interpretation of Cultures: Selected Essays.* New York: Basic Books.

Geissler, P. Wenzel, ed. 2015. *Para-States and Medical Science: Making African Global Health.* Durham, NC: Duke University Press.

George, Abosede. 2013. "Getting the Hang of It." *Scholar and Feminist Online* 11 (1–2).

Ghana Statistical Service. 2012. *2010 Population and Housing Census, Summary Report of Final Results.* Accra: Ghana Statistical Service.

Gilbert, Michelle. 2006. "Things Ugly: Ghanaian Popular Painting." In *Beautiful Ugly: African and Diaspora Aesthetics,* edited by Sarah Nuttall. Durham, NC: Duke University Press.

Glazebrook, Trish. 2011. "Women and Climate Change: A Case-Study from Northeast Ghana." *Hypatia* 26 (4): 762–82.

Gocking, Roger. 2000. "A Chieftaincy Dispute and Ritual Murder in Elmina, Ghana, 1945–6." *Journal of African History* 41 (2): 197–219.

Goldstone, Brian. 2012. "The Miraculous Life: Scenes from the Charismatic Encounter in Northern Ghana." PhD diss., Department of Anthropology, Duke University, Durham, NC.

Gosselin, Claudie. 2000. "Handing over the Knife: *Numu* Women and the Campaign against Excision in Mali." In Shell-Duncan and Hernlund 2000a, 193–214.

Grant, Richard, and J. A. N. Nijman. 2004. "The Re-Scaling of Uneven Development in Ghana and India." *Tijdschrift voor Economische en Sociale Geografie* 95 (5): 467–81.

Greenhouse, Carol J. 1989. *Praying for Justice: Faith, Order, and Community in an American Town.* Ithaca, NY: Cornell University Press.

Grewal, Inderpal. 1999. "'Women's Rights as Human Rights': Feminist Practices, Global Feminism, and Human Rights Regimes in Transnationality." *Citizenship Studies* 3 (3): 337–54.

Grewal, Inderpal. 2014. "American Humanitarian Citizenship: The Soft Power of Empire." In *Gender, Globalization, and Violence: Postcolonial Conflict Zones,* edited by Sandra Ponzanesi, 64–81. New York: Routledge.

Griaule, Marcel. 1970. *Conversations with Ogotemmeli: An Introduction to Dogon Religious Ideas.* Oxford: Oxford University Press.

Grischow, Jeff D. 2006. *Shaping Tradition: Civil Society, Community and Development in Colonial Northern Ghana, 1899–1957.* African Social Studies Series. Boston: Brill.

Gruenbaum, Ellen. 1996. "The Cultural Debate over Female Circumcision: The Sudanese Are Arguing This One Out for Themselves." *Medical Anthropology Quarterly* 10 (4): 455–75.

Gruenbaum, Ellen. 2001. *The Female Circumcision Controversy: An Anthropological Perspective.* Philadelphia: University of Pennsylvania Press.

Gruenbaum, Ellen. 2009. "Honorable Mutilation? Changing Responses to Female Genital Cutting in Sudan." In *Anthropology and Public Health,* 2d ed., edited by Robert A. Hahn and Marcia Inborn, 397–421. Oxford: Oxford University Press.

Gunning, Isabelle R. 2002. "Female Genital Surgeries: Eradication Measures at the Western Local Level—A Cautionary Tale." In *Genital Cutting and Transnational Sisterhood: Disputing US Polemics,* edited by Stanlie M. James and Claire C. Robertson, 114–25. Urbana: University of Illinois Press.

Gupta, Akhil. 1998. *Postcolonial Developments: Agriculture in the Making of Modern India.* Durham, NC: Duke University Press.

Guyer, Jane I. 1993. "Wealth in People and Self-realization in Equatorial Africa." *Man* 28 (2): 243–65.

Hahn, Robert A., and Marcia Claire Inhorn. 2009. *Anthropology and Public Health: Bridging Differences in Culture and Society.* New York: Oxford University Press.

Hale, Sondra. 1994. "A Question of Subjects: The 'Female Circumcision' Controversy and the Politics of Knowledge." *Ufahamu: A Journal of African Studies* 22 (3): 26–35.

Halley, Janet, Prabha Kotiswaran, Hila Shamir, and Chantal Thomas. 2006. "From the International to the Local in Feminist Legal Responses to Rape, Prostitution/ Sex Work, and Sex Trafficking: Four Studies in Contemporary Governance Feminism." *Harvard Journal of Law & Gender* 29:335–423.

Hamdy, Sherine F. 2008. "When the State and Your Kidneys Fail: Political Etiologies in an Egyptian Dialysis Ward." *American Ethnologist* 35 (4): 553–69.

Harsch, Ernest. 2008. "Closing Ghana's National Poverty Gap." *Africa Renewal Online,* October 2008, www.un.org/africarenewal/magazine/october-2008 /closing-ghana%E2%80%99s-national-poverty-gap.

Hart, Keith. 1973. "Informal Income Opportunities and Urban Employment in Ghana." *Journal of Modern African Studies* 11 (1): 61–89.

Hartman, Saidiya V. 2007. *Lose Your Mother: A Journey along the Atlantic Slave Route.* New York: Farrar, Straus and Giroux.

Hasty, Jennifer. 2005a. "The Pleasures of Corruption: Desire and Discipline in Ghanaian Political Culture." *Cultural Anthropology* 20 (2): 271–301.

Hasty, Jennifer. 2005b. *The Press and Political Culture in Ghana.* Bloomington: Indiana University Press.

Hawkins, Sean. 2002. *Writing and Colonialism in Northern Ghana: The Encounter between the LoDagaa and "The World on Paper."* Toronto: University of Toronto Press.

Hayden, Cori. 2007. "Taking as Giving." *Social Studies of Science* 37 (5): 729–58.

Hayes, Rose Oldfield. 1975. "Female Genital Mutilation, Fertility Control, Women's Roles, and the Patrilineage in Modern Sudan: A Functional Analysis." *American Ethnologist* 2 (4): 617–33.

Hernlund, Ylva. 2000. "Cutting without Ritual and Ritual without Cutting: Female 'Circumcision' and the Re-ritualization of Initiation in the Gambia." In Shell-Duncan and Hernlund 2000a, 235–52.

Hernlund, Ylva, and Bettina Shell-Duncan, eds. 2007. *Transcultural Bodies: Female Genital Cutting in Global Context.* New Brunswick, NJ: Rutgers University Press.

Hetherington, Penelope. 1998. "The Politics of Female Circumcision in the Central Province of Colonial Kenya, 1920–30." *Journal of Imperial and Commonwealth History* 26 (1): 93–126.

Hibou, Beatrice. 2015. *The Bureaucratization of the World in the Neoliberal Era: An International and Comparative Perspective.* New York: Palgrave Macmillan.

Hodgson, Dorothy L. 2001. *Once Intrepid Warriors: Gender, Ethnicity, and the Cultural Politics of Maasai Development.* Bloomington: Indiana University Press.

Hodžić, Saida. 2009. "Unsettling Power: Domestic Violence, Gender Politics, and Struggles over Sovereignty in Ghana." *Ethnos* 74 (3): 331–60.

Hodžić, Saida. 2010. "The Logics of Controversy: Gender Violence as a Site of Frictions in Ghanian Advocacy." In *Domestic Violence and the Law in Colonial and Postcolonial Africa,* edited by Emily Burrill, Richard Roberts, and Elizabeth Thornberry, 220–38. Athens: Ohio University Press.

Hodžić, Saida. 2011. "Seduced by Information, Contaminated by Power: Women's Rights as a Global Panopticon." In *Confronting Global Gender Justice: Women's Lives, Human Rights,* edited by Debra Bergoffen, Paula Ruth Gilbert, Tamara Harvey, and Connie L. McNeely, 215–30. New York: Routledge.

Hodžić, Saida. 2013. "Ascertaining Deadly Harms: Aesthetics and Politics of Global Evidence." *Cultural Anthropology* 28 (1): 86–109.

Hodžić, Saida. 2014. "Feminist Bastards: Towards a Post-humanist Critique of NGOization." In *Theorizing NGOs: States, Feminisms, and Neoliberalism,* edited by Inderpal Grewal and Victoria Bernal. Durham, NC: Duke University Press.

Holsey, Bayo. 2008. *Routes of Remembrance: Refashioning the Slave Trade in Ghana.* Chicago: University of Chicago Press.

Hunt, Alan, and Gary Wickham. 1994. *Foucault and Law: Towards a Sociology of Law as Governance.* London: Pluto Press.

ICF Macro. 2010a. *Gender and Health Indicators in Ghana, Data from the 2008 Demographic and Health Survey.* Calverton, MD: ICF Macro.

ICF Macro. 2010b. *Nutrition of Children and Women in Ghana: A New Look at Data from the 2008 Ghana Demographic and Health Survey.* Calverton, MD: ICF Macro.

Inda, Jonathan Xavier, ed. 2005a. "Analytics of the Modern: An Introduction." In Inda 2005b, 1–22.

Inda, Jonathan Xavier. 2005b. *Anthropologies of Modernity: Foucault, Governmentality, and Life Politics.* Malden, MA: Blackwell.

International Monetary Fund. 2006. *Ghana: Poverty Reduction Strategy Paper.* Washington, DC: International Monetary Fund.

Jackson, Elizabeth F., Patricia Akweongo, Evelyn Sakeah, Abraham Hodgson, Rofina Asuru, and James F. Phillips. 2003. "Inconsistent Reporting of Female Genital Cutting Status in Northern Ghana: Explanatory Factors and Analytical Consequences." *Studies in Family Planning* 34 (3): 200–10.

Johnsdotter, Sara. 2004. "Female Genital Cutting among Immigrants in European Countries: Are Risk Estimations Reasonable?" Paper presented at the conference Mutilazioni Genitali Femminili in Europa, Rome, December 10–11.

Johnsdotter, Sara. 2009. *Discrimination of Certain Ethnic Groups? Ethical Aspects of Implementing FGM Legislation in Sweden.* Malmö, Sweden: Malmö University Faculty of Health and Society.

Johnsdotter, Sara, and Birgitta Essén. 2004. "Sexual Health among Young Somali Women in Sweden: Living with Conflicting Culturally Determined Sexual Ideologies." Paper presented at the conference Advancing Knowledge on Psycho-Sexual Effects of FGM/C: Assessing the Evidence, Alexandria, Egypt, October 10–12.

Johnsdotter, Sara, and Birgitta Essén. 2015. "Cultural Change after Migration: Circumcision of Girls in Western Migrant Communities." *Best Practice & Research Clinical Obstetrics & Gynaecology* 32:1–11.

Johnson, Michelle. 2000. "Becoming a Muslim, Becoming a Person: Female "Circumcision," Religious Identity, and Personhood in Guinea-Bissau." In Shell-Duncan and Hernlund 2000a, 215–34.

Johnson, Michelle. 2007. "Making Mandinga or Making Muslims?" In Hernlund and Shell-Duncan 2007, 202–23.

Johnson-Hanks, Jennifer. 2002. "On the Limits of Life Stages in Ethnography: Toward a Theory of Vital Conjunctures." *American Anthropologist* 104 (3): 865–80.

Kanogo, Tabitha. 2005. *African Womanhood in Colonial Kenya, 1900–1950.* Athens: Ohio University Press.

Kenyatta, Jomo. (1938) 1965. *Facing Mount Kenya.* New York: Vintage.

Knudsen, Oware Christiana. 1994. *The Falling Dawadawa Tree: Female Circumcision in Developing Ghana.* Hojbjerg, Denmark: Intervention Press.

Konadu-Agyemang, Kwadwo. 2000. "The Best of Times and the Worst of Times: Structural Adjustment Programs and Uneven Development in Africa: The Case of Ghana." *Professional Geographer* 52 (3): 469–83.

Kramer, Fritz. 1993. *The Red Fez: Art and Spirit Possession in Africa.* London: Verso.

Kratz, Corinne A. 1993. *Affecting Performance: Meaning, Movement, and Experience in Okiek Women's Initiation.* Washington, DC: Smithsonian Institution Press.

Kratz, Corinne A. 2007. "Seeking Asylum, Debating Values, and Setting Precedents in the 1990s: The Cases of Kassindja and Abankwah in the United States." In Hernlund and Shell-Duncan 2007, 167–201.

Langwick, Stacey A. 2008. "Articulate(d) Bodies: Traditional Medicine in a Tanzanian Hospital." *American Ethnologist* 35 (3): 428–39.

Langwick, Stacey A. 2011. *Bodies, Politics, and African Healing: The Matter of Maladies in Tanzania.* Bloomington: Indiana University Press.

Latour, Bruno. 1987. *Science in Action.* Cambridge, MA: Harvard University Press.

Laube, Wolfram. 2007. *Changing Natural Resource Regimes in Northern Ghana: Actors, Structures and Institutions.* Münster, Germany: LIT Verlag.

Lefebvre, Henri. 2010. *Everyday Life in the Modern World.* New York: Continuum.

Lentz, Carola. 1999. "Colonial Ethnography and Political Reform: The Works of AC Duncan-Johnstone, RS Rattray, J. Eyre-Smith and J. Guiness on Northern Ghana." *Ghana Studies* 2:119–69.

Lentz, Carola. 2003. "'This Is Ghanaian Territory!': Land Conflicts on a West African Border." *American Ethnologist* 30 (2): 273–89.

Lentz, Carola. 2006. *Ethnicity and the Making of History in Northern Ghana.* Edinburgh: Edinburgh University Press.

Lentz, Carola, and Paul Nugent, eds. 2000. *Ethnicity in Ghana: The Limits of Invention.* New York: Macmillan.

Leonard, Lori. 2009. "Experiments with 'Modernism': The Allure and the Dangers of Genital Surgeries in Southern Chad." *Medische Anthropologie* 21 (1): 93–106.

Lightfoot-Klein, Hanny. 1989. *Prisoners of Ritual: An Odyssey into Female Genital Circumcision in Africa.* New York: Harrington Park Press.

Lindsey, Lisa A. 2007. "Working with Gender: The Emergence of the 'Male Breadwinner' in Colonial Southwestern Nigeria." In *Africa after Gender?,* edited by Catherine M. Cole, Takyiwaa Manuh, and Stephan Miescher, 241–52. Bloomington: Indiana University Press.

Lobnibe, Isidore. 2008. "Between Aspirations and Realities: Northern Ghanaian Migrant Women and the Dilemma of Household (Re)Production in Southern Ghana." *Africa Today* 55 (2): 53–74.

Lobnibe, Isidore. 2010. "Of Jong Migrants and Jongsecans: Understanding Contemporary Rural Out-migration from Northwest Ghana." *Journal of Dagaare Studies* 7 (10): 1–21.

Lund, Christian. 2013. "The Past and Space: On Arguments in African Land Control." *Africa* 83 (1): 14–35.

MacGaffey, Wyatt. 2010. "The Residue of Colonial Anthropology in the History and Political Discourse of Northern Ghana: Critique and Revision." *History Compass* 8 (6): 431–39.

Macharia, Keguro. 2012. "'How Does a Girl Grow into a Woman?' Girlhood in Ngugi wa Thiong'o's *The River Between*." *Research in African Literatures* 43 (2): 1–17.

Macklin, Audrey. 2006. "The Double-Edged Sword: Using the Criminal Law against Female Genital Mutilation." In *Female Circumcision: Multicultural Perspectives,* edited by Rogaia Mustafa Abusharaf, 207–23. Philadelphia: University of Pennsylvania Press.

Mahmood, Saba. 2005. *Politics of Piety: The Islamic Revival and the Feminist Subject.* Princeton, NJ: Princeton University Press.

Mahmood, Saba. 2008. "Feminism, Democracy, and Empire: Islam and the War on Terror." In *Women's Studies on the Edge,* edited by Joan Wallach Scott, 81–114. Durham, NC: Duke University Press.

Mamdani, Mahmood 1996. *Citizen and Subject: Contemporary Africa and the Legacy of Late Colonialism.* Princeton, NJ: Princeton University Press.

Mani, Lata. 1998. *Contentious Traditions: The Debate on Sati in Colonial India.* Berkeley: University of California Press.

Manuh, Takyiwaa. 1989. "A Study of Selected Voluntary Development Organizations in Ghana." *Women as Agents and Beneficiaries of Development Assistance,* edited by Patricia McFadden and Ndèye Sow, 119–51. Dakar, Senegal: Association of African Women for Research and Development.

Manuh, Takyiwaa. 2007. "Doing Gender Work in Ghana." In *Africa After Gender?,* edited by Catherine M. Cole, Takyiwaa Manuh, and Stephan Miescher, 125–49. Bloomington: Indiana University Press.

Masquelier, Adeline. 2011. "The Bloodstain: Spirit Possession, Menstruation, and Transgression in Niger." *Ethnos* 76 (2): 157–82.

Mathers, Kathryn. 2010. *Travel, Humanitarianism, and Becoming American in Africa.* New York: Palgrave Macmillan.

Mbembe, Achille. 1992. "Provisional Notes on the Postcolony." *Africa* 62 (1): 3–37.

Mbembe, Achille. 2001. *On the Postcolony.* Berkeley: University of California Press.

McClintock, Anne. 1995. *Imperial Leather: Race, Gender and Sexuality in the Colonial Contest.* New York: Routledge.

Meier, Barbara. 1999. "'Doglientiri': An Institutionalised Relationship between Women among the Bulsa of Northern Ghana." *Africa: Journal of the International African Institute* 69 (1): 87–107.

Merry, Sally Engle. 2008. Review of *Law and Disorder in the Postcolony* by Jean Comaroff and John L. Comaroff. *Law & Society Review* 42 (3): 683–85.

Meyer, Birgit. 1998. "'Make a Complete Break with the Past.' Memory and Postcolonial Modernity in Ghanaian Pentecostalist Discourse." *Journal of Religion in Africa* 28 (3): 316–49.

Meyer, Birgit. 2003. "Visions of Blood, Sex, and Money: Fantasy Spaces in Popular Ghanaian Cinema." *Visual Anthropology* 16 (1): 15–41.

Miers, Suzanne. 2003. *Slavery in the Twentieth Century: The Evolution of a Global Problem.* Lanham, MD: Rowman & Littlefield.

Miers, Suzanne, and Igor Kopytoff, eds. 1979. *Slavery in Africa: Historical and Anthropological Perspectives.* Madison: University of Wisconsin Press.

Mills, David. 2008. *Difficult Folk?: A Political History of Social Anthropology.* New York: Berghahn Books.

Mitchell, Timothy. 2002. *Rule of Experts: Egypt, Techno-politics, Modernity.* Berkeley: University of California Press.

Miyazaki, Hirokazu, and Annelise Riles. 2005. "Failure as an Endpoint." In *Global Assemblages: Technology, Politics, and Ethics as Anthropological Problems,* edited by Aihwa Ong and Stephen J. Collier, 320–32. Malden, MA: Blackwell.

Mohan, Giles. 2002. "The Disappointments of Civil Society: The Politics of NGO Intervention in Northern Ghana." *Political Geography* 21:125–54.

Mol, Annemarie. 2002. *The Body Multiple: Ontology in Medical Practice.* Durham, NC: Duke University Press.

Moore, Donald S. 2005. *Suffering for Territory: Race, Place, and Power in Zimbabwe.* Durham, NC: Duke University Press.

Moore, Henrietta L., and Todd Sanders, eds. 2003. *Magical Interpretations, Material Realities: Modernity, Witchcraft and the Occult in Postcolonial Africa.* New York: Routledge.

Moran, Mary H. 2011. Review of *Law and Disorder in the Postcolony* by Jean Comaroff and John L. Comaroff. *PoLAR* 34 (1): 192–95.

Morsy, Soheir A. 1991. "Safeguarding Women's Bodies: The White Man's Burden Medicalized." *Medical Anthropology Quarterly* 5 (1): 19–23.

Muñoz, José Esteban. 1999. *Disidentifications: Queers of Color and the Performance of Politics.* Minneapolis: University of Minnesota Press.

Nader, Laura. 1990. *Harmony Ideology: Justice and Control in a Mountain Zapotec Village.* Stanford, CA: Stanford University Press.

Newton, Sam, Victor Doku, Wenzel Geissler, Kwaku Poku Asante, and Simon Cousens. 2009. "Drawing Blood from Young Children: Lessons Learned from a Trial in Ghana." *Transactions of the Royal Society of Tropical Medicine and Hygiene* 103 (5): 497–99.

Nguyen, Vinh-Kim. 2010. *The Republic of Therapy: Triage and Sovereignty in West Africa's Time of AIDS.* Durham, NC: Duke University Press.

Nnaemeka, Obioma. 2005a. "African Women, Colonial Discourses, and Imperialist Interventions: Female Circumcision as Impetus." In Nnaemeka 2005c, 27–46.

Nnaemeka, Obioma. 2005b. "The Challenges of Border-Crossing: African Women and Transnational Feminisms." In Nnaemeka 2005c, 3–20.

Nnaemeka, Obioma, ed. 2005c. *Female Circumcision and the Politics of Knowledge: African Women in Imperialist Discourses.* Westport, CT: Praeger.

Nordstrom, Carolyn. 2009. "Fault Lines." In *Global Health in Times of Violence,* edited by Barbara Rylko-Bauer, Paul Farmer, and Linda M. Whiteford, 63–88. Santa Fe, NM: School for Advanced Research Press.

Northcott, Henry Ponting. (1899) 2011. *Report on the Northern Territories of the Gold Coast: From Reports Furnished by Officers of the Administration.* Gloucester, UK: British Library Historical Print Editions.

Nugent, Paul. 1995. *Big Men, Small Boys and Politics in Ghana: Power, Ideology and the Burden of History, 1982–1994.* London: Pinter.

Obeng, Samuel Gyasi. 2002. "Metaphors in Ghanaian Political Communication." In *Surviving through Obliqueness: Language of Politics in Emerging Democracies,* edited by Samuel Gyasi Obeng and Beverly Hartford, 83–99. New York: Nova Science.

Oduro, A. R., P. Ansah, A. Hodgson, T. M. Afful, F. Baiden, P. Adongo, and K. A. Koram. 2006. "Trends in the Prevalence of Female Genital Mutilation and Its Effect on Delivery Outcomes in the Kassena-Nankana District of Northern Ghana." *Ghana Medical Journal* 40 (3): 87–92.

Ortner, Sherry B. 1984. "Theory in Anthropology since the Sixties." *Comparative Studies in Society and History* 26 (1): 126–66.

Osei-Asare, Yaw Bonsu, and Mark Eghan. 2013. "Food Price Inflation and Consumer Welfare in Ghana." *International Journal of Food and Agricultural Economics* 1 (1): 27–39.

Osseo-Assare, Abena Dove. 2008. "Bioprospecting and Resistance: Transforming Poisoned Arrows into Strophanthin Pills in Colonial Gold Coast, 1885–1922." *Social History of Medicine* 21 (2): 269–90.

Parker, John. 2006. "Northern Gothic: Witches, Ghosts and Werewolves in the Savanna Hinterland of the Gold Coast, 1900s–1950s." *Africa: The Journal of the International African Institute* 76 (3): 352–80.

Passaro, Joanne. 1997. " 'You Can't Take the Subway to the Field!': 'Village' Epistemologies in the Global Village." In *Anthropological Locations: Boundaries and Grounds of a Field Science,* edited by Akhil Gupta and James Ferguson, 147–62. Berkeley: University of California Press.

Pedersen, Susan. 1991. "National Bodies, Unspeakable Acts: The Sexual Politics of Colonial Policy-making." *Journal of Modern History* 63 (4): 647–80.

Pellow, Deborah. 2011. "Internal Transmigrants: A Dagomba Diaspora." *American Ethnologist* 38 (1): 132–47.

Pellow, Deborah. 2015. "Multiple Modernities: Kitchens for an African Elite." *Home Cultures* 12 (1): 55–81.

Perry, Donna L. 2009. "Fathers, Sons, and the State: Discipline and Punishment in a Wolof Hinterland." *Cultural Anthropology* 24 (1): 33–67.

Petryna, Adriana. 2007. "Clinical Trials Offshored: On Private Sector Science and Public Health." *Biosocieties* 2:21–40.

Pierre, Jemima. 2013. *The Predicament of Blackness: Postcolonial Ghana and the Politics of Race.* Chicago: University of Chicago Press.

Pigg, Stacy Leigh. 1996. "The Credible and the Credulous: The Question of 'Villagers' Beliefs' in Nepal." *Cultural Anthropology* 11 (2): 160–201.

Pigg, Stacy Leigh. 1997. "Found in Most Traditional Societies: Traditional Medical Practitioners between Culture and Development." In *International Development and the Social Sciences,* edited by Frederick Cooper and Randall M. Packard, 259–90. Berkeley: University of California Press.

Pigg, Stacy Leigh. 2001. "Languages of Sex and AIDS in Nepal: Notes on the Social Production of Commensurability." *Cultural Anthropology* 16:481–541.

Pigg, Stacy Leigh. 2005. "Globalizing the Facts of Life." In *Sex in Development,* edited by Vincanne Adams and Stacy Leigh Pigg, 39–67. Durham, NC: Duke University Press.

Pigg, Stacy Leigh, and Vincanne Adams. 2005. Introduction to Adams and Pigg, *Sex in Development,* 1–38.

Piot, Charles. 1999. *Remotely Global: Village Modernity in West Africa.* Chicago: University of Chicago Press.

Piot, Charles. 2010. *Nostalgia for the Future: West Africa after the Cold War.* Chicago: University of Chicago Press.

Plange, Nii-K. 1979. "Underdevelopment in Northern Ghana: Natural Causes or Colonial Capitalism?" *Review of African Political Economy* 6 (15): 4–14.

Povinelli, Elizabeth A. 1998. "The State of Shame: Australian Multiculturalism and the Crisis of Indigenous Citizenship." *Critical Inquiry* 24 (2): 575–610.

Povinelli, Elizabeth A. 2002. *The Cunning of Recognition: Indigenous Alterities and the Making of Australian Multiculturalism.* Durham, NC: Duke University Press.

Povinelli, Elizabeth A. 2011a. *Economies of Abandonment: Social Belonging and Endurance in Late Liberalism.* Durham, NC: Duke University Press.

Povinelli, Elizabeth A. 2011b. "The Governance of the Prior." *Interventions* 13 (1): 13–30.

Povinelli, Elizabeth A. 2015. "The Rhetorics of Recognition in Geontopower." *Philosophy & Rhetoric* 48 (4): 428–42.

Povinelli, Elizabeth A. 2016. *Geontologies.* Durham, NC: Duke University Press.

Pratt, Mary Louise. 1986. "Fieldwork in Common Places." In *Writing Culture: The Poetics and Politics of Ethnography,* edited by James Clifford and George E. Marcus, 27–50. Berkeley: University of California Press.

Rabinow, Paul. 2005. "Midst Anthropology's Problems." In *Global Assemblages: Technology, Politics, and Ethics as Anthropological Problems,* edited by Aihwa Ong and Stephen J. Collier, 40–54. Malden, MA: Blackwell.

Rabinow, Paul, and Nikolas Rose. 2003. Introduction to *The Essential Foucault,* edited by Paul Rabinow and Nikolas Rose, vii–xxxv. New York: New Press.

Rancière, Jacques. 2010. *Dissensus: On Politics and Aesthetics.* Translated by Steven Corcoran. London: Continuum.

Rancière, Jacques. 2013. *The Politics of Aesthetics: Distribution of the Sensible.* London: Bloomsbury.

Rathbone, Richard. 1989. "A Murder in the Colonial Gold Coast: Law and Politics in the 1940s." *Journal of African History* 30 (3): 445–61.

Rathbone, Richard. 2000. *Nkrumah & the Chiefs: The Politics of Chieftaincy in Ghana, 1951–60.* Athens: Ohio University Press.

Redfield, Peter. 2013. *Life in Crisis: The Ethical Journey of Doctors Without Borders.* Berkeley: University of California Press.

Riles, Annelise. 1998. "Infinity within the Brackets." *American Ethnologist* 25 (3): 378–98.

Riles, Annelise. 2001. *The Network Inside Out.* Ann Arbor: University of Michigan Press.

Rogers, Juliet. 2007. "Managing Cultural Diversity in Australia: Legislating Female Circumcision, Legislating Communities." In Hernlund and Shell-Duncan 2007, 135–56.

Roitman, Janet. 2013. *Anti-crisis.* Durham, NC: Duke University Press.

Rose, Nikolas. 1999. *Powers of Freedom: Reframing Political Thought.* Cambridge: Cambridge University Press.

Rutherford, Danilyn. 2012. *Laughing at Leviathan: Sovereignty and Audience in West Papua.* Chicago: University of Chicago Press.

Saaka, Yakubu. 2001. *Regionalism and Public Policy in Northern Ghana, Society and Politics in Africa.* New York: Peter Lang.

Sanderson, Lilian M. Passmore. 1995. "The Role of the Sudan in the Work for the Eradication of Female Genital Mutilation." *Sudan Studies* 17:23–29.

Scheper-Hughes, Nancy. 1991. "Virgin Territory: The Male Discovery of the Clitoris." *Medical Anthropology Quarterly* 5 (1): 25–28.

Scheper-Hughes, Nancy. 1993. *Death without Weeping: The Violence of Everyday Life in Brazil.* Berkeley: University of California Press.

Scheper-Hughes, Nancy, and Margaret M. Lock. 1987. "The Mindful Body: A Prolegomenon to Future Work in Medical Anthropology." *Medical Anthropology Quarterly* 1 (1): 6–41.

Schildkrout, Enid. 1970. "Strangers and Local Government in Kumasi." *Journal of Modern African Studies* 8 (2): 251–69.

Scott, David. 1995. "Colonial Governmentality." *Social Text* (43): 191–220.

Scott, James C. 2012. *Two Cheers for Anarchism: Six Easy Pieces on Autonomy, Dignity, and Meaningful Work and Play.* Princeton, NJ: Princeton University Press

Scott, James C. 2014. *The Art of Not Being Governed: An Anarchist History of Upland Southeast Asia.* New Haven, CT: Yale University Press.

Sharma, Aradhana. 2008. *Logics of Empowerment: Development, Gender, and Governance in Neoliberal India.* Minneapolis: University of Minnesota Press.

Shell-Duncan, Bettina, and Ylva Hernlund, eds. 2000a. *Female "Circumcision" in Africa: Culture, Controversy, and Change.* Boulder, CO: Lynne Rienner.

Shell-Duncan, Bettina, and Ylva Hernlund. 2000b. "Female 'Circumcision' in Africa: Dimensions of the Practice and Debates." In Shell-Duncan and Hernlund 2000a, 1–40.

Shell-Duncan, Bettina, and Ylva Hernlund. 2007. "Are There "Stages of Change" in the Practice of Female Genital Cutting? Qualitative Research Finding from Senegal and the Gambia." *African Journal of Reproductive Health* 10 (2): 57–71.

Shell-Duncan, Bettina, Katherine Wander, Ylva Hernlund, and Amadou Moreau. 2011. "Dynamics of Change in the Practice of Female Genital Cutting in Senegambia: Testing Predictions of Social Convention Theory." *Social Science & Medicine* 73 (8): 1275–83.

Shell-Duncan, Bettina, Katherine Wander, Ylva Hernlund, and Amadou Moreau. 2013. "Legislating Change? Responses to Criminalizing Female Genital Cutting in Senegal." *Law & Society Review* 47 (4): 803–35.

Shepherd, Andrew E. Gyimah-Boadi, Sulley Gariba, Sophie Plagerson, and Abdul Wahab Musa. 2004. "Bridging the North-South Divide in Ghana." Background paper prepared for the 2005 World Development Report. Draft summary available at http://siteresources.worldbank.org/INTWDRS/Resources/477365-1327693659766/8397901-1327773323392/Bridging_the_North_South_Divide_in _Ghana.pdf.

Shipley, Jesse Weaver. 2012. *Living the Hiplife: Celebrity and Entrepreneurship in Ghanaian Popular Music.* Durham, NC: Duke University Press.

Singh, Bhrigupati. 2012. "The Headless Horseman of Central India: Sovereignty at Varying Thresholds of Life." *Cultural Anthropology* 27 (2): 383–407.

Skinner, Elliott Percival. 1964. *The Mossi of the Upper Volta: The Political Development of a Sudanese People.* Stanford, CA: Stanford University Press.

Smith, Daniel Jordan. 2008. *A Culture of Corruption: Everyday Deception and Popular Discontent in Nigeria.* Princeton, NJ: Princeton University Press.

Smith, Daniel Jordan. 2014. *AIDS Doesn't Show Its Face: Inequality, Morality, and Social Change in Nigeria.* Chicago: University of Chicago Press.

Snorton, C. Riley. 2014. *Nobody Is Supposed to Know: Black Sexuality on the Down Low.* Minneapolis: University of Minnesota Press.

Songsore, Jacob. 2003. *Regional Development in Ghana: The Theory and the Reality.* Accra: Woeli.

Spivak, Gayatri. 1999. *A Critique of Postcolonial Reason: Toward a History of the Vanishing Present.* Cambridge, MA: Harvard University Press.

Stoler, Ann Laura. 2008. "Imperial Debris: Reflections on Ruins and Ruination." *Cultural Anthropology* 23 (2): 191–219.

Strathern, Marilyn. 1991. *Partial Connections.* Walnut Creek, CA: Altamira.

Sutton, Inez. 1989. "Colonial Agricultural Policy: The Non-Development of the Northern Territories of the Gold Coast." *International Journal of African Historical Studies* 22 (4): 637–69.

Talle, Aud. 1993. "Transforming Women into Pure Agnates: Aspects of Female Infibulation in Somalia." In *Carved flesh/Cast Selves: Gendered Symbols and Social Practices,* edited by Vigdis Broch-Due, Ingrid Rudie, and Tone Bleie, 83–106. London: Bloomsbury.

Tambiah, Stanley J., Mitzi Goheen, Alma Gottlieb, Jane I. Guyer, Emelie A. Olson, Charles Piot, Klaas W. Van Der Veen, and Trudeke C. Vuyk. 1989. "Bridewealth and Dowry Revisited: The Position of Women in Sub-Saharan Africa and North India [and Comments and Reply]." *Current Anthropology* 30 (4): 413–35.

Tankebe, Justice. 2008. "Colonialism, Legitimation, and Policing in Ghana." *International Journal of Law, Crime and Justice* 36 (1): 67–84.

Taylor, Janelle. 2005. "Surfacing the Body Interior." *Annual Review of Anthropology* 34:741–56.

Taylor, Janelle. 2014. "The Demise of the Bumbler and the Crock: From Experience to Accountability in Medical Education and Ethnography." *American Anthropologist* 116 (3): 523–34.

Thomas, Lynn M. 2003. *Politics of the Womb: Women, Reproduction, and the State in Kenya*. Berkeley: University of California Press.

Thomas, Roger G. 1973. "Forced Labour in British West Africa: The Case of the Northern Territories of the Gold Coast 1906–1927." *Journal of African History* 14 (1): 79–103.

Thomas, Roger G. 1974. "Education in Northern Ghana, 1906–1940: A Study in Colonial Paradox." *International Journal of African Historical Studies* 7 (3): 427–67.

Ticktin, Miriam. 2011. *Casualties of Care: Immigration and the Politics of Humanitarianism in France*. Berkeley: University of California Press.

Ticktin, Miriam. 2014. "Transnational Humanitarianism." *Annual Review of Anthropology* 43: 273–89.

Tilly, Charles. 2009. *Credit and Blame*. Princeton, NJ: Princeton University Press.

Trinh, T. Minh-Ha. 1989. *Woman, Native, Other: Writing Postcoloniality and Feminism*. Bloomington: Indiana University Press.

Tsing, Anna Lowenhaupt. 1993. *In the Realm of the Diamond Queen: Marginality in an Out-of-the-way Place*. Princeton, NJ: Princeton University Press.

Tsing, Anna Lowenhaupt. 2005. *Friction: An Ethnography of Global Connection*. Princeton, NJ: Princeton University Press.

UNICEF. 2004. *Report of the Review of the Accelerated Child Survival and Development Programme in the Upper East Region of Ghana*. November.

UNICEF. 2008. "At a Glance: Ghana." UNICEF, April 20, 2008, www.unicef.org /infobycountry/ghana.html.

UNICEF. 2013. *Female Genital Mutilation/Cutting: A Statistical Overview and Exploration of the Dynamics of Change*. New York: UNICEF.

University of Ghana Population Impact Project. 2000. "Editorial: The Case Against Female Genital Mutilation." *Population, Environment & Development in Ghana Research Update* 4 (1): 1–14.

Van de Poel, Ellen, Ahmad Hosseinpoor, Caroline Jehu-Appiah, Jeanette Vega, and Niko Speybroeck. 2007. "Malnutrition and the Disproportional Burden on the Poor: The Case of Ghana." *International Journal for Equity in Health* 6 (1), www .biomedcentral.com/content/pdf/1475-9276-6-21.pdf.

Visweswaran, Kamala. 1994. *Fictions of Feminist Ethnography*. Minneapolis: University of Minnesota Press.

Wainaina, Binyavanga. 2005. "How to Write About Africa." *Granta* 92:91.

Wardlow, Holly. 2012. "The Task of the HIV Translator: Transforming Global AIDS Knowledge in an Awareness Workshop." *Medical Anthropology* 31 (5): 404–19.

Warren, Kay B. 2012. "Troubling the Victim/Trafficker Dichotomy in Efforts to Combat Human Trafficking: The Unintended Consequences of Moralizing Labor Migration." *Indiana Journal of Global Legal Studies* 19 (1): 105–20.

wa Thiong'o, Ngũgĩ. 1965. *The River Between.* Oxford: Heineman.

wa Thiong'o, Ngũgĩ. 1994. *Decolonising the Mind: The Politics of Language in African Literature.* London: East African Publishers.

Watkins, Susan Cotts, and Ann Swidler. 2013. "Working Misunderstandings: Donors, Brokers, and Villagers in Africa's AIDS Industry." *Population and Development Review* 38:197–218.

Weiss, Brad, ed. 2004. *Producing African Futures: Ritual and Reproduction in a Neoliberal Age.* Leiden, Netherlands: Brill.

White, Luise. 2000. *Speaking with Vampires: Rumor and History in Colonial Africa.* Berkeley: University of California Press.

Whitehead, Ann. 2002. "Tracking Livelihood Change: Theoretical, Methodological and Empirical Perspectives from North-East Ghana." *Journal of Southern African Studies* 28 (3): 575–98.

Whitehead, Ann. 2006. "Persistent Poverty in North East Ghana." *Journal of Development Studies* 42 (2): 278–300.

Wilson, Ara. 2010. "NGOs as Erotic Sites." In *Development, Sexual Rights and Global Governance,* edited by Amy Lind, 86–98. New York: Routledge.

World Health Organization. 1979. *Traditional Practices Affecting the Health of Women and Children: Female Circumcision, Childhood Marriage, Nutritional Taboos, Etc.* WHO/EMRO Technical Publication No. 2. Alexandria, Egypt: WHO/EMRO.

World Health Organization. 2001. *Female Genital Mutilation: A Student's Manual.* Department of Gender and Women's Health. WHO/FCH/GWH/01.4; WHO/RHR/01.17. Geneva: World Health Organization.

World Health Organization. 2016. "Female Genital Mutilation: Fact Sheet." www.who.int/mediacentre/factsheets/fs241/en/.

World Health Organization Study Group on Female Genital Mutilation and Obstetric Outcome. 2006. "Female Genital Mutilation and Obstetric Outcome: WHO Collaborative Prospective Study in six African Countries." *Lancet* 367 (9525): 1835–41.

Yarrow, Thomas. 2008a. "Life/History: Personal Narratives of Development amongst NGO Workers and Activists in Ghana." *Africa* 78 (03): 334–58.

Yarrow, Thomas. 2008b. "Negotiating Difference: Discourses of Indigenous Knowledge and Development in Ghana." *PoLAR* 31 (2): 224–42.

INDEX

Abampoka. *See* Mbawini, Abampoka

abandonment by the state: circumcisers positioned in terms of, 134, 169; and desire for humanitarian hero, 128–129; and Othering of northern Ghana, 15; and political agency of villagers, 127–128, 345n23, 350n19; rural women's critique of, via blood narrative, 211, 218, 221, 222, 238–239, 240–243, 334, 350n19. *See also* neoliberalism; scarcity; survival vs. thriving

Abilba, Martin III, 4–5, 182

abstinence-only campaigns, 159

Adjei, Dr. (pseudonym). *See* RHI (Rural Help Integrated)

affect: distant, 82–83; of feminist ethnographers, 34–35; production of, in GAWW workshops, 105, 107, 111–113, 215; simulated, taught to nurses, 109; sympathetic, 69, 70–71. *See also* sensibilities

Africa: *African*, as term intertwined with the West, 25; African Charter for Human Rights, 340n19; "Africa Rising" paradigm, 345n19; deficit view of, 9–10, 153, 249; ICC as targeting only, 351n4; and international law, global reach of, 250; lawlessness as integral to depictions of, 249; new constitutions in states of, 250; and proofs of rationality, demand for, 26–28, 340n14; as scale of study, 37–38.

See also anthropology of Africa; colonial Africa; from the South analysis; migrants to global North, and anticutting campaigns; NGOs (African)

African Americans: down-low discourse and, 144–145; homeless men, distrust for, 145; right of residence in Ghana, 13

agents of governmentality. *See* NGO workers

agriculture: anthropological analysis of difficulty with, 345n16; development projects for, 126; and double bind of NGO workers, 130; food shortages and, 222, 227; harmful traditions blamed for troubles with, 119, 121; market liberalization and destruction of rice production, 114, 344n11; subsistence, government discourse on, 114–115, 116, 344n12

Aidoo, Ama Ata, *Our Sister Killjoy*, 27, 150, 159–160, 237, 310, 335

Alhassan (pseudonym). *See* Center for Human Rights Education and Advocacy

Allman, Jean, 72–73, 76, 87, 117, 163, 170, 343n38, 346n10

ancestor reverence and worship, as primary mechanism of securing order, 294. *See also* gods

anemia, 222–223, 229, 237

animism. *See* traditional religion

"denial paper," 139; as public knowledge, 184, 286; stringent punishments of reformed law, 246–247, 270–271, 273–274, 301–302; treatment of cut women/girls in process of, 278, 298, 304–305, 306; watchdog/eradication committees, 288–294, 295–299, 303–308, 318. *See also* circumcisers; Dari, Fefe; Mbawini, Abampoka; reversal of punitive rationality

articulated subjects, 17

Aryee, Gloria, 16, 19, 246, 338n1

asylum claims, and cutting, x, 13–14, 136, 142–143

Atholl, Dutchess of, 55, 56, 62, 69, 70–71, 82

Australia, 144, 271–272

authority: liberal ideals of noncoercion vs. forms of NGO practice, 201–203; of RHI, and knowledge production, 185, 188–190, 195–196, 201–203

Awedoba, Albert K., 14, 150, 157–158, 159, 223–224

Bacchi, Carol, 8, 10

Banga, Emma Hellen, 16, 95, 246, 263–264, 338n1

Basu, Srimati, 253, 353–354n5

Bateson, Gregory, 31

Bawku District, cutting as continuing in, 145–146

Benjamin, Walter, 7, 288, 330

Berlant, Lauren, 213, 243

Biehl, João, 6, 25, 30–31, 213, 239, 331–332, 349n14

Billionaires Club (film), 233–235, 236

biopolitical governance, 229, 231, 243

Bledsoe, Caroline, 162, 219, 220–221

blood: blood loss as hemorrhagic crisis, anticutting campaigns and focus on, 214–218, *216*; research requiring drawing of, 236–237, 349n16; as resource for wealth accumulation, 210. *See also* occult economy, discourses of

blood and health: analogous to immune system, 219; as central concept, 219; as universal symbol, 348n3

blood narrative (end of cutting due to chronic blood shortage): and abandonment by government, 211, 218, 221, 222, 238–239, 240–243, 334, 350n19; calculus of blood loss, and lifelong susceptibility to ill health, 212, 219–220; at critical distance from anticutting interventions and governance by extraction, 212–213, 224, 227–229, 240–241, 348n5; cutting as unworthy of blood loss, 212; death as not defining, 213–214, 243; definition of, 210–212; as disrupting analytics, 228, 239–243, 350nn21–24; drought and, 103, 118, 227; as emerging in the wake of cutting's end, 214; food shortages and, 212, 220, 221, 222–223, 225–226; as historically and temporally situated, 211–212, 214, 225–228; and menstruation, 218; and moral economies of obligation and belonging, 211, 240–243; narratives about, 210, 218, 220; reproductive lives of women, blood loss of, 218, 220–221; scarcity as chronic and need to protect the blood, 160, 212, 221–223, 227; scientific and popular discourses as context of, 103, 228–231; slow harm of blood loss, 213–214, 218, 224–225, 226, 243, 246; traction of, 211–212, 228–229, 243; women's vitality weakening, 211, 214, 238, 243

blood shortages (collective blood supply): blood drives, 229; blood transfusion contractors, 229–230; cost of transfusions, 229–230, 237, 349n11; and critiques of governance, 230; family blood donations, 209, 229; gendered character of blood donations, 221, 230, 348n4; health cost of donating blood, 209; National Blood Service, 230–231, 349n10; national health insurance and, 230–231; transfusion demand as increasing, 229

blood tonics (herbal), 222–223, 229

Boddy, Janice, 21, 49, 52, 53, 55, 67–68, 70, 224, 337n1, 340n11, 341n2, 348n3

Bongo District, 145–150

Convention on the Elimination of All Forms of Discrimination Against Women (CEDAW), 268
Convention on the Rights of the Child, 268
cosmetic surgery, 26
criminality, Othering of northern Ghana and, 15
criminalization and feminism. *See* feminist theory; fetishization of law (postcolonial Ghana); GAWW and criminalization of cutting (reform of 2007); Western feminist activism
criminalization of cutting: colonial officers' opposition to, and ethnographic style of reports, 52, 66, 81, 82; Criminal Code (Amendment) Act (2007), 247; education assumed to be necessary to supplement, 258–259; hyperawareness of those subject to laws, 197–198, 246, 306–307; Kenyatta and opposition to, 20–21, 68–69; lack of voice for opposition to, 271–273, 276–278, 310, 313–314, 352–353n15; Navrongo Health Research Center and opposition to, 203, 264; NGO implication in, 198; passage of 1994 law, 33, 246, 258, 259; politician expressing opposition to, 325–326; and problematization, stakes of, 10; RHI as opposing and excluding mention of, 197–198, 203, 264–266, 288, 328; "underground resistance" discourse as inciting further, 81, 135, 143–145, 258, 346n4. *See also* arrest and punishment of circumcisers; GAWW and criminalization of cutting (reform of 2007); global North, anticutting campaigns in; reversal of punitive rationality
critical theory, as immanent in life, 30. *See also* feminist theory; from the South
critiques by subjects of NGO governmentality: as immanent critique, 34, 340n16; as lived critique, 34; problematization and, 10–11; scarcity, rural women's understanding of, 123–129, 345nn21,23; as unintended consequence of NGO projects, 7–8, 207. *See also* blood narrative (end of

cutting due to chronic blood shortage); reversal of punitive rationality
Crowley, Joe, 40, 41, 42
cultural meaning: dictum of understanding of, prior to interventions, 6–7, 9, 325. *See also* harmful traditional practices; harsh culture (cultural pathology and patriarchy constructed as source of problems); tradition
cultural triage, 91–92, 98, 101, 154
cutting: active voice used to refer to, 347n5; age for, 64, 106, 158, 300; alternate forms of, in Sudan, 49, 55–56; anatomical model of, 107, *108*, 215; as foreign, 93–94, 107, 112–113; imperatives to disavow, 17–18, 141, 339n10; as mapped onto blackness, 339n3; as mapped onto class, ethnicity, and rural-urban divide, 17–18, 339n10; as mapped onto Muslims, 94, 107, 176, 339n3; as mapped onto the North, 93; as silence, 140–141. *See also* anticutting campaigns; blood narrative (end of cutting due to chronic blood shortage); circumcisers; criminalization of cutting; cut women; ending of cutting; FGM as discursive concept; northern Ghana, Othering of
cut women: agency of, and reversal of punitive rationality, 314–317; bundling of, vs. age appropriate times, 300; care for, lack of, 96, 130; "denial paper" and, 138–141, 142; enforcement of law and shaming of, 277–278; framed as untrustworthy, 139–140, 141–143; lack of voice in anticutting laws, 271–273, 352–353n15; law reform and calls for punishment of, 271, 275, 314–316, 352n14; nostalgia for cutting not expressed by, 134, 160, 334; positioning of, 17–18, 83; recuperation following cutting, 225–226, 319; shame and last generation of, 18, 141; treatment of, during arrests of circumcisers, 278, 298, 304–305, 306. *See also* blood narrative (end of cutting due to chronic blood shortage)

Dagbon state, 72

Dari, Fefe: arrest of, 288, 297–299; early release of, 287; false confession of, 299–300; GAWW involvement in arrest of, 290, 292, 297–300; GAWW regret of arrest/imprisonment of, and reversal of punitive rationality, 299–302, 321, 322, 326–327; lack of legal representation, 302; no pseudonym used for, 338n1; sentence and imprisonment of, 293, 298, 299, 299–302, 309; and "underground resistance" discourse, 136

death: colonial northern Ghana and incidental, 76, 79; infant/child mortality rates, 117, 223, 345n16; northern Ghana laborers and, 79; portrayal in RHI anticutting film, 191–192, 196; slavery and slave trade and, 76; as ultimate effect of harmful traditions, 98, 111; the West as associated with, 237

decolonial analysis, defined, 340n13

deconstruction, distinguished from problematization, 8

Deleuze, Gilles, 31

development: goal of poverty elimination, adjustments to, 131; humanitarian emergency relief as new paradigm of, 131; management of harsh culture as goal of, 116, 129; projects to alleviate scarcity, 124, 126–127, 131; as recursive process, 198; sensitization preferred over redistribution of material resources, 116, 121, 130–131, 164. *See also* donors; governance; neoliberalism; NGOs; NGO workshops; sensitization

diet. *See* food and diet

Dirie, Waris, 11, 111, 203

disabilities, people with, and voter education workshop, 152, 154

disidentification: definition of, 34, 329; fetishism of law leading to, 248; of NGO workers, and claiming of kinship, 328–329; of NGO workers, and reversal of punitive rationality, 287; of NGO workers from shared worlds (sensibilities), 6, 36

distribution of the sensible, 82

divination. *See* soothsaying (divination)

domestic violence: opposition to criminalization of, in context of refusal to enforce anticutting laws, 322–325, 353n4; and power of law to compel vs. punish, 257, 352n8

Domestic Violence Act (Ghana), 256, 323, 352–354n15

Domestic Violence and Victim Support Unit (DOVVISU, Ghana), 257, 352n8

donors: cultural sensitivity as priority of, 201–202; educational workshops preferred by, over redistribution of resources, 130–131, 168; evidence as key for, 138, 306; funding for GAWW, 16, 20, 52, 204, 245, 258, 259, 290–291; funding for RHI, 16–17, 181, 187, 201–202, 233; interest in research about ending cutting, 138; law enforcement as priority of, 292–293; liberal ideals of horizontal dialog and, 201–203; priorities of, and educational outreach, 187; success stories as preferred by, 259

Dorkenoo, Efua, 39, 90, 95–96, 102–103, 118, 340n19

Douglass, Frederick, 340n14

down-low discourse, 144–145

drought: cutting as threatening survival of women in face of scarcity and, 103, 118, 227; harsh environment and, 345n16; as persistent since 1970s, 114, 119, 227; rain dances, 119–120. *See also* scarcity

Dukureh, Jaha, 41–42, 144, 333

duty, sense of, 314

education: as alternative to criminalization of cutting, 20–21, 68, 272–273, 325; as assumed to be necessary to supplement criminalization, 258–259; and colonial rule of northern Ghana, 68, 77, 79; independence of Ghana and, 113–114; in northern Ghana, 113–114, 115, 124, 344n10, 345n23; production of patriarchal values and noneducation of girls, 155; and strategic essentialisms, use of, 154. *See also* sensitization

feminism. *See* feminist anthropology and anthropologists; feminist ethnography; feminist theory; Ghanaian feminism; Western feminist activism

feminist anthropology and anthropologists: critique from a distance and, 82–83; and fallback position, 23–24; "hands off" dictum and, 21–22, 24; "head on" analysis, 24, 38; and theories of the social and governmental as entangled vs. opposed, 339n5; and waning of cutting vs. discourse of "intractable FGM," xii. *See also* feminist ethnography

feminist ethnography: affect of ethnographer, 34–35; multitude of perspectives in, 33, 34–35, 83; positioning of ethnographer, 83; as unruly, 32; writing nearby as commitment of, 29, 34, 83, 255

feminist theory: against certainty of critique of governance feminism in, 32–36, 82, 248–249, 252–255, 351n3; the body as process, 240; center-periphery axis and, 254, 352n6; and critique from a distance, 51, 82–83, 255; fallback position embraced by, 23–24; hermeneutical injustice, 228; left legalism, 32–33, 248, 253–254, 352n6–7; as motivated to strengthen and defend feminism, 324; and politics vs. the political, entanglement of, 252–253, 352n5; productive power of law and, 248–249, 351n3; from the South analysis, 254–255; white women's burden of challenging globalist feminism, 24. *See also* feminist anthropology and anthropologists; feminist ethnography; Western feminist activism

Ferguson, James, 22, 37, 38, 81, 88, 116, 119, 131, 177, 232, 235, 247, 296, 345n18

Ferme, Mariane, 73, 199–200

fetishization of law (postcolonial Ghana): faith in new constitutions as manifestation of, 250, 256; feminist aesthetics and form of law, 266–268, 281; feminist left legalism and, 32–33,

248, 253–254, 352n6–7; instability inherent in, 248; and judicialization of political processes, 250, 251; neoliberal austerity measures and, 256; NGOs and, 250–251, 256; order and disorder dialectic and, 250, 257–258, 262–263; overview, 249; and politics vs. the political, entanglement of, 252–253; and power of law to compel, not to punish, 256–257, 278, 278–283; productive power of law and, 248, 254–255, 279; proliferating sites of adjudication and, 250; and sovereign violence, 248; as term, 345n2; weakness of state and demand for more laws, 257–258, 261–262. *See also* GAWW and criminalization of cutting (reform of 2007); Ghanaian feminism (gender workers); law as communicative and instructive vs. punishing (Ghanaian logic of discipline)

FGM as discursive concept: as abject and inhuman, 111–113; colonial taxonomies used to construct, 63–66, 105–107; errors of cultural information as deliberate in, and knowledge formation, 177–179, 194–196, 198–201, 206–207; four types of, 107, *108*; incommensurability with regional forms of cutting, 174, 176, 200, 207; *ludo* game version developed by GAWW to teach, 204, *205*; patterns given at the start of, 178; and terminology change to FGM, 269–270, 352n13; and terminology of FGM/C, 270; as violent and harmful, 110–112. *See also* anti-FGM discourses, Western; criminalization of cutting; cutting; ending of cutting; harmful traditional practices (cutting); intractability of FGM, as discourse; underground resistance, as discourse; zero tolerance of FGM

film screenings: by GAWW, 215. *See also* RHI film screenings

fistulas, 110, 344n9

floods of 2007, 119, 121

Fluehr-Lobban, Carolyn, 49, 81, 341n1

kinship: disavowed, 72, 79; patriarchy
reinforced via, 323, 353–354n5; and
reversal of punitive rationality, 322,
326–329

knowledge, governmental: defined, 338–
339n2; lack of cultural knowledge as
source of failure, 176–178, 206, 351n1;
lack of cultural knowledge employed in
interventions as deliberate and
producing success on NGO's own
terms, 177–178, 194–196, 206–207;
of NGOs, tactical decisions based on,
178, 263; public initiation ritual as,
153–154

knowledge production: the concealed vs.
visible and, 199–200, 207, 347nn6–7;
errors in cultural knowledge creating
success in, 177–179, 194–196, 198–201,
206–207; as recursive process, 198;
rhetorical contestation and, 189;
spectacle and, 189–190, 197, 200–201;
stories and, 194; translation/discussion/
narrative deliberately minimized and,
174, 178, 187–189, 204; universalizing
and particularizing marks required for,
175, 200–201

Kouyata, Morissanda, 270, 352n13

Kumasi. See Ghana; northern Ghana as
migrant labor pool

Kusaal language, 187–188

Langwick, Stacey A., 17, 165

Latour, Bruno, 26, 237

Laube, Wolfram, 121

law: positivist formula of jurisprudence,
279. See also criminalization and
feminism; criminalization of cutting;
law as communicative and instructive
vs. punishing (Ghanaian logic of
discipline); law enforcement; punitive
rationality

law as communicative and instructive vs.
punishing (Ghanaian logic of
discipline): and concepts of the langue
(letter) vs. parole (spirit) of the law,
278–279, 280, 282–283, 287, 302;
deterrence as central to, 279, 282, 287;
discussion of the law as central to, 281;

feminist lawyers (Ghanaian) as sharing
belief in, 280–281, 282–283; GAWW
and, 292, 302; and human rights
commission as soft power, 256–257,
352n8; and lack of corporeal punishment
in child raising, 279; precolonial society
and, 294; and pressure on girls to cut,
146; and reversal of punitive rationality,
287–288, 302, 311–312, 316–317;
surveillance-oriented watchdog
committees and, 289; transgression of
law viewed as failure of law, 279. See also
fetishization of law (postcolonial
Ghana)

law enforcement: colonial police forces,
295; end of arrests of circumcisers, 33,
286, 287, 318, 353n1; and letter of the
law, 287; Native Authority Forces, 295;
police force resistance to enforcement
of anticutting laws, 304, 305–306, 313,
315, 318; police forces and (performed)
incapacity, 296, 297–298, 322–323,
324–325, 352n8; postindependence
police forces, 295. See also paraformal
law enforcement; punitive rationality;
sovereign violence

Leach, Melissa, 68, 122, 219, 350n17

Lee, Sheila Jackson, 40

left legalism, 32–33, 248, 253–254, 352n6–7.
See also feminist theory

Legal Aid, 317–318, 331

Lentz, Carola, 74, 80, 136, 340n17,
343n38

liberalism: anxiety of mistaken
intolerance, 28, 41; cultural sensitivity
as concern of, 4, 110, 201–202, 302;
dilemma of, 22; and formal
terminology change to FGM, 269–
270; ideals of dialogue of, vs. actual
NGO practice, 201–203; lack of
ethnographies of, 337n2; latent violence
of, 12, 334; "learning to question"
pedagogy of, 103; relativism and
performance of, 25

Lightfoot-Klein, Hanny, 23

Limann, Hilla, 15

Linnander, Margareta, 20, 52

Lugard, Lord, 63

superstition, harmful traditions denounced as, 98

surveillance: by nurses, workshops explaining process for, 109; and sovereign violence of global North, 40–42; "underground resistance" discourse as inciting increased, 143–145. *See also* paraformal law enforcement

survival vs. thriving: biopolitical governance and, 231, 243; concentration camp metaphor for, 319; humanitarianism's revised goals and, 131; rural women's critique of, 238–239, 241, 243, 350n19

Sutton, Inez, 74, 76–77

Sweden, 144

sympathetic affect, 69, 70–71

Taylor, Janelle, 31, 51, 240

teenage pregnancy, 97

Tévoedjrè, Isabelle, 19–20

third-person pronouns in NGO discourse, 321–322

Thomas, Roger G., 74, 75, 77, 79

Ticktin, Miriam, 71, 130, 131, 143–144, 203, 252, 315

Togo, 93, 189–190, 199

Tongnaab shrine, 87

Tongo, 120

Tostan, xi

Toubia, Nahid, 95

tradition: Appreciative Inquiry approach to, 152–153; colonial governance and preservation of, 71, 77–79, 170–171, 343n41; dictum of need to understand meaning of, before intervening, 6–7, 9, 325; disidentification with, by NGO workers, 36; extended family, nostalgia for, 170–171; patriarchy in Africa, as constructed by colonialists, 63, 159–160; precolonial governance, 159–160, 294, 329–332, 341n3; seen as inimical to development, 88. *See also* blood narrative (end of cutting due to chronic blood shortage); harmful traditional practices; kinship; law as communicative and instructive vs. punishing (Ghanaian logic of discipline); marriage; nostalgia

for cutting; patriarchy; traditional birth attendants; traditional medicine; traditional religion

traditional birth attendants (TBAs), as harmful tradition, 99, 165, 191

traditional medicine: blood tonics (herbal), 222–223, 229; occult representations in film and demonization of, 349n15. *See also* traditional religion

traditional religion: blood ritual and, 232, 349n12; colonialist ambivalence toward, 78; enumerated as harmful tradition, 98; and fetish, as term, 351n2; occult representations in film and demonization of, 349n15; opposition to cutting in, 146; and Othering of northern Ghana, 14; rain dance, 119–120. *See also* gods (ancestor spirits and); soothsaying (divination); witchcraft

translation of public health concepts: and critical anthropology, importance of credible knowledge via, 175; deliberate mistakes in, 179; HIV/AIDS, 175; refusals of, as deliberate tactic, 174, 178, 187–189, 204; underlying assumptions about the body, sexuality, and subjectivity as necessary to, 175

tribal markings: blood narrative and ending of, 210, 220; as harmful tradition, 97, 98; independence of Ghana and ending of, 113, 145, 330; and non-intervention colonialists, 66–67

Trinh, T. Minh-Ha, 29, 34

trokosi, law prohibiting, 266, 267–268, 270–271, 275, 352n11

truth regime, 150

Tsing, Anna Lowenhaupt, ii, 15, 22, 30, 32, 178, 227, 339n5

Twumasi, Dr. Patrick, 263

underground resistance, as discourse: anthropology adopting uncritically, 81, 143; awareness of and desire to combat, by rural women and men, 148–150; border crossings and, 135–136, 137, 262; colonial northern Ghana and, 68, 81, 135; criminalization, surveillance, and

CPSIA information can be obtained
at www.ICGtesting.com
Printed in the USA
LVOW10s0141300917
549717LV00007B/5/P